Immunotherapy for Pediatric Malignancies

Juliet C. Gray • Aurélien Marabelle
Editors

Immunotherapy for Pediatric Malignancies

Springer

Editors
Juliet C. Gray
Cancer Sciences Unit
University of Southampton
Southampton, UK

Aurélien Marabelle
Département d'Innovation Thérapeutique et d'Essais Précoces
University of Paris-Saclay Gustave Roussy
Villejuif, France

ISBN 978-3-319-43484-1 ISBN 978-3-319-43486-5 (eBook)
https://doi.org/10.1007/978-3-319-43486-5

Library of Congress Control Number: 2017956752

Printed on acid-free paper

This Springer imprint is published by Springer Nature
The registered company is Springer International Publishing AG
The registered company address is: Gewerbestrasse 11, 6330 Cham, Switzerland

Contents

List of Contributors

John Anderson, B.A., Ph.D. Department of Paediatric Oncology, Great Ormond Street Hospital and Institute of Child Health, University College London, London, UK

Matthew J. Barth, M.D. Pediatric Hematology and Oncology, Women and Children's Hospital of Buffalo/Roswell Park Cancer Institute, Buffalo, NY, USA

Mitchell S. Cairo, M.D. Department of Pediatrics, New York Medical College, Valhalla, NY, USA

Nathalie Chaput, PharmD., Ph.D. Biotherapy, Gustave Roussy, Villejuif, France

Kenneth DeSantes, M.D. Department of Pediatrics, University of Wisconsin, American Family Children's Hospital, Madison, WI, USA

Nader Kim El-Mallawany, M.D. Pediatric Hematology, Oncology, and Stem Cell Transplantation, Maria Fareri Children's Hospital, New York Medical College, Valhalla, NY, USA

Jonathan Fisher, BM(Hons), BSc, MClinRes, Ph.D. Cancer Section, GOSH/UCL Institute of Child Health, London, UK

Juliet C. Gray, M.A., FRCPCH, Ph.D. Cancer Sciences Unit, University of Southampton, Southampton, UK

Department of Paediatric Oncology, Southampton Children's Hospital, Southampton, UK

Rupert Handgretinger, Ph.D. Hematology/Oncology, University Children's Hospital Tübingen, Tübingen, Germany

Jessica Hochberg, M.D. Division Pediatric Hematology, Oncology & Stem Cell Transplant, Westchester Medical Center, Valhalla, NY, USA

Theodore S. Johnson, M.D. Department of Pediatrics, Children's Hospital of Georgia, Augusta, GA, USA

Peter Lang, Ph.D. Hematology/Oncology, University Children's Hospital Tübingen, Tübingen, Germany

Holger N. Lode, M.D. Pediatric Hematology and Oncology, University Medicine Greifswald, Greifswald, Germany

Aurélien Marabelle, M.D., Ph.D. Département d'Innovation Thérapeutique et d'Essais Précoces, Gustave Roussy, Université Paris-Saclay, Villejuif F-94805, France

INSERM U1015, Gustave Roussy, Université Paris-Saclay, Villejuif F-94805, France

Kimberly A. McDowell, M.D., Ph.D. Pediatrics, Division of Pediatric Hematology, Oncology and Bone Marrow Transplant, University of Wisconsin, American Family Children's Hospital, Madison, WI, USA

Véronique Minard-Colin, M.D. Department Child and Adolescent Cancer, Institut Gustave Roussy, Villejuif, France

Shakeel Modak, M.D., M.R.C.P. Department of Pediatrics, Memorial Sloan Kettering Cancer Center, New York, NY, USA

David H. Munn, M.D. Department of Pediatrics, Children's Hospital of Georgia, Augusta, GA, USA

Miho Nakajima, M.D. Department of Pediatrics, Memorial Sloan Kettering Cancer Center/Weill Cornell Medical Center, New York, NY, USA

Claudia Pasqualini, M.D. Paediatric and Adolescent Oncology Unit, Gustave Roussy, Villejuif Cedex, France

Vito Pistoia, M.D. Immunology Area, Bambino Gesù Pediatric Hospital, Rome, Italy

Ignazia Pringione, Ph.D. Translational Research and Laboratory Medicine, Istituto Giannina Gaslini, Genoa, Italy

Lizzia Raffaghello, Ph.D. Translational Research and Laboratory Medicine, Istituto Giannina Gaslini, Genoa, Italy

Claudia Rossig, M.D. Pediatric Hematology and Oncology, University Children's Hospital Muenster, Muenster, Germany

Patrick Schlegel, M.D. Hematology/Oncology, University Children's Hospital Tübingen, Tübingen, Germany

Christian Seitz, M.D. Hematology/Oncology, University Children's Hospital Tübingen, Tübingen, Germany

Michaela Semeraro Hôpital Necker-Enfants malades, Paris, France

Paul M. Sondel, M.D., Ph.D. Departments of Pediatrics, Human Oncology, and Genetics, University of Wisconsin, American Family Children's Hospital, Madison, WI, USA

About the Editors

Juliet Gray is an Associate Professor in Paediatric Oncology at the Cancer Immunology Centre, University of Southampton. She leads a translational research group focused on novel antibody immunotherapies for neuroblastoma, including preclinical evaluation of novel combinational therapies as well as early phase clinical trials. She is a member of the UK NCRI Childhood Cancer and Leukaemia and Neuroblastoma groups, and an executive member of the European Neuroblastoma Research Network (SIOPEN).

Aurélien Marabelle is currently the Clinical Director of the Cancer Immunotherapy Program at Gustave Roussy Cancer Center in Villejuif, France. Dr. Marabelle is an immunologist and a pediatric oncologist by training. His clinical practice is currently dedicated to Early Phase Clinical trials in Cancer Immunotherapy and his translational research is focused on mechanisms of action of immune targeted therapies. He works as a senior medical oncologist and an investigator in the Drug Development Department (DITEP) directed by Prof. Jean-Charles Soria. He is coordinating a team focusing on cancer immunotherapy translational research projects in the INSERM U1015 lab directed by Prof. Laurence Zitvogel. Dr. Marabelle is a member of the European Society of Medical Oncology (ESMO), the American Society of Clinical Oncology (ASCO), the European Academy of Tumor Immunology (EATI), and the American Association of Cancer Research (AACR).

Chapter 1
Introduction to Pediatric Cancer Immunotherapy

Aurélien Marabelle and Claudia Rossig

Abstract Cancer immunotherapy comes of age for adult malignancies. Immune targeted antibodies aiming at disrupting immunosuppressive pathways such as the checkpoints PD-1/PD-L1 and CTLA-4/B7 are providing durable responses and overall survival benefits in multiple relapsing/refractory adult cancer types. Novel immunotherapies such as oncolytic viruses and adoptive CAR-T cells are also becoming approved immune therapies and revolutionize the world of drug development. These therapeutic innovations are currently fostering an unprecedented research effort in adult tumor immunology. Pediatric cancers have major histological, biological and developmental differences with adult cancers. Although the fundamental immunological rules remain the same between adults and children, the limited data currently available suggest that the immune cells and the immunosuppressive pathways that are at stake in pediatric cancers might be different than the ones acting in adult cancers. Clinical results of passive immunotherapy with tumor targeting antibodies, cytokines, bispecific T-cell engaging antibodies and CAR-T cells have recently demonstrated that pediatric cancers can be treated with immunotherapy. However, the benefits of these novel treatments are limited to a small fraction of pediatric cancers. Fundamental and translational research efforts are currently eagerly needed to better decipher what drives the immune surveillance and editing of pediatric cancers.

Keywords Pediatric tumors • Pediatric cancer • Immunotherapy • Immune system • Immune cells

A. Marabelle, M.D., Ph.D. (✉)
Département d'Innovation Thérapeutique et d'Essais Précoces, Gustave Roussy, Université Paris-Saclay, Villejuif F-94805, France

INSERM U1015, Gustave Roussy, Université Paris-Saclay, Villejuif F-94805, France
e-mail: aurelien.marabelle@gustaveroussy.fr

C. Rossig, M.D.
Pediatric Hematology and Oncology, University Children's Hospital Muenster, Muenster, Germany

J.C. Gray, A. Marabelle (eds.), *Immunotherapy for Pediatric Malignancies*,
https://doi.org/10.1007/978-3-319-43486-5_1

1.1 Introduction

During their evolution over the last 3 billion years, multicellular organisms have developed tissues and organs with refined specificities to allow better survival and interbreeding. Among the subsets of tissues which compose a vertebrate living organism, the immune system can be defined as the subsets of cells that are produced by the hematopoietic stem cells in the bone marrow but do not belong to the red blood cell and platelet lineages. These so called "white blood cells" or leucocytes are present throughout the body, either staying in tissues as resident cells since the early embryogenesis, or circulating through the tissues, blood vessels and lymphatic vessels of the body. They can directly contribute to the structure of specific organs of the body known as the primary and secondary lymphoid organs. Primary lymphoid organs include the bone marrow and the thymus where immune cells (lymphocytes for the thymus) are formed and mature. Secondary lymphoid organs include structures such as lymph nodes, tonsils, spleen, Peyer's patches and mucosa associated lymphoid tissue (MALT). These white blood cells, their protein products (cytokines, chemokines, antibodies), and their related organs are key elements of mammalians natural defenses against pathogens (virus, fungus, bacteria).

1.2 Overview of the Components of the Immune System

Immune cells can be divided in two subsets of cells: the innate immune cells and the adaptive immune cells (Fig. 1.1). Innate immune cells are granulocytes (neutrophils, basophils and eosinophils), monocytes/macrophages, mast cells and dendritic cells. They can react fast against pathogens in a stereotypic, pathogen non-specific manner and are devoid of memory features. Adaptive immune cells are B-cells and T-cells. These lymphocytes react more slowly than innate immune cells. They have memory features which allow them to react in a pathogen specific manner, and to increase this reaction over time. Some immune cells such as γδ T-cells and NK-T cells share some common features of both the innate and adaptive immune system as they can respond in an antigen specific and non-specific manner. All these immune cells act in coordination with each other over time and at the different sites of the body in order to maintain the homeostasis of the host. Communications between immune cells and other cellular components of the body is performed through cell-cell interactions, cytokines and chemokines. Detailed aspects of the composition and function of the immune system have been extensively reviewed in the literature, notably in the context of cancer [1].

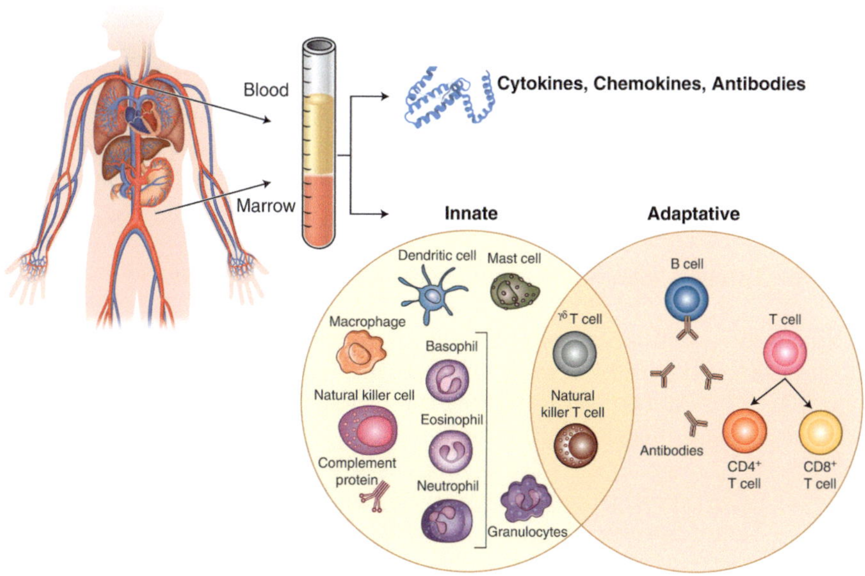

Fig. 1.1 Components of the immune system. The main effectors of the immune system have been described in the blood and bone marrow although specific tissue resident immune cells are not present in these compartment (e.g. some subsets of gamma deltaT-cells). Innate immune cells have rapid, stereotypic responses to dangers signals such as pathogens but are devoided of memory features. Alternatively, it takes a couple of weeks to the adaptive immune cells to generate a novel antigen-specific response, but its memory features provides more rapid and potent responses upon subsequent exposures

1.3 Role of the Immune System in Cancer Biology

1.3.1 Tumor Infiltrating Immune Cells and Immune-Editing

Besides cancer cells and stromal cells, the tumor micro-environment can be infiltrated by subsets of immune cells. Some of these immune cells can contribute to the anti-tumor immune response against cancer cells. These effector cells can be cytotoxic CD8+ T-cells, type 1T-helper cells (so called "Th1"), type 1 macrophages (so-called "M1"), B-cells (including differentiated, antibody producing, plasmocytes), natural killer cells (NK cells), NKT-cells, and γδ T-cells. Our understanding of cancer biology has evolved over the last 15 years thanks to the description of subsets of immune cells which protect cancer cells from anti-tumor "auto-reactive" immune cells. Indeed, because cancer cells "belong to the immunological "self", they can evade the immune system by using pathways and effectors that generate immune tolerance. Tolerogenic immune effectors are regulatory FOXP3-positive CD4+

T-cells (Tregs), type 2 macrophages (so-called "M2"), and other types of more undifferentiated myeloid cells also called myeloid derived suppressor cells (or "MDSC"). The balance between immune rejection and immune tolerance of cancer cells, and the subsequent Darwinian pressure of selection of the fittest sub-clones of cancer cells over time has been coined with the concept of tumor "immuno-editing" [2]. Pediatric tumors typically have only sparse infiltrates of lymphocytes [3], but CD8+ T cells capable of effector memory responses were found e.g. in neuroblastomas [4].

1.3.1.1 Tumor Antigens and Immunogenicity of Pediatric Tumors

Although tumor cells are immunologically "self", they can differ from healthy cells by the aberrant expression of molecules that can be recognized by the immune system (Fig. 1.2). On the other hand, they can secrete molecules or express ligands which can hamper immune cell functions.

1.3.1.2 Tumor-Specific Antigens of Pediatric Tumors

Somatic point mutations in the cancer cell DNA can lead to the expression of aberrant proteins. Peptides from these proteins can behave as neo-antigens when they become presented to T-cells via MHC molecules. Such neo-epitopes are

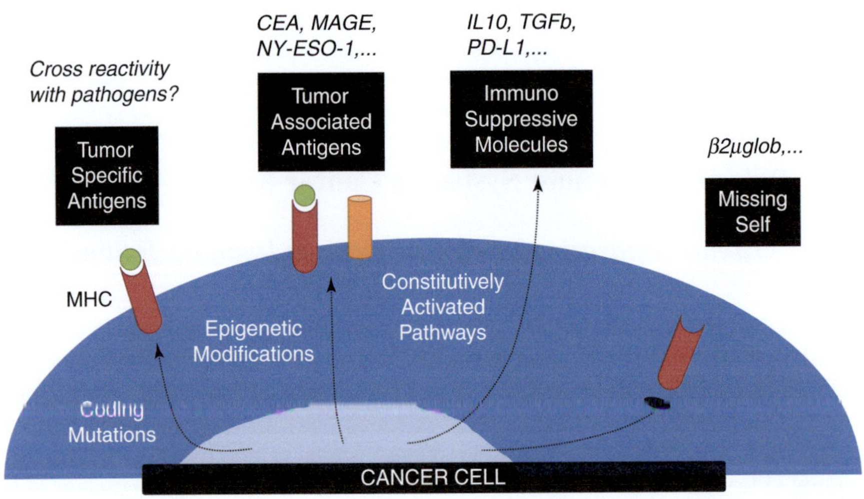

Fig. 1.2 Impact of genomic and epigenetic abnormalities on cancer cells immunogenicity. Cancer cells are "self" cells and can therefore use many physiological pathways to prevent an "auto" immune reaction (e.g. PD-L1 upregulation). However, the multiple genomic alterations happening in the cancer cell genome and the epigenetic changes have an impact on the overall immunogenicity of tumors. Some alterations can increase the cancer cell immunogenicity (e.g. tumor specific antigens presented by the MHC molecules upon somatic point mutations in the cancer cell genome). Others can dampen the recognition of cancer cells by the immune system (e.g. mutations in the beta2-microglobulin preventing functional presentation of MHC-I molecules)

tumor-specific antigens (TSA) and can generate tumor-specific T-cell responses. This phenomenon has been recently well described, and seems to play a significant role in the response to checkpoint blockade (CTLA-4, PD-1) immunotherapy in some adult cancers but also in biallelic mismatch repair deficiency hypermutant pediatric glioblastoma [5–8]. However, we do not know if it plays a significant role in the immunogenicity of other pediatric cancers. Pediatric cancers often carry chromosome rearrangements [9, 10], but generally have a low frequency of somatic point mutations [11–13]. Still, in some subsets of patients, notably of poor prognosis, the mutation rate can be higher. Indeed, it has been recently demonstrated that high-risk neuroblastomas have a higher level of somatic point mutations than neuroblastomas with a good prognosis [14]. Specifically, the neuroblastoma genome can undergo chromothripsis, a phenomenon where some areas of a given genome can undergo thousands of chromosome rearrangements in limited regions of some chromosomes [14]. Besides somatic point mutations, the analysis of pediatric tumor genomes has also revealed that they have frequent chromosome rearrangements [9, 10]. These chromosome rearrangements could in theory generate truncated or translocated abnormal proteins which could become TSA. This hypothesis remains to be explored.

1.3.1.3 Tumor-Associated Antigens of Pediatric Tumors

Besides somatic genome aberrations, cancer cells can undergo epigenetic modifications which can result to the aberrant expression of some molecules. For instance, cancer cells can express high levels of proteins that are usually only expressed during embryonic development or in limited subsets of cells related to germ cells. These so called "carcino-embryonic" or "cancer-testis" antigens, such as NY-ESO-1, CEA, MAGE, and many others (see [15] for review) can be highly expressed on cancer cells, either by membrane expression of the full length protein (with possible alternate splicing), and/or via MHC presentation of peptides. T-cell or B-cell (antibody) specific responses to these TAA have been described in detail in adult cancers over the last 20 years. Interestingly, IgG antibodies against NY-ESO-1 as well as CD4/CD8 T-cell specific responses to HLA-A2-restricted peptide NY-ESO-$_{1157-167}$ were found in children with NY-ESO-1 positive neuroblastoma [16]. Also, immunization with an autologous interleukin-2 gene transduced neuroblastoma tumor cell vaccine has been shown to generate specific antibody responses against neuroblastoma cells [17].

Epigenetic changes in cancer cells can also end up in modifications of ganglioside expression. Gangliosides are sialic-acid-containing glycosphingolipids expressed on all vertebrate plasma membrane cells. Human healthy tissues usually do not express glycolylneuraminic acid containing gangliosides, but this molecule is expressed in tumors and in human fetal tissues [18]. Therefore, gangliosides are another type of onco-fetal TAA. Reminiscent of their neuroectodermal tissue origin, neuroblastomas express the ganglioside GD2 at high density. GD2 can also be overexpressed in Ewing sarcomas [19–21]. GD2 expression in neuroblastoma cells was suggested to contribute to tumor immune escape by negatively affecting the differentiation and capacity of dendritic cells to prime the proliferation of T-cells [22].

Anti-GD2 antibody therapy has been developed in the clinic and is becoming part of the standard of care of high-risk neuroblastoma [23–25]. More recently, GD2 is evaluated as an immune target also of redirected T cells (see Chap. 10).

Genetic and epigenetic changes in cancer cells can also result in the aberrant expression of intra-cellular proteins which can become TSA while being presented through the physiological MHC-I route. For instance, genomic alterations such as p53 inactivation can result in the upregulation of an intracytoplamic anti-apoptotic molecule called survivin. Interestingly, survivin-specific CD8+ T-cells have been detected in the blood of children with high risk neuroblastoma [26]. However, very few tumor infiltrating T-cells were found in the same patients, suggesting that immune cell infiltration into pediatric tumors may be a critical limitation to effective anticancer immune responses [26].

1.3.1.4 Immune Tolerance of Pediatric Cancer Cells

MHC Expression

Besides TSA and TAA, cancer cells can express molecules with immune-inhibitory function which contribute to their overall low immunogenicity. First, the downregulation or absence of expression of MHC-I molecules has been a classical mechanism of immune escape by preventing cancer cells to be recognized by CD8+ cytotoxic T-cells. Low or no MHC-I expression has been widely described in pediatric cancers [27]. However, downregulation of MHC-I is often reversible, and inflammatory conditions such as exposure to interferon-γ can upregulate MHC-I in most pediatric cancer cell lines [27, 28]. Sometimes, the absence of expression of MHC-I is a consequence of mutations in the beta-2 microglobulin, a protein which is part of the MHC-I complex. For instance, this has been recently described in about 70% of Hodgkin lymphomas [29]. The absence of MHC-I expression should in theory activate NK cells ("missing self" theory). Indeed, in neuroblastoma, where MHC-I molecules are often not expressed, NK cells were suggested to play a significant role in immune surveillance. One example is the recent finding that expression of distinct isoforms of the NK receptor NKp30, which can functionally interact with B7-H6 present in the serum of the patients in its soluble form and at the surface of tumor cells, is associated with survival in high-risk neuroblastoma patients [30].

Cytokines and Chemokines Expression

Cancer cells can further secrete cytokines either in an autocrine or paracrine manner which create a pro-tumoral inflammatory micro-environment. For instance, interleukin-6 (IL-6) has been found to be expressed by glioblastoma and neuroblastoma cells [31] but also by stromal cells in metastatic niches such as the bone marrow [32, 33]. IL-6 receptor (IL-6R) can also be expressed by neuroblastoma cells, and IL-6 from either cancer cells or metastatic bone-marrow on IL-6R positive neuroblastoma cells can sustain their proliferation and prevent them from chemotherapy (etoposide)-induced apoptosis [33]. Also, IL-6 acts on myeloid derived osteoclast cells which can contribute to the development of metastatic bone marrow sites [33]. Accordingly, the circulating blood levels of IL-6 have been shown to be significantly higher in high-risk neuroblastoma [34], and the single nucleotide polymorphism rs1800795 in the promoter of the IL-6 gene (also known as the as the IL-6 "174" polymorphism) has been shown to have a prognostic value both in event-free and overall survival in children with high-risk neuroblastoma [35]. Also, interleukin-8 seem to play a role in neuroblastoma as both IL-8 and its receptor can be expressed on cancer cells [36]. Interestingly, treatment of neuroblastoma cells by retinoic acid (which is part of the standard of care of high risk neuroblastoma) stimulates IL-8 secretion by neuroblastoma cells and promote neutrophil and lymphocyte chemotaxis [37]. Both G-CSF and its receptor have been shown to be expressed by Ewing tumors, and osteosarcoma, and G-CSF has been shown to support Ewing xenograft tumor growth through both angiogenesis and leukocyte recruitment into tumors [38, 39]. However this data has been generated in immunocompromised xenograft models and might not be physiological. Subsequent concerns that G-CSF administration to promote granulocyte recovery post chemotherapy may be unsafe in Ewing sarcoma patients have not been substantiated, arguing against a relevant role of this pathway and GCSF remains part of the supportive care of Ewing sarcoma [40].

Chemokines can be critical for the infiltration of immune cells into the tumor microenvironment. In Ewing sarcoma, chemokine and chemokine receptor profiling revealed an association between an inflammatory immune microenvironment with infiltration by CD8+ T cells [41]. Genomic changes occurring in cancer cells can affect expression of chemokines. E.g., the oncogene MYCN, a hallmark of high-risk neuroblastoma, has been shown to repress the expression of CCL2 by neuroblastoma cells, a chemokine that can attract immune effector cells [42].

1.3.1.5 Immunosuppressive Pathways

Immunosuppressive ligands can be expressed on cancer cells. These so-called "immune checkpoints" can interact specifically with molecules expressed by immune cells and block their activation, induce tolerance and exhaustion. Programmed-death ligand-1 (PD-L1) is the most extensively studied immune checkpoint molecules in adult cancers. It interacts with the co-inhibitory receptor PD-1 which is expressed on lymphocytes. PD-L1 expression was also found in pediatric cancers such as neuroblastoma, nephroblastoma (Wilms tumor) and osteosarcoma [43–46]. Another potential tolerogenic immune checkpoint called B7-H3, and its isoform 4Ig6B7-H3, have been shown to be expressed in osteosarcoma and neuroblastoma, respectively [47, 48].

Tryptophane is a critical amino acid for the metabolism of immune cells, notably T-cells. The enzyme indoleamine 2,3-dioxygenase (usually called IDO) depletes tryptophan in the tumor micro-environment, and IDO expression has been described as a key immunosuppressive pathway in many adult cancer types, notably under interferon-γ exposure. IDO has been shown to be expressed by osteosarcoma cell lines exposed to IL-12 and IL-18, suggesting a possible role in that pediatric cancer [49].

1.4 Conclusion

Overall, although the level of somatic point mutations remains low in pediatric cancer cell genomes, the cells can be immunogenic by other genomic and epigenetic alterations. Future research will have to identify the most relevant immune escape mechanisms in the biology of pediatric cancers to allow for effective intervention by immunotherapy. The subsequent chapters of this book will detail the immune contexture of pediatric cancers, the prognostic role of the different immune subsets and how they differ from adult cancers. Also, this book will provide a comprehensive overview of the various immunotherapy strategies under current development that aim to exploit the immune system to treat pediatric cancers.

References

1. Dranoff G. Cytokines in cancer pathogenesis and cancer therapy. Nat Rev Cancer. 2004;4:11–22. doi:10.1038/nrc1252.
2. Schreiber RD, Old LJ, Smyth MJ. Cancer immunoediting: integrating immunity's roles in cancer suppression and promotion. Science. 2011;331:1565–70. doi:10.1126/science.1203486.
3. Vakkila J, Jaffe R, Michelow M, Lotze MT. Pediatric cancers are infiltrated predominantly by macrophages and contain a paucity of dendritic cells: a major nosologic difference with adult tumors. Clin Cancer Res. 2006;12:2049–54. doi:10.1158/1078-0432.CCR-05-1824.
4. Carlson L, De Geer A, Sveinbjørnsson B, Orrego A, Martinsson T, Kogner P, et al. The microenvironment of human neuroblastoma supports the activation of tumor-associated T lymphocytes. Oncoimmunology. 2013;2:e23618. doi:10.4161/onci.23618.
5. Bouffet E, Larouche V, Campbell BB, Merico D, de Borja R, Aronson M, et al. Immune checkpoint inhibition for hypermutant glioblastoma multiforme resulting from germline biallelic mismatch repair deficiency. J Clin Oncol. 2016;34(19):2206–11. doi:10.1200/JCO.2016.66.6552.
6. Boussiotis VA. Somatic mutations and immunotherapy outcome with CTLA-4 blockade in melanoma. N Engl J Med. 2014;371:2230–2. doi:10.1056/NEJMe1413061.
7. Rizvi NA, Hellmann MD, Snyder A, Kvistborg P, Makarov V, Havel JJ, et al. Mutational landscape determines sensitivity to PD-1 blockade in non-small cell lung cancer. Science. 2015;348(6230):124–8. doi:10.1126/science.aaa1348.
8. McGranahan N, Furness AJS, Rosenthal R, Ramskov S, Lyngaa R, Saini SK, et al. Clonal neoantigens elicit T cell immunoreactivity and sensitivity to immune checkpoint blockade. Science. 2016;351:1463–9. doi:10.1126/science.aaf1490.
9. Janoueix-Lerosey I, Schleiermacher G, Michels E, Mosseri V, Ribeiro A, Lequin D, et al. Overall genomic pattern is a predictor of outcome in neuroblastoma. J Clin Oncol. 2009;27:1026–33. doi:10.1200/JCO.2008.16.0630.

10. Schleiermacher G, Janoueix-Lerosey I, Ribeiro A, Klijanienko J, Couturier J, Pierron G, et al. Accumulation of segmental alterations determines progression in neuroblastoma. J Clin Oncol. 2010;28:3122–30. doi:10.1200/JCO.2009.26.7955.
11. Lee R, Stewart C, Carter S. A remarkably simple genome underlies highly malignant pediatric rhabdoid cancers. J Clin Invest. 2012;122:2983–8. doi:10.1172/JCI64400DS1.
12. Downing JR, Wilson RK, Zhang J, Mardis ER, Pui C-H, Ding L, et al. The pediatric cancer genome project. Nat Genet. 2012;44:619–22. doi:10.1038/ng.2287.
13. Pugh TJ, Morozova O, Attiyeh EF, Asgharzadeh S, Wei JS, Auclair D, et al. The genetic landscape of high-risk neuroblastoma. Nat Genet. 2013;45:279–84. doi:10.1038/ng.2529.
14. Molenaar JJ, Koster J, Zwijnenburg DA, van Sluis P, Valentijn LJ, van der Ploeg I, et al. Sequencing of neuroblastoma identifies chromothripsis and defects in neuritogenesis genes. Nature. 2012;483:589–93. doi:10.1038/nature10910.
15. Gnjatic S, Nishikawa H, Jungbluth AA, Güre AO, Ritter G, Jäger E, et al. NY-ESO-1: review of an immunogenic tumor antigen. Adv Cancer Res. 2006;95:1–30. doi:10.1016/S0065-230X(06)95001-5.
16. Rodolfo M, Luksch R, Stockert E, Chen YT, Collini P, Ranzani T, et al. Antigen-specific immunity in neuroblastoma patients: antibody and T-cell recognition of NY-ESO-1 tumor antigen. Cancer Res. 2003;63:6948–55.
17. Rossig C, Nuchtern JG, Brenner MK. Selection of human antitumor single-chain Fv antibodies from the B-cell repertoire of patients immunized against autologous neuroblastoma. Med Pediatr Oncol. 2000;35:692–5.
18. Krengel U, Bousquet PA. Molecular recognition of gangliosides and their potential for cancer immunotherapies. Front Immunol. 2014;5:325. doi:10.3389/fimmu.2014.00325.
19. Schulz G, Cheresh DA, Varki NM, Yu A, Staffileno LK, Reisfeld RA. Detection of ganglioside GD2 in tumor tissues and sera of neuroblastoma patients. Cancer Res. 1984;44:5914–20.
20. Dobrenkov K, Ostrovnaya I, Gu J, Cheung IY, Cheung N-KV. Oncotargets GD2 and GD3 are highly expressed in sarcomas of children, adolescents, and young adults. Pediatr Blood Cancer. 2016;63(10):1780–5. doi:10.1002/pbc.26097.
21. Kailayangiri S, Altvater B, Meltzer J, Pscherer S, Luecke A, Dierkes C, et al. The ganglioside antigen GD2 is surface-expressed in Ewing sarcoma and allows for MHC-independent immune targeting. Br J Cancer. 2012;106:1123–33. doi:10.1038/bjc.2012.57.
22. Shurin GV, Shurin MR, Bykovskaia S, Shogan J, Lotze MT, Barksdale EM. Neuroblastoma-derived gangliosides inhibit dendritic cell generation and function. Cancer Res. 2001;61:363–9.
23. Yu AL, Gilman AL, Ozkaynak MF, London WB, Kreissman SG, Chen HX, et al. Anti-GD2 antibody with GM-CSF, interleukin-2, and isotretinoin for neuroblastoma. N Engl J Med. 2010;363:1324–34. doi:10.1056/NEJMoa0911123.
24. Simon T, Hero B, Faldum A, Handgretinger R, Schrappe M, Klingebiel T, et al. Long term outcome of high-risk neuroblastoma patients after immunotherapy with antibody ch14.18 or oral metronomic chemotherapy. BMC Cancer. 2011;11:21. doi:10.1186/1471-2407-11-21.
25. Gilman AL, Ozkaynak MF, Matthay KK, Krailo M, Yu AL, Gan J, et al. Phase I study of ch14.18 with granulocyte-macrophage colony-stimulating factor and interleukin-2 in children with neuroblastoma after autologous bone marrow transplantation or stem-cell rescue: a report from the Children's Oncology Group. J Clin Oncol. 2009;27:85–91. doi:10.1200/JCO.2006.10.3564.
26. Coughlin CM, Fleming MD, Carroll RG, Pawel BR, Hogarty MD, Shan X, Vance BA, Cohen JN, Jairaj S, Lord EM, Wexler MH, Danet-Desnoyers GH, Pinkus JL, Pinkus GS, Maris JM, Grupp SA, Vonderheide RH. Immunosurveillance and survivin-specific T-cell immunity in children with high-risk neuroblastoma. J Clin Oncol. 2006;24:5725–34. doi:10.1200/JCO.2005.05.3314.
27. Haworth KB, Arnold MA, Pierson CR, Leddon JL, Kurmashev DK, Swain HM, et al. Characterization of MHC class I and β-2-microglobulin expression in pediatric solid malignancies to guide selection of immune-based therapeutic trials. Pediatr Blood Cancer. 2016;63:618–26. doi:10.1002/pbc.25842.

28. Reid GSD, Shan X, Coughlin CM, Lassoued W, Pawel BR, Wexler LH, et al. Interferon-gamma-dependent infiltration of human T cells into neuroblastoma tumors in vivo. Clin Cancer Res. 2009;15:6602–8. doi:10.1158/1078-0432.CCR-09-0829.
29. Reichel J, Chadburn A, Rubinstein PG, Giulino-Roth L, Tam W, Liu Y, et al. Flow-sorting and exome sequencing reveals the oncogenome of primary Hodgkin and Reed-Sternberg cells. Blood. 2015;12:1061–72. doi:10.1182/blood-2014-11-610436.
30. Semeraro M, Rusakiewicz S, Minard-Colin V, Delahaye NF, Enot D, Vély F, et al. Clinical impact of the NKp30/B7-H6 axis in high-risk neuroblastoma patients. Sci Transl Med. 2015;7:283ra55. doi:10.1126/scitranslmed.aaa2327.
31. Stephanou A, Knight RA, Annicchiarico-Petruzzelli M, Finazzi-Agrò A, Lightmann SL, Melino G. Interleukin-1 beta and interleukin-6 mRNA are expressed in human glioblastoma and neuroblastoma cells respectively. Funct Neurol. 1992;7:129–33.
32. Silverman AM, Nakata R, Shimada H, Sposto R, DeClerck YA. A galectin-3-dependent pathway upregulates interleukin-6 in the microenvironment of human neuroblastoma. Cancer Res. 2012;72:2228–38. doi:10.1158/0008-5472.CAN-11-2165.
33. Ara T, Song L, Shimada H, Keshelava N, Russell HV, Metelitsa LS, et al. Interleukin-6 in the bone marrow microenvironment promotes the growth and survival of neuroblastoma cells. Cancer Res. 2009;69:329–37. doi:10.1158/0008-5472.CAN-08-0613.
34. Egler RA, Burlingame SM, Nuchtern JG, Russell HV. Interleukin-6 and soluble interleukin-6 receptor levels as markers of disease extent and prognosis in neuroblastoma. Clin Cancer Res. 2008;14:7028–34. doi:10.1158/1078-0432.CCR-07-5017.
35. Lagmay JP, London WB, Gross TG, Termuhlen A, Sullivan N, Axel A, et al. Prognostic significance of interleukin-6 single nucleotide polymorphism genotypes in neuroblastoma: rs1800795 (promoter) and rs8192284 (receptor). Clin Cancer Res. 2009;15:5234–9. doi:10.1158/1078-0432.CCR-08-2953.
36. Ferrer FA, Pantschenko AG, Miller LJ, Anderson K, Grunnet M, McKenna PH, et al. Angiogenesis and neuroblastomas: interleukin-8 and interleukin-8 receptor expression in human neuroblastoma. J Urol. 2000;164:1016–20.
37. Yang KD, Cheng SN, Wu NC, Shaio MF. Induction of interleukin-8 expression in neuroblastoma cells by retinoic acid: implication of leukocyte chemotaxis and activation. Pediatr Res. 1993;34:720–4. doi:10.1203/00006450-199312000-00005.
38. Lisignoli G, Toneguzzi S, Cattini L, Pozzi C, Facchini A. Different expression pattern of cytokine receptors by human osteosarcoma cell lines. Int J Oncol. 1998;12:899–903.
39. Morales-Arias J, Meyers PA, Bolontrade MF, Rodriguez N, Zhou Z, Reddy K, et al. Expression of granulocyte-colony-stimulating factor and its receptor in human Ewing sarcoma cells and patient tumor specimens: potential consequences of granulocyte-colony-stimulating factor administration. Cancer. 2007;110:1568–77. doi:10.1002/cncr.22964.
40. Ladenstein R, Pötschger U, Le Deley MC, Whelan J, Paulussen M, Oberlin O, et al. Primary disseminated multifocal Ewing sarcoma: results of the Euro-EWING 99 trial. J Clin Oncol. 2010;28:3284–91. doi:10.1200/JCO.2009.22.9864.
41. Berghuis D, Santos SJ, Baelde HJ, Taminiau AH, Egeler RM, Schilham MW, et al. Pro-inflammatory chemokine-chemokine receptor interactions within the Ewing sarcoma micro-environment determine CD8(+) T-lymphocyte infiltration and affect tumour progression. J Pathol. 2011;223:347–57. doi:10.1002/path.2819.
42. Song L, Ara T, Wu H-W, Woo C-W, Reynolds CP, Seeger RC, et al. Oncogene MYCN regulates localization of NKT cells to the site of disease in neuroblastoma. J Clin Invest. 2007;117:2702–12. doi:10.1172/JCI30751.
43. Dondero A, Pastorino F, Della Chiesa M, Corrias MV, Morandi F, Pistoia V, et al. PD-L1 expression in metastatic neuroblastoma as an additional mechanism for limiting immune surveillance. Oncoimmunology. 2015;5:e1064578. doi:10.1080/2162402X.2015.1064578.
44. Lussier DM, O'Neill L, Nieves LM, McAfee MS, Holechek SA, Collins AW, et al. Enhanced T-cell immunity to osteosarcoma through antibody blockade of PD-1/PD-L1 interactions. J Immunother. 2015;38:96–106. doi:10.1097/CJI.0000000000000065.

45. Routh JC, Grundy PE, Anderson JR, Retik AB, Kurek KC. B7-h1 as a biomarker for therapy failure in patients with favorable histology Wilms tumor. J Urol. 2013;189:1487–92. doi:10.1016/j.juro.2012.11.012.
46. Routh JC, Ashley RA, Sebo TJ, Lohse CM, Husmann DA, Kramer SA, et al. B7-H1 expression in Wilms tumor: correlation with tumor biology and disease recurrence. J Urol. 2008;179:1954–60. doi:10.1016/j.juro.2008.01.056.
47. Wang L, Zhang Q, Chen W, Shan B, Ding Y, Zhang G, et al. B7-H3 is overexpressed in patients suffering osteosarcoma and associated with tumor aggressiveness and metastasis. PLoS One. 2013;8:e70689. doi:10.1371/journal.pone.0070689.
48. Castriconi R, Dondero A, Augugliaro R, Cantoni C, Carnemolla B, Sementa AR, et al. Identification of 4Ig-B7-H3 as a neuroblastoma-associated molecule that exerts a protective role from an NK cell-mediated lysis. Proc Natl Acad Sci U S A. 2004;101:12640–5. doi:10.1073/pnas.0405025101.
49. Liebau C, Baltzer AWA, Schmidt S, Roesel C, Karreman C, Prisack JB, et al. Interleukin-12 and interleukin-18 induce indoleamine 2,3-dioxygenase (IDO) activity in human osteosarcoma cell lines independently from interferon-gamma. Anticancer Res. 2002;22:931–6.

Chapter 2
Overcoming Immune Suppression in the Tumor Microenvironment: Implications for Multi-modal Therapy

Theodore S. Johnson and David H. Munn

Abstract Effective immunotherapy, whether by checkpoint blockade, vaccines or adoptive cell therapy, is limited in most patients by a fundamental barrier: the immunosuppressive tumor microenvironment. This problem is more than just the suppression of effector T cells, but also includes profound defects in the inflammatory milieu and immunogenic antigen-presenting cells that are required to drive T cell activation. To date, much of the field of immunotherapy has focused on downstream checkpoints that regulate activated T cells, or on vaccination and T cell adoptive transfer to expand the T cell pool. Relatively less attention has been given to regulatory pathways that govern cross-presentation and response to endogenous tumor antigens. But these "upstream" pathways become particularly important in settings where immunotherapy is combined with standard-of-care chemotherapy or radiation therapy, both of which release a wave of tumor antigens. The choice of whether to treat these antigens as tolerizing or immunizing is fundamental to generating an effective immune response against the tumor. In this chapter we consider immunosuppressive mechanisms in the tumor microenvironment from the perspective of factors that that may impact the response to antigens from dying tumor cells.

Keywords Indoleamine 2,3-dioxygenase • IDO • Tolerance • Tumor microenvironment • Tumor • Immunotherapy • Checkpoint • Chemotherapy • Radiation

T.S. Johnson, M.D. (✉) • D.H. Munn, M.D.
Department of Pediatrics, Children's Hospital of Georgia, Augusta, GA, USA
e-mail: thjohnson@augusta.edu

J.C. Gray, A. Marabelle (eds.), *Immunotherapy for Pediatric Malignancies*,
https://doi.org/10.1007/978-3-319-43486-5_2

2.1 Introduction

In this chapter, we will focus on two aspects of tumor immunotherapy that are particularly relevant to pediatrics, but which often receive somewhat less attention in the field. First, our emphasis will be less on the downstream checkpoints that affect activated T cells, and more on the fundamental upstream factors that control the cross-presentation of tumor antigens to T cells in the first place. It is increasingly being realized that this key endogenous antigen-presentation step needs to elicit robust T cell immunity in order for immunotherapy to be successful [1]. Unfortunately, however, the default response in the tumor is frequently T cell suppression and tolerance, rather than an aggressive response to tumor antigens. Thus, one of the important goals of tumor immunotherapy must be to re-configure the suppressive and tolerogenic tumor microenvironment so that it becomes robustly immunogenic for tumor antigen [2, 3].

The second, and conceptually related, focus of this chapter will be on ways in which immunotherapy can be integrated with standard-of-care chemotherapy and radiation-therapy treatment. In adult oncology, the combination of immunotherapy with chemo/radiation therapy is increasingly recognized as a potential opportunity (although currently under-utilized) for achieving valuable synergy [2, 4–6]. In pediatrics, however, it is virtually a requirement that immunotherapy be integrated in combination with the existing standard-of-care treatments. This is because in pediatrics the standard-of-care therapies are often highly effective, and even in relapsed or high-risk disease can still offer significant (albeit reduced) benefit. Thus, if immunotherapy is going to have a major near-term impact on the treatment of children, it will need to extend and enhance the efficacy of our existing treatments, not attempt to replace them. Fortunately, emerging preclinical evidence suggests that both chemotherapy and radiation are not only feasible for combination with immunotherapy, but can be highly synergistic.

2.2 Exploiting Immunotherapy to Create Synergy with Cytotoxic Therapy

2.2.1 Chemo-Immunotherapy: Beyond Synergy to True Synthetic Lethality

For a number of years it has been recognized that chemotherapy creates effects that can be exploited to enhance the immune response to tumors [7]. One obvious effect is the release of tumor antigens from dying cells; but, in addition, certain chemotherapy drugs may deplete regulatory T cells [8], or create lymphopenic conditions that favor T cell proliferation and expansion [9]. However, these effects are essentially passive: creating a general milieu in which vaccines or other immunotherapy may work better. A more active role for chemotherapy was revealed with the discovery of so-called "immunogenic cell death" (ICD) [10–12]. When certain preclinical mouse tumor models are treated with particular chemotherapy drugs, the tumor cells die in a fashion that triggers a spontaneous immune response. Not only does this help prime the immune system against the tumor, but (at least in these particular model/drug combinations) a substantial component of the efficacy of the chemotherapy itself is actually contributed by the immune system [12]. While this was a ground-breaking discovery, in practical terms there are relatively few drugs that elicit ICD, and the effect is highly model-dependent [13]. Thus, while the underlying concept is important, the high-impact clinical role for immunogenic cell death is likely to be in combination with immunomodulatory agents that can enhance and exploit the effect [14]. As we will discuss, when the underlying inhibitory pathways are removed by active immunotherapy, then many chemotherapy drugs may prove to be immunogenic [4].

Ultimately, the goal in combining immunotherapy with chemotherapy is not merely "synergy" in the pharmacologic sense, but rather to generate authentic *synthetic lethality* by the combination. Synthetic lethality describes a combination in which the two agents together recruit an entirely new set of molecular mechanisms, which would not come into play with either agent alone [15, 16]. Thus, for example, in pre-clinical models, our own group has shown that combining a normally ineffective dose of chemotherapy with a specific immune-activating agent (i.e., an agent that blocks a tolerogenic checkpoint to dying tumor cells), allows the ineffective chemotherapy to now cause potent and rapid tumor regression [17]. The mechanism of anti-tumor effect was almost entirely immunologic (T cell dependent), but these immune mechanisms were only triggered if the tumor was also treated with chemotherapy.

2.2.2 *The Importance of Endogenous Tumor Antigens*

One of the surprising findings of the past several years has been the importance of endogenous tumor antigens in cancer immunotherapy [18]. Prior to the advent of checkpoint-blockade agents, the focus of immunotherapy was often on supplying antigens and T cells exogenously—e.g., via defined vaccines, TIL infusions, TCR-transgenic T cells, or CAR T cells. However, as increasing numbers of patients have been treated with blockade of the CTLA-4 and PD-1/PD-L1 pathways, it has become evident that the best responses are seen in those patients who have many mutational neoantigens in the tumor, and who already have a robust spontaneous immune response prior to treatment [19, 20].

In part this may simply be an artifact of early trials, which use only single-agent checkpoint blockade. In this setting, it is perhaps logical that only those patients who were already spontaneously pre-activated could respond to removing a single checkpoint. This effect may disappear as more powerful combination regimens are employed [21]. But the key take-home point is that the tumor's own endogenous antigens, cross-presented by the patient's own APCs to the endogenous T cell repertoire, were the critical factor that drove the anti-tumor response. This emphasizes the importance of endogenous tumor antigens, and the ability to cross-present them in an immunogenic fashion.

This has obvious importance for the immune response to chemotherapy or radiation, which release a wave of endogenous tumor antigens. But even in the case of an exogenous immune intervention, such as an antigen-specific vaccine or T cell adoptive transfer (CAR T cells, etc.), a successful long-term outcome may still depend on generating a response to endogenous tumor antigens [1]. Transferred T cells or defined vaccines are directed against just one or a few antigens. The initial response may be dramatic, but eventual emergence of escape variants is almost inevitable. If, however, during the initial period of robust inflammation and tumor killing, the endogenous host immune system becomes primed to endogenous tumor antigens, then the danger of escape variants is minimized, and long-term tumor control becomes a possibility.

2.2.3 Immunogenic Cell Death Versus Tolerogenic Cell Death: Overcoming Natural Pathways of Tolerance

The preceding general discussion does not tell us how—specifically—to render chemotherapy immunogenic in the clinic. In part this reflects the fact that much still needs to be discovered about the molecular mechanisms of combination chemo-immunotherapy. Also, our current options for immune intervention in the clinic are still somewhat limited, comprising primarily blocking agents against CTLA-4 or the PD-1/PD-L1 pathways, and blockade of the indoleamine 2,3-dioxygenase (IDO) pathway. However, the field is expanding rapidly and the armamentarium is quickly increasing. Thus, a better understanding of the molecular events that regulate the immune response following chemotherapy, in order to exploit this for therapy, has become a subject of some urgency.

In this regard, one fundamental insight emerging recently is the fact that the immune response to dying cells—even normal, non-malignant self cells—is not fixed and inherent. Rather, it reflects a combination of signals generated by the manner in which the cells die (ICD, apoptosis, necrosis etc.), combined with signals from the milieu in which the dying cells are cross-presented by the immune system. These local environmental signals are a very active—and changeable—process. Blocking even one of the tolerogenic signals elicited by apoptotic cells may render dying cells suddenly immunogenic instead. Thus, for example, the tolerogenic IDO pathway is strongly up-regulated by exposure to apoptotic cells [22]. When challenged with apoptotic self cells, normal IDO-sufficient mice remained tolerant, but mice lacking the IDO1 gene rapidly developed lethal lupus-like autoimmunity against self antigens [22–24]. Thus, it was not the nature of the antigens themselves that determined immunity versus tolerance, nor the type of cell death; but rather the ability of the apoptotic cells to elicit the immunosuppressive IDO signal. If this IDO pathway was blocked, then the same cells, and the same self antigens, now became immunogenic.

The relevance of this concept for cancer treatment is that chemotherapy and radiation release a wave of tumor antigens, many of which are potentially immunogenic

[18, 25]. The problem is that these antigens are released into a tumor milieu that is overwhelmingly dominated by immunosuppressive mechanisms. Thus, even though dying tumor cells are potentially immunogenic [6] the actual outcome is usually tolerance and anergy, due to these dominant suppressive mechanisms. If, however, the tolerogenic pathways used by the tumor (such as IDO, Tregs or others) can be identified and blocked at the time of chemotherapy, then the antigens thus released may be treated as immunizing instead of tolerizing. This concept is now well accepted in principle [1, 2], and relevant preclinical studies are beginning to emerge [17], but much of the underlying molecular machinery still remains to be discovered. However, even with our current limited state of knowledge, it is possible to begin to design clinical trials aimed at exploiting the immunogenicity of chemotherapy.

2.3 Negative Regulation in the Tumor Microenvironment

In this section we will briefly discuss several of the key suppressive pathways operating in the tumor. Many of these are discussed in detail elsewhere in this volume, so our focus here is specifically how these inhibitory pathways may affect the cross-presentation and immune response to tumor antigens.

2.3.1 Regulatory T Cells: Recruitment and Activation

Regulatory T cells (Tregs) in tumors are an important suppressive population [26]. Physically depleting Tregs [27] or inhibiting the signals that they require [28] rescues anti-tumor immune surveillance. However, it is still unclear how Tregs exert their suppressive function. One important mechanism may be their ability to inhibit tumor-associated antigen-presenting cells [29, 30]. This would be a key leverage point for control of antigen cross-presentation to T cells.

One important unanswered question in the field is why Treg activity is so excessive in the tumor. Many of the Tregs in tumors appear to recognize the same self antigens as in normal tissues [31], but there is a greater degree of constitutive functional activation of Tregs in tumors [32]. Several upstream pathways are known to activate tumor-associated Tregs, includes IDO [32] and neuropilin-1 [33]. Recently, it was shown that when Tregs are activated by IDO they up regulate the PD-1 receptor; PD-1 signaling then maintains the suppressive Treg phenotype long-term, via activation of the downstream PTEN phosphatase [17]. Neuropilin-1 also activates PTEN in Tregs [33], and PTEN has been recently implicated in maintaining normal function and stability of Tregs in the normal immune system [34, 35]. Thus, PTEN may be a centrally-positioned pathway in tumor-induced activation of Tregs. In tumor-bearing mice, ablation or inhibition of the PTEN pathway in Tregs prevented tumors from creating their usual immunosuppressive microenvironment, and this markedly enhanced the immune response to dying tumor cells following chemotherapy [17].

2.3.2 CTLA-4 and PD-1 Pathways: The Classic T Cell Checkpoints

CTLA-4 and PD-1 are inhibitory molecules expressed by activated T cells. Clinically, antibodies against these molecules may dramatically enhance the ability of patient's T cells to attack their own tumors, especially in patients who already have a pre-existing anti-tumor T cell response at diagnosis. Anti-CTLA-4 was the first checkpoint-inhibitor to be approved [36]. While responses to single-agent therapy have been limited, combination with PD-1 blockade is encouraging [21]. Clinical benefit was greatest in patients with a high mutational burden in their tumor genome, and a large number of predicted mutational neoantigens [37, 38]. But the effect of CTLA-4 is not limited to tumor-specific neoantigens; patients also showed a significant increase in the frequency of T cells against self antigens associated with melanoma [39]. Thus, blocking CTLA-4 may enhance the ability of the host immune system to respond to endogenous tumor antigens, including even breaking tolerance to shared self/tumor antigens. Therefore, a key take-home message from these studies is that the T cell response to endogenous tumor antigens is not fixed, and can be increased if the relevant suppressive mechanisms can be blocked.

The mechanism of action of CTLA-4 blockade is still unclear [40]. It may lower the activation threshold for effector T cells, and/or it may inhibit or deplete regulatory T cells (Tregs) [40, 41]. Since Tregs can suppress the function of antigen-presenting cells in the tumor [29, 30], blocking CTLA-4 may indirectly enhance cross-presentation of tumor antigens.

PD-1 is a second inhibitory molecule expressed on activated T cells. Some tumor cells constitutively express PD-L1, the counter-ligand for PD-1, and other tumor cells may up-regulate PD-L1 in response to inflammatory signals. In addition, host APCs (dendritic cells (DCs), Myeloid Derived Suppressor Cells (MDSCs) and macrophages) can express constitutive or inducible PD-L1 or PD-L2, and this may be a biologically important source of inhibition [42]. In certain tumors, blocking PD-1 or PD-L1 can trigger striking clinical responses in a subset of patients. Like CTLA-4 blockade, response to single-agent therapy is more likely in patients who have many neoantigens and a strong spontaneous anti-tumor immune response at baseline [20, 42, 43].

Although there is little published literature on attempts to combine CTLA-4 or PD-1/PD-L1 blockade with chemotherapy, this strategy to date has not met with much obvious success [44]. In this regard it may be important to note that both CTLA-4 and PD-1 are expressed by T cells, and become relevant when the T cells are activated. In the setting of chemotherapy, however, the fundamental immunologic defect may occur much earlier than this, at the level of the tolerogenic milieu and the initial antigen-presentation step. If antigen-presentation is defective or tolerogenic, then the CTLA-4 and PD-1 checkpoints may not even come into play. Thus, CTLA-4 and PD-1 may not be the optimal targets for combination with chemotherapy, because they are too far downstream. That said, if the antigen-presenting milieu after chemotherapy can be improved by blocking upstream checkpoints such as IDO, then the CTLA-4 and PD-1 checkpoints on T cells may now become relevant and useful for combinatorial therapy.

2.3.3 *Targeting the IDO Pathway*

Indoleamine 2,3-dioxygenase (IDO) is a tryptophan-degrading enzyme expressed by cells in the immune system; it can also be expressed by inflamed tissues (epithelial cells and fibroblasts) and by some tumor cells (reviewed in ref. [45]). The immunologic function of the IDO pathway is both counter-regulatory (suppressing excessive inflammation) and tolerogenic (creating de novo antigen-specific tolerance in T cells). In preclinical models, when the IDO pathway is interrupted mice experience multiple defects in tolerance, including maternal tolerance to the fetus during pregnancy [46–48]; mucosal and other forms of acquired peripheral tolerance [49–56]; and tolerance to apoptotic cells [22, 24]. Conversely, artificial overexpression of IDO can create systemic tolerance de novo [24, 56–58]. IDO also controls inflammation, acting to enhance the tissue-reparative effects of inflammation while limiting the tissue-destructive effects [59–66]. In all of these models, the role of IDO is focused and selective; and IDO-deficient mice do not have the broad, spontaneous defects in self-tolerance that are seen with mice lacking CTLA-4 or Treg cells. (This may be an important consideration in understanding the mild toxicity profile of IDO-inhibitor drugs in the clinic.) However, in settings where IDO is important, it can be a crucial and non-redundant mechanism of immune regulation.

IDO degrades the essential amino acid tryptophan to kynurenine. The IDO gene family includes IDO1 (the main subject of this section) and a related gene, IDO2 [67–69] which is much less well studied. In this chapter, we will use the term "IDO" to refer to IDO1, or to the collective functional IDO enzyme activity. Depletion of local tryptophan by IDO can activate the amino-acid sensitive stress-kinase GCN2. Activation of GCN2 in T cells can inhibit effector T cell proliferation and function, and increase the suppressor function of Tregs [70–72]. In antigen-presenting cells, GCN2 inhibits inflammatory signals [73], and it can profoundly bias antigen-presenting cells toward tolerance induction [24]. In addition to activating GCN2, IDO produces diffusible soluble factors (kynurenine and downstream metabolites) that bind to the aryl hydrocarbon receptor (AhR) [74]. The AhR can enhance Treg function [72, 74], suppress acute inflammatory cytokines such as IL-12 and IL-6 [22, 24, 75] and bias dendritic cells and macrophages toward an immunosuppressive phenotype [24, 75–78]. Taken together, this means that IDO expression can have a profound effect on the nature of the antigen-presentation process in a local tissue site: rendering it tolerogenic when IDO is active, or immunogenic when IDO is blocked [22, 24, 70, 79–81].

2.3.3.1 Activation of Treg Cells by IDO

IDO controls an important activation pathway in Tregs. Resting Tregs are not suppressive, and they must undergo activation in order to become functionally active [82]. This activation step requires both TCR engagement [83] and modulating signals from the local microenvironment [84]. When Tregs are activated by an

IDO-expressing APC, they become highly suppressive [32]. IDO affects Treg activation by inhibiting mTORC2 and Akt signaling in the Treg [17]. This results in up-regulation of PD-1 expression by the Tregs, which then activates the PTEN lipid phosphatase. The PD-1 → PTEN pathway then continues the inhibition of Akt, thus forming a positive feedback loop that maintains on-going Treg suppressor activity as long as the milieu contains PD-ligands. IDO is not the only pathway that can activate PTEN in Tregs: neuropilin-1 (Nrp1) can have a similar activating effect [33]. But IDO may be particularly important in the tumor following chemotherapy or other insult, because it appears that IDO may directly link exposure to apoptotic cells with activation of the potent PTEN-expressing Tregs [17], as discussed in the next section.

2.3.3.2 IDO and Tolerance to Apoptotic Cells

In the normal immune system, IDO is strongly induced by apoptotic cells [22] and appears to play an important role in maintaining tolerance to apoptotic cells. When normal mice are challenged with large numbers of apoptotic thymocytes they remain tolerant, and will even create de novo tolerance to foreign antigens introduced on the apoptotic cells [22, 24]. However, if IDO1 is blocked then mice cannot create tolerance to apoptotic cells, and rapidly develop lupus-like autoimmunity against self antigens [22, 24].

In the case of tumors, challenge with apoptotic tumor cells was found to up-regulate IDO, which in turn elicited PTEN-expressing Tregs. These then inhibited immune response to antigens from the apoptotic cells [17]. Even in mice without tumors, targeted deletion of the PTEN gene in Tregs caused loss of self-tolerance when challenged with apoptotic cells (a phenotype essentially identical to mice lacking IDO) [17]. It is still speculative whether these same molecular pathways are operative in human tumors following chemotherapy; but it is clear that tumors are constantly faced with the need to suppress immune recognition of the highly abnormal dying tumor cells. Thus, tumors may "hijack" the normal IDO and PTEN-Treg pathways that inhibit responses to dying cells, and exaggerate them to render dying tumor cells tolerogenic.

2.3.3.3 IDO, PTEN-Tregs and Immunogenic Cell Death

The concept that specific regulatory mechanisms such as IDO and PTEN-Tregs are actively up-regulated by dying cells, and thus prevents the immune system from responding, has significant implications for tumor immunotherapy. In principle, tumor cells should be much more immunogenic than normal cells, since they possess mutational neoantigens, and can also aberrantly over-express self antigens in an immunogenic fashion [18, 25]. It is well known that certain forms of chemotherapy, in the right tumor models, can create sufficient inflammation to elicit T cell immune responses (immunogenic cell death, as reviewed in ref. [10]). Unfortunately, in most tumors, most chemotherapy drugs do not appear to elicit a robust immune response—at least by themselves. However, this may be an artifact of the exaggerated levels of counter-regulatory suppression, such as IDO and activated Tregs, which are present in the tumor. If these suppressive pathways can be blocked, then immunogenic cell death may actually be much more widespread than currently recognized. Figure 2.1 summarizes the possibility that, during tumor cell death, two sets of signals are created simultaneously: some death occurs by apoptosis, and thus elicits mechanisms of tolerance; while some death is disordered and immunogenic. In the suppressive tumor milieu, however, the inhibitory pathways are exaggerated, and the immunogenic component is therefore dominantly suppressed. If these suppressive signals are blocked, however, then the immune system becomes able to respond to the underlying immunogenic cell death.

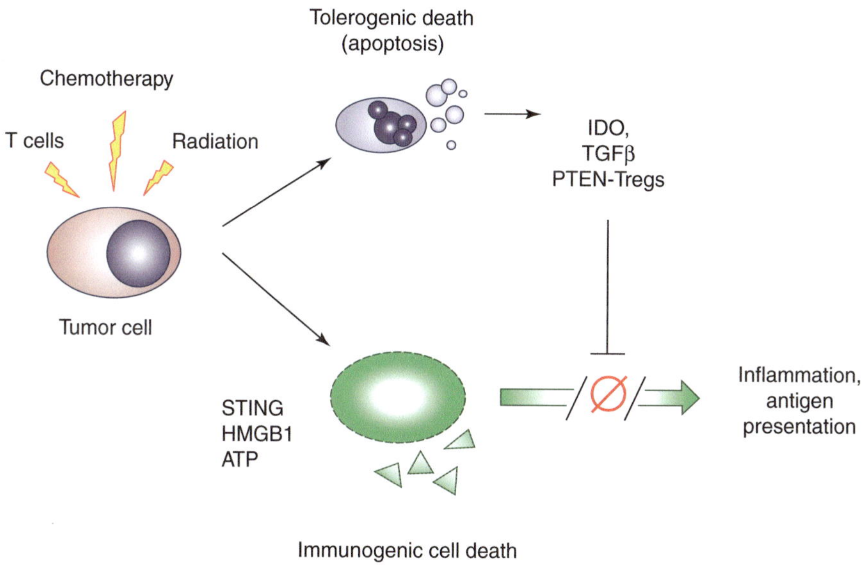

Fig. 2.1 Two possible responses to dying tumor cells. When tumor cells die following exposure to chemotherapy, radiation or killing by cytotoxic T cells, they may be treated by the immune system in one of two ways. Either they die in an immunogenic fashion, releasing inflammatory mediators and triggering cross-presentation of tumor antigens to T cells; or, alternatively, they may die in a tolerogenic fashion, eliciting suppressive signals such as IDO, TGFβ and activated Tregs. In the model shown, we propose that both forms of cell death usually co-exist in the tumor following therapy, but that the tolerogenic pathways are dominant unless they can be blocked or circumvented by immunotherapy

2.3.3.4 Clinical Trials of IDO-Inhibitor Drugs

Inhibitors of the IDO pathway do not kill tumor cells directly. Their role is to permit and enhance immune responses following chemotherapy, radiation or other immunotherapy. Table 2.1 gives a partial listing of current clinical trials of inhibitors of the IDO pathway. Most of the trials are based on either indoximod (1-methyl-D-tryptophan, NewLink Genetics, Inc.) [85–88] or epacadostat (INCB024360, Incyte Pharmaceuticals, Inc.) [89–91]. One of these trials (NCT02502708) is in pediatric

Table 2.1 Clinical trials of IDO-inhibitor drugs

Strategy	Drug	Patients	Trial design	Trial number
Combination with chemotherapy	Indoximod (NewLink Genetics)	Adult	With taxanes in breast cancer	NCT01792050
	Indoximod	Adult	With temozolomide ± radiation in refractory glioblastoma brain tumors	NCT02052648
	Indoximod	Pediatric	With temozolomide ± radiation in pediatric brain tumors	NCT02502708
	Indoximod	Adult	With gemcitabine/abraxane in pancreatic cancer	NCT02077881
	Epacadostat (Incyte)	Adult	With Jak1 inhibitor or PI3Kδ inhibitor	NCT02559492
Combination with checkpoint inhibitors	Epacadostat	Adult	With anti-CTLA-4 (ipilimumab)	NCT01604889
	Indoximod	Adult	With anti-CTLA-4 (ipilimumab)	NCT02073123
	Epacadostat	Adult	With anti-PD-1 (pembrolizumab)	NCT02178722
	Epacadostat	Adult	With anti-PD-L1 (atezolizumab)	NCT02298153
	Epacadostat	Adult	With anti-PD-L1 (MEDI4736)	NCT02318277
	GDC-0919 (Genentech Roche)	Adult	With anti-PD-L1 (atezolizumab)	NCT02471846
Combination with vaccines	Epacadostat	Adult	With NY-ESO-1 vaccine in ovarian cancer	NCT02166905
	Indoximod	Adult	With Hyperacute vaccine (NewLink Genetics) + docetaxel in lung cancer	NCT02460367
	Epacadostat	Adult	With peptide vaccine in melanoma	NCT01961115
	Epacadostat	Adult	With Listeria mesothelin vaccine in ovarian cancer	NCT02575807

patients. No final results have yet been published, so it is too early to assess the benefits of these strategies, but anecdotal results and meeting reports have been encouraging. Additional IDO inhibitors are in the development pipeline, as well as agents that may target IDO2 [92] or TDO [93, 94], two other tryptophan-catabolizing enzymes that may affect tumor immunity [95].

2.3.4 *Tumor-Associated Macrophages and Myeloid-Derived Suppressor Cells (MDSCs)*

Tumor-associated macrophages (TAMs) are key coordinators of tumor-promoting angiogenesis, fibrous stroma deposition and metastasis formation [96]. In addition, TAMs are also actively suppressive for T cell responses [97]. In part, this immunosuppressive phenotype may simply recapitulate the "reparative" phenotype of macrophages during tissue remodeling [98]. While it is usual to think of wounds as inflammatory, a sterile healing wound (i.e., without a superimposed infection) is actually not a receptive milieu for antigen-specific T cell activation. Sterile wounds are indeed inflammatory, but this is all chronic innate immunity, and any antigens present are purely self antigens. Thus, T cell responses are undesirable, and they are actively suppressed by signals such as TGFβ and VEGF, which are high during tissue repair. Tumors resemble "wounds that do not heal" [99], and share many of these features of chronic inflammation with T cell immunosuppression. In addition, tumors contain abnormal signals such as acidosis and hypoxia which may further drive the immunosuppressive phenotype of the associated macrophages [100]. The molecular mechanisms by which TAMs suppress T cell activation in tumors are not yet well defined, but likely include production of VEGF and TGFβ, as mentioned above. Whatever the mechanism, destabilization of the intra-tumoral macrophage pool, e.g., by blocking the CSF-1-receptor, significantly impairs tumor growth and enhances anti-tumor immune responses [101, 102].

While TAMs may superficially resemble normal macrophages, in reality the myeloid cells in the tumor are all profoundly disordered [96, 103]. In tumor-bearing hosts, bone-marrow myelopoiesis is altered by factors secreted from the tumor, such as GM-CSF and IL-6, which affects both the monocytic and granulocytic lineages [104, 105]. These abnormal circulating cells become further altered when they are recruited into the tumor microenvironment, with its chronic low-grade inflammation, free-radical flux and constant metabolic stress [106]. The presence of IDO and activated Tregs in the tumor may further enhance the recruitment of these cells, and render them even more suppressive [86]. Once in place, this heterogeneous population of myeloid-derived suppressor cells (MDSCs) creates an immunosuppressive milieu via elaboration of nitric oxide, arginase and reactive oxygen species [96, 107]. Much of the preclinical work on MDSCs has been performed in mouse models, but analogous cells exist in human tumors [108]. The suppressive nature of MDSCs in tumors is completely different from their inflammatory, highly immunogenic counterparts that would normally be created at the site of an infection (inflammatory monocytes, macrophages and myeloid DCs) [104, 105]. Currently, it is unclear exactly how this abnormal, suppressive state of the myeloid cells in tumors can be reversed. Certain forms of chemotherapy may reduce the number of MDSCs [109]; but, paradoxically, chemotherapy may also elicit a rebound increase in MDSCs [110]. Reducing suppression by MDSCs is a subject of ongoing investigation. Ultimately, however, the most effective approach may be to create a robust pro-inflammatory microenvironment within the tumor by means of immunotherapy: under these conditions the myeloid-lineage cells may now be able to follow their normal, beneficial pathway of differentiation into immunogenic APCs [104].

2.3.5 Overcoming Therapy-Induced Counter-Regulation

The immune system provides potent protection against infection, but it can also be lethal if its activation is not controlled. Hence, the normal immune system contains multiple built-in regulatory feedback loops that control inflammation and limit excessive activation. Thus, for example, pro-inflammatory IFNγ simultaneously up-regulates anti-inflammatory PD-L1 and IDO [111]; while T cell activation spontaneously recruits corresponding suppressive Tregs [84, 112]. In the tumor milieu, these same counter-regulatory mechanisms are operative, and they are often pathologically exaggerated and dominant. As discussed above, this becomes relevant when the immune system must make the decision between immunity and tolerance to apoptotic tumor cells. In addition, pathways of inducible counter-regulation may become important when successful immunotherapy (e.g., a vaccination or CAR T cells) begins to create beneficial inflammation in the tumor. The presence of this desirable inflammation may elicit exaggerated and undesirable counter-regulation, e.g., by up-regulating PD-ligands or IDO [43, 111]. Thus, the efficacy of the initiating therapy is unwittingly compromised by its own success, unless agents are added to block this inducible counter-regulation.

2.4 Implications for the Clinic: Using Chemotherapy as an Immune Adjuvant

2.4.1 Bi-directional Synergy: Chemotherapy as a Vaccine, and the Immune System as a Cytolytic Agent

Based on the forgoing discussion of mechanisms, the field of immunotherapy has a growing opportunity to exploit the synergy (synthetic lethality) between chemotherapy and immunotherapy. As mentioned above, it is now well accepted that chemotherapy has the potential to function as an endogenous "vaccine" when it releases antigens from dying tumor cells [2, 4, 6]. By itself, conventional chemotherapy is typically not highly immunogenic [13]; but as we begin to better understand—and thus become able to block—the inhibitory mechanisms that suppress immune responses after chemotherapy, our standard chemotherapy agents may become much more immunogenic as part of a combined regimen.

A second, less appreciated aspect of the synergy between chemotherapy and immunotherapy is that the immune system can become a potent downstream effector mechanism for conventional chemotherapy. Historically, when immunogenic cell death was first discovered, there was some speculation that all chemotherapy—even without immunotherapy—might rely on the immune system to cause tumor regression [113]. This turned out to be over-optimistic, and probably applies more to mouse models of transplantable tumor cell lines [114]. However, the situation becomes much different when chemotherapy is combined with active immunotherapy into a dual regimen. Now the immune system is being actively recruited and empowered to provide additional anti-tumor effector mechanisms, which would not normally come into play with standard chemotherapy alone. Thus, the immune system becomes, in effect, a downstream effector arm for the chemotherapy. This effect has been modeled in preclinical mouse systems [17, 115], and there are some encouraging suggestions that it may be translatable into the clinic as well [116, 117].

2.4.2 *Targeted Therapies Can Also Release Antigen*

The armamentarium of the oncologist is increasing beyond standard chemotherapy, and now includes antibodies, antibody-drug conjugates (ADCs) and selective kinase inhibitors. ADCs target chemotherapy drugs preferentially to tumor cells; they may be very cytolytic and immune-activating, and prime the tumor milieu for response to immunotherapy [118]. The immunologic response to targeted kinase inhibitors is not yet well understood, but when used against a tumor that is heavily dependent on the specific pathway being targeted, then these drugs can cause dramatic tumor regression (although subsequent resistance is a problem). It is not yet known if these targeted agents are as stimulatory for immune responses as conventional chemotherapy, but there is mounting evidence that many (perhaps all) of these agents can be immunogenic [6]. However, because these targeted agents at present play less of a role in pediatrics, our focus will be primarily on conventional cytotoxic chemotherapy.

2.4.3 *How Immunosuppressive Is Chemotherapy … Really?*

Every oncologist has a healthy respect for the myelosuppressive potential of chemotherapy; thus, it seems somewhat counter-intuitive to combine chemotherapy with immunotherapy. However, myelosuppression does not necessarily imply a corresponding degree of T cell suppression (which is the relevant attribute for response to immunotherapy). Thus, for example, most chemotherapy regimens for solid tumors—even dose-intensive pediatric regimens—do not require prophylaxis against Pneumocystis or invasive fungal infections, in the way that a T cell-immunocompromised patient would require. While patients may transiently have a low circulating T cell after chemotherapy, their lymph nodes and spleen do not go away, nor do the T cells in the tumor. Indeed, given the chance, the antigen-specific T cells associated with the tumor may be the first to rebound after chemotherapy, because they are responding to the wave of tumor antigens that have been released [119].

The timing and dosage of chemotherapy relative to the timing of immunotherapy must be optimized so as not to suppress the T cell response produced, but appropriate regimens can be designed to accomplish this [120]. Such regimens may be helped by the fact that antigen-specific T cells in the tumor may be non-proliferating at the time of chemotherapy (because they are anergic, or suppressed by the tumor microenvironment), and are thus protected from the effects of chemotherapy. Tumor-associated T cells may only become activated and proliferating later, after the chemotherapy is eliminated and gone. Thus, far from being inimical to immunotherapy, chemotherapy is in fact a ready-made opportunity to be exploited [2, 4].

2.4.4 The Late-Responder Paradox: Immune-Related Response Criteria

When patients are treated with conventional chemotherapy, they typically show one of three patterns: either they respond and are cured; or they fail to respond at all; or they respond for a period of time and then progress despite therapy (i.e., they become resistant). In those patients who do respond, the benefit of conventional chemotherapy is invariably front-loaded: the best response occurs in the initial cycles, and once the tumor begins to progress on therapy (becomes resistant) there is no further benefit from that particular agent or regimen.

In contrast, when tumors are treated with immunotherapy, there can be additional, less familiar patterns of response (Fig. 2.2). The immune system inherently displays memory and recall. Thus, as we know from childhood immunizations, an immune response can become progressively stronger the more times it is exposed to antigen (prime and boost). Therefore, some patients treated with anti-tumor immunotherapy may experience paradoxical late responses, occurring only after many months of treatment. Indeed, there can even be a period of early progression, sometimes lasting several cycles of therapy, before the immune system becomes sufficiently activated to cause tumor regression. This pattern of apparent resistance followed by late regression is essentially never seen with chemotherapy alone. (The specialized case of transient pseudoprogression in brain tumors is actually an effect of successful treatment, not progression [121]). The exact mechanism of these late immunologic responses is still a subject of investigation. It may simply represent progressive "boosting" with repeated treatment; but it also seems likely that late responses reflect a complex shift in the equilibrium between the suppression and immunity in the tumor milieu [1, 122]. Whatever the mechanism, it is important to bear in mind the possibility of late responses when designing clinical trials and stopping rules. This means, for example, the use of appropriate immune-related response criteria [123], which allow for a limited period of initial progression before removing patients from the study.

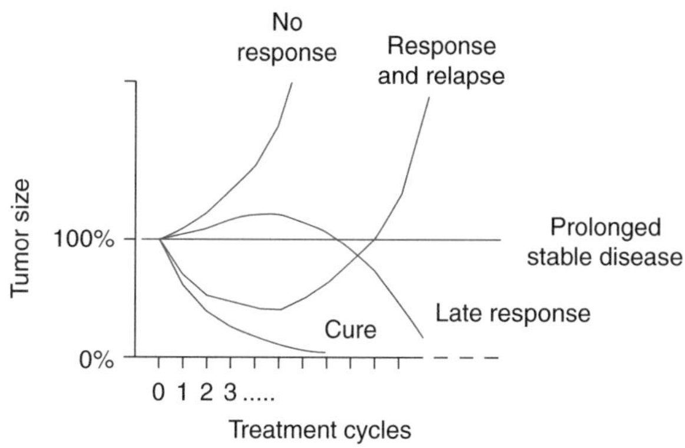

Fig. 2.2 Late responses and stable disease as potential outcomes with immunotherapy. Traditionally, responses to conventional chemotherapy or radiation tend to occur early, if they occur at all. With chemotherapy, for example, the traditional response patterns are either progressive remission induction leading to cure, or an early response followed by subsequent relapse (i.e., the tumor becomes resistant). However, when the immune system participates in the anti-tumor response, due to the addition of immunotherapy to the treatment regimen, then additional patterns of response become possible. Because the immune system can show increasing activation with repeated antigen exposure (immunologic memory), patients receiving immunotherapy may show late responses—sometimes even after multiple cycles of apparent non-response, or even transient progression. Alternatively, the immune system may establish an apparent "equilibrium" state with the tumor, during which residual disease remains, but is prevented from growing by the on-going immune attack. This results in a pattern of long-term stable disease, even though residual tumor is still present. Neither of these latter two patterns would be expected with conventional chemotherapy or radiation, but they are recognized patterns with immunotherapy

As a variant of the late-response pattern, immunotherapy may sometimes simply produce a prolonged period of stable disease, without complete regression (or a pattern of mixed regression of only some lesions). On the occasions when these stable lesions have been biopsied, they often contain an active, on-going immune response. Obviously, in pediatric patients the ultimate goal is cure. But it is important to bear in mind that stable disease in the setting of immunotherapy may actually be a signal of robust immune activation, and an on-going, almost-successful effort at tumor control.

2.4.5 *Using Immunotherapy to Reduce the Dose of Chemotherapy*

Pediatric malignancies tend to be chemotherapy-responsive, and the cure rate in pediatrics is much higher than in adults. However, this success is often purchased at the price of higher dose-intensity, especially in patients with high-risk or relapsed disease. Indeed, much of the acute and long-term morbidity and impact on quality of life relates to the side effects of chemotherapy—and, specifically, to the need for higher dose-intensity in many settings. But the use of more dose-intense and toxic regimens has been largely driven by the need to extract more efficacies from chemotherapy regimens used by themselves. Now that immunotherapy agents are becoming available for combination regimens, it may be possible to leverage the immunotherapy to reduce the dose of the conventional chemotherapy. Whether this approach will be successful in the clinic remains to be seen, but preclinical models would suggest that it does not take ultra-high doses of chemotherapy to release immunologically useful amounts of antigen; and, indeed, higher doses of chemotherapy may actually suppress the immune response of interest. Clinically, the dose-reduction needed to reduce side-effects and increase quality of life may not be huge: even a 25–33% dose-reduction from the MTD may be significantly less toxic. One would not intentionally trade loss of efficacy for fewer side-effects, but if adding immunotherapy allows greater efficacy at lower doses, then this would be an important advance for pediatric patients.

2.4.6 Combination Chemo-Immunotherapy Is Particularly Well-Suited to the Pediatric Population

Because childhood malignancies are typically more responsive to chemotherapy, there is more opportunity to treat even relapsed or metastatic disease with curative intent, rather than just for palliation (as often occurs in adults). Thus, second-line or even third-line regimens in children may have a percentage of patients (albeit perhaps small) who can legitimately hope for cure. This is almost never the case in adults. But the consequence of this superior responsiveness to chemotherapy is that it would be inappropriate in children to attempt to forego standard-of-care chemotherapy, and replace it with immunotherapy alone. This may well be appropriate in adults, where immunotherapy often is used in place of chemotherapy [36], because of the dismal prognosis with chemotherapy. However, in children chemotherapy often still holds prospect of benefit. Thus, in order to offer optimal benefit of immunotherapy to the pediatric population, it is important to seamlessly integrate immunotherapy with standard-of-care chemotherapy. This not only allows immunotherapy to be used earlier in the course of the disease, when the patient's immune system is less compromised by extensive pre-treatment and widespread burden of disease; but it also holds the prospect of enhancing the efficacy of the standard chemotherapy itself, and perhaps reducing the dose-intensity and toxicity.

2.5 Rethinking the Possibilities of Radiation: Using Local Radiation to Create an Endogenous Vaccine

2.5.1 Local Radiation and Systemic Immune Responses: The Abscopal Effect

Radiation kills tumor cells by damaging DNA, via a process that depends heavily on generating oxygen free radicals. The effects of radiation are highly inflammatory, and the dying tumor cells are potentially immunogenic [124]. Because radiation is so pro-inflammatory (whereas most systemic chemotherapy is not); local irradiation may serve as a valuable adjunct to chemo-immunotherapy. By releasing a wave of tumor antigens and creating local inflammation, ablative radiation may serve as an effective "vaccine" against endogenous tumor antigens [125]. However, just as with cell death after chemotherapy, radiation by itself is rarely able to break tolerance to tumor antigens. However, the tolerogenic and suppressive checkpoints after radiation appear very similar to the checkpoints that restrict response to chemotherapy [126]. Thus, when combined with active immunotherapy, the immunologic effects of radiation may become much more pronounced and exploitable [2].

As an example, in 2012, Wolchok and colleagues reported a serendipitous observation in a patient with metastatic melanoma being treated with CTLA-4 blockade, who also happened to receive concurrent palliative local radiation to a single lesion for relief of spinal-cord compression [127]. Unexpectedly, this patient underwent widespread involution of metastatic lesions outside the field of radiation (the so-called "abscopal" effect), with systemic tumor-specific immune activation. Similar anecdotal abscopal effects have been reported with other immunotherapy, and follow-on clinical trials have been initiated in a variety of indications [128]. In another approach, local irradiation of isolated tumor lesions has been combined with intralesional injection of an immune adjuvant (TLR-ligand), and this can actively elicit abscopal responses at distant sites [129].

Thus—at least in principal—local irradiation, with its intense inflammation and endogenous "vaccine" effect, has the potential to make an important and non-redundant contribution to multi-modal immunotherapy regimens.

2.5.2 Designing Radiation Strategies for Maximal Immune Effect

If radiation is intended as an immune-activating component of a combination immunotherapy regimen (rather than as a single-agent treatment), then the design considerations become somewhat different. Radiation is highly toxic to normal tissues, yet radiation alone can only be curative if every tumor cell is included in the field. Thus, under conventional strategies, radiation fields must deliberately incorporate a margin of normal tissue so as to include microscopic infiltrating tumor cells. It is this need to irradiate margins of normal tissue that accounts for almost all of the acute and long-term toxicities of radiation. Radiating only the middle of the tumor would have little toxicity, but it would also never be curative, since the residual tumor would rapidly regrow. However, as a component of immunotherapy, irradiating only the lesion itself (without margins of normal tissue) is a perfectly usable source of tumor antigens and the "endogenous vaccine" effect. And, if the immunotherapy works at all, it will work on microscopic residual disease, so there is no need to increase the toxicity of radiation in an attempt to secure extensive margins. As a source of antigens and inflammation, hypofractionated radiation (stereotactic radiosurgery, or stereotactic body radiotherapy) may be more inflammatory and immunogenic than a less toxic hyper-fractionated schedule [125].

When radiation is used as a single agent, the decision whether to use it at all is restricted by considerations of toxicity and futility. Thus, re-irradiation must be undertaken with caution (and often may not be possible); and stereotactic radiation of a lesion is futile (other than for palliation) if other metastatic lesions are present. However, when radiation is used as an integral component of active immunotherapy, then the calculus is changed. Toxicity may be much reduced because margins are not necessary; and it is no longer necessary to include every lesion in the radiation field (since the whole goal is the abscopal effect) [127]. Finally, irradiating a key, life-threatening lesion may de-bulk the tumor and buy valuable time to allow the immune system to generate a subsequent response.

Obviously, all of this new hypothetical calculus depends entirely on the ability of the immunotherapy or chemo-immunotherapy to deliver the necessary efficacy. (If not, then the radiation is indeed futile.) However, the experience in multiple adult immunotherapy trials has been that the immune system is indeed capable of delivering very potent anti-tumor effects—including regression of widespread metastatic disease; and it can work in very aggressive and refractory tumors. Thus, the problem is not the inherent potency of the immune system, but rather inducing that efficacy become a reality in all patients. This is the rationale for adding immunogenic radiation to multi-modal immunotherapy.

2.6 Possibilities of Surgery: Can Immunotherapy Help Downstage Tumors for Definitive Resection?

Finally, we consider surgery. Pediatric surgery has reached a superb level of technical competence, but the role for additional surgical intervention in the face of recurrent or metastatic disease remains limited by the problem of futility. However, if immunotherapy is added to the traditional modalities of chemotherapy and radiation, this may also change the calculus for surgery. First, since the immune system is better at dealing with microscopic disease than with bulky disease, up-front de-bulking surgery (even in relapsed disease) may improve the chances of an immune response. And second, regimens that incorporate immunotherapy may create a situation of prolonged stable disease—e.g., a lesion that does not shrink, but does not spontaneously re-grow either (see Fig. 2.2, above). At what point does it become in the patient's interest to resect this remaining stable lesion(s)? In our own immunotherapy trials, we do not yet have an unambiguous answer to this question. The best approach will have to be empirically determined through clinical trials, and may be a judgment call for each patient. But the addition of an immune effector arm, with its potential for late responses and prolonged stable equilibrium, has raised new potential roles for surgery in the management of patients who show evidence of response.

Acknowledgments The authors gratefully acknowledge the generous support of the Alex's Lemonade Stand Foundation (to TSJ), and the Beloco Foundation (to DHM).

References

1. Chen DS, Mellman I. Oncology meets immunology: the cancer-immunity cycle. Immunity. 2013;39:1–10.
2. Medler TR, Cotechini T, Coussens LM. Immune response to cancer therapy: mounting an effective antitumor response and mechanisms of resistance. Trends Cancer. 2015;1:66–75.
3. Munn DH, Bronte V. Immune suppressive mechanisms in the tumor microenvironment. Curr Opin Immunol. 2016;39:1–6.
4. Belvin M, Mellman I. Is all cancer therapy immunotherapy? Sci Transl Med. 2015;7:315fs48.
5. Lesokhin AM, Callahan MK, Postow MA, Wolchok JD. On being less tolerant: enhanced cancer immunosurveillance enabled by targeting checkpoints and agonists of T cell activation. Sci Transl Med. 2015;7:280sr1.
6. Galluzzi L, Buqué A, Kepp O, Zitvogel L, Kroemer G. Immunological effects of conventional chemotherapy and targeted anticancer agents. Cancer Cell. 2015;28:690–714.
7. Machiels JP, Reilly RT, Emens LA, Ercolini AM, Lei RY, Weintraub D, Okoye FI, Jaffee EM. Cyclophosphamide, doxorubicin, and paclitaxel enhance the antitumor immune response of granulocyte/macrophage-colony stimulating factor-secreting whole-cell vaccines in HER-2/neu tolerized mice. Cancer Res. 2001;61:3689–97.
8. Sistigu A, Viaud S, Chaput N, Bracci L, Proietti E, Zitvogel L. Immunomodulatory effects of cyclophosphamide and implementations for vaccine design. Semin Immunopathol. 2011;33:369–83.
9. Klebanoff CA, Khong HT, Antony PA, Palmer DC, Restifo NP. Sinks, suppressors and antigen presenters: how lymphodepletion enhances T cell-mediated tumor immunotherapy. Trends Immunol. 2005;26:111–7.
10. Kroemer G, Galluzzi L, Kepp O, Zitvogel L. Immunogenic cell death in cancer therapy. Annu Rev Immunol. 2013;31:51–72.
11. Obeid M, Tesniere A, Ghiringhelli F, Fimia GM, Apetoh L, Perfettini JL, Castedo M, Mignot G, Panaretakis T, Casares N, Metivier D, Larochette N, van Endert P, Ciccosanti F, Piacentini M, Zitvogel L, Kroemer G. Calreticulin exposure dictates the immunogenicity of cancer cell death. Nat Med. 2007;13:54–61.
12. Apetoh L, Ghiringhelli F, Tesniere A, Obeid M, Ortiz C, Criollo A, Mignot G, Maiuri MC, Ullrich E, Saulnier P, Yang H, Amigorena S, Ryffel B, Barrat FJ, Saftig P, Levi F, Lidereau R, Nogues C, Mira JP, Chompret A, Joulin V, Clavel-Chapelon F, Bourhis J, Andre F, Delaloge S, Tursz T, Kroemer G, Zitvogel L. Toll-like receptor 4-dependent contribution of the immune system to anticancer chemotherapy and radiotherapy. Nat Med. 2007;13:1050–9.
13. Coffelt SB, de Visser KE. Immune-mediated mechanisms influencing the efficacy of anticancer therapies. Trends Immunol. 2015;36:198–216.
14. Bezu L, Gomes-de-Silva LC, Dewitte H, Breckpot K, Fucikova J, Spisek R, Galluzzi L, Kepp O, Kroemer G. Combinatorial strategies for the induction of immunogenic cell death. Front Immunol. 2015;6:187.
15. McLornan DP, List A, Mufti GJ. Applying synthetic lethality for the selective targeting of cancer. N Engl J Med. 2014;371:1725–35.
16. Kaelin WG Jr. The concept of synthetic lethality in the context of anticancer therapy. Nat Rev Cancer. 2005;5:689–98.
17. Sharma MD, Shinde R, McGaha T, Huang L, Holmgaard RB, Wolchok JD, Mautino MR, Celis E, Sharpe A, Francisco LM, Powell DJ Jr, Yagita H, Mellor AL, Blazar BR, Munn DH. The PTEN pathway in Tregs is a critical driver of the suppressive tumor microenvironment. Sci Adv. 2015;1:e1500845.
18. Schumacher TN, Schreiber RD. Neoantigens in cancer immunotherapy. Science. 2015;348:69–74.
19. McGranahan N, Furness AJS, Rosenthal R, Ramskov S, Lyngaa R, Saini SK, Jamal-Hanjani M, Wilson GA, Birkbak NJ, Hiley CT, Watkins TBK, Shafi S, Murugaesu N, Mitter R, Akarca AU, Linares J, Marafioti T, Henry JY, Van Allen EM, Miao D, Schilling B, Schadendorf

D, Garraway LA, Makarov V, Rizvi NA, Snyder A, Hellmann MD, Merghoub T, Wolchok JD, Shukla SA, Wu CJ, Peggs KS, Chan TA, Hadrup SR, Quezada SA, Swanton C. Clonal neoantigens elicit T cell immunoreactivity and sensitivity to immune checkpoint blockade. Science. 2016;351(6280):1463–9. doi:10.1126/science.aaf1490.
20. Rizvi NA, Hellmann MD, Snyder A, Kvistborg P, Makarov V, Havel JJ, Lee W, Yuan J, Wong P, Ho TS, Miller ML, Rekhtman N, Moreira AL, Ibrahim F, Bruggeman C, Gasmi B, Zappasodi R, Maeda Y, Sander C, Garon EB, Merghoub T, Wolchok JD, Schumacher TN, Chan TA. Mutational landscape determines sensitivity to PD-1 blockade in non-small cell lung cancer. Science. 2015;348:124–8.
21. Larkin J, Chiarion-Sileni V, Gonzalez R, Grob JJ, Cowey CL, Lao CD, Schadendorf D, Dummer R, Smylie M, Rutkowski P, Ferrucci PF, Hill A, Wagstaff J, Carlino MS, Haanen JB, Maio M, Marquez-Rodas I, McArthur GA, Ascierto PA, Long GV, Callahan MK, Postow MA, Grossmann K, Sznol M, Dreno B, Bastholt L, Yang A, Rollin LM, Horak C, Hodi FS, Wolchok JD. Combined nivolumab and ipilimumab or monotherapy in untreated melanoma. N Engl J Med. 2015;373:23–34.
22. Ravishankar B, Liu H, Shinde R, Chandler P, Baban B, Tanaka M, Munn DH, Mellor AL, Karlsson MC, McGaha TL. Tolerance to apoptotic cells is regulated by indoleamine 2,3-dioxygenase. Proc Natl Acad Sci U S A. 2012;109:3909–14.
23. Ravishankar B, Shinde R, Liu H, Chaudhary K, Bradley J, Lemos HP, Chandler P, Tanaka M, Munn DH, Mellor AL, McGaha TL. Marginal zone CD169+ macrophages coordinate apoptotic cell-driven cellular recruitment and tolerance. Proc Natl Acad Sci U S A. 2014;111:4215–20.
24. Ravishankar B, Liu H, Shinde R, Chaudhary K, Xiao W, Bradley J, Koritzinsky M, Madaio MP, McGaha TL. The amino acid sensor GCN2 inhibits inflammatory responses to apoptotic cells promoting tolerance and suppressing systemic autoimmunity. Proc Natl Acad Sci U S A. 2015;112:10774–9.
25. Coulie PG, Van den Eynde BJ, van der Bruggen P, Boon T. Tumour antigens recognized by T lymphocytes: at the core of cancer immunotherapy. Nat Rev Cancer. 2014;14:135–46.
26. Nishikawa H, Sakaguchi S. Regulatory T cells in cancer immunotherapy. Curr Opin Immunol. 2014;27:1–7.
27. Bos PD, Plitas G, Rudra D, Lee SY, Rudensky AY. Transient regulatory T cell ablation deters oncogene-driven breast cancer and enhances radiotherapy. J Exp Med. 2013;210:2435–66.
28. Ali K, Soond DR, Pineiro R, Hagemann T, Pearce W, Lim EL, Bouabe H, Scudamore CL, Hancox T, Maecker H, Friedman L, Turner M, Okkenhaug K, Vanhaesebroeck B. Inactivation of PI(3)K p110delta breaks regulatory T-cell-mediated immune tolerance to cancer. Nature. 2014;510:407–11.
29. Joshi NS, Akama-Garren EH, Lu Y, Lee DY, Chang GP, Li A, DuPage M, Tammela T, Kerper NR, Farago AF, Robbins R, Crowley DM, Bronson RT, Jacks T. Regulatory T cells in tumor-associated tertiary lymphoid structures suppress anti-tumor T cell responses. Immunity. 2015;43:579–90.
30. Bauer CA, Kim EY, Marangoni F, Carrizosa E, Claudio NM, Mempel TR. Dynamic Treg interactions with intratumoral APCs promote local CTL dysfunction. J Clin Invest. 2014;124:2425–40.
31. Malchow S, Leventhal DS, Nishi S, Fischer BI, Shen L, Paner GP, Amit AS, Kang C, Geddes JE, Allison JP, Socci ND, Savage PA. Aire-dependent thymic development of tumor-associated regulatory T cells. Science. 2013;339:1219–24.
32. Sharma MD, Baban B, Chandler P, Hou DY, Singh N, Yagita H, Azuma M, Blazar BR, Mellor AL, Munn DH. Plasmacytoid dendritic cells from mouse tumor-draining lymph nodes directly activate mature Tregs via indoleamine 2,3-dioxygenase. J Clin Invest. 2007;117:2570–82.
33. Delgoffe GM, Woo SR, Turnis ME, Gravano DM, Guy C, Overacre AE, Bettini ML, Vogel P, Finkelstein D, Bonnevier J, Workman CJ, Vignali DA. Stability and function of regulatory T cells is maintained by a neuropilin-1-semaphorin-4a axis. Nature. 2013;501:252–6.
34. Huynh A, DuPage M, Priyadharshini B, Sage PT, Quiros J, Borges CM, Townamchai N, Gerriets VA, Rathmell JC, Sharpe AH, Bluestone JA, Turka LA. Control of PI(3) kinase in Treg cells maintains homeostasis and lineage stability. Nat Immunol. 2015;16:188–96.

35. Shrestha S, Yang K, Guy C, Vogel P, Neale G, Chi H. Treg cells require the phosphatase PTEN to restrain Th1 and Tfh cell responses. Nat Immunol. 2015;16:178–87.
36. Postow MA, Callahan MK, Wolchok JD. Immune checkpoint blockade in cancer therapy. J Clin Oncol. 2015;33:1974–82.
37. Snyder A, Makarov V, Merghoub T, Yuan J, Zaretsky JM, Desrichard A, Walsh LA, Postow MA, Wong P, Ho TS, Hollmann TJ, Bruggeman C, Kannan K, Li Y, Elipenahli C, Liu C, Harbison CT, Wang L, Ribas A, Wolchok JD, Chan TA. Genetic basis for clinical response to CTLA-4 blockade in melanoma. N Engl J Med. 2014;371:2189–99.
38. Van Allen EM, Miao D, Schilling B, Shukla SA, Blank C, Zimmer L, Sucker A, Hillen U, Geukes Foppen MH, Goldinger SM, Utikal J, Hassel JC, Weide B, Kaehler KC, Loquai C, Mohr P, Gutzmer R, Dummer R, Gabriel S, Wu CJ, Schadendorf D, Garraway LA. Genomic correlates of response to CTLA4 blockade in metastatic melanoma. Science. 2015;350:207–11.
39. Kvistborg P, Philips D, Kelderman S, Hageman L, Ottensmeier C, Joseph-Pietras D, Welters MJ, van der Burg S, Kapiteijn E, Michielin O, Romano E, Linnemann C, Speiser D, Blank C, Haanen JB, Schumacher TN. Anti-CTLA-4 therapy broadens the melanoma-reactive CD8+ T cell response. Sci Transl Med. 2014;6:254ra128.
40. Walker LS, Sansom DM. Confusing signals: recent progress in CTLA-4 biology. Trends Immunol. 2015;36:63–70.
41. Simpson TR, Li F, Montalvo-Ortiz W, Sepulveda MA, Bergerhoff K, Arce F, Roddie C, Henry JY, Yagita H, Wolchok JD, Peggs KS, Ravetch JV, Allison JP, Quezada SA. Fc-dependent depletion of tumor-infiltrating regulatory T cells co-defines the efficacy of anti-CTLA-4 therapy against melanoma. J Exp Med. 2013;210:1695–710.
42. Herbst RS, Soria JC, Kowanetz M, Fine GD, Hamid O, Gordon MS, Sosman JA, McDermott DF, Powderly JD, Gettinger SN, Kohrt HE, Horn L, Lawrence DP, Rost S, Leabman M, Xiao Y, Mokatrin A, Koeppen H, Hegde PS, Mellman I, Chen DS, Hodi FS. Predictive correlates of response to the anti-PD-L1 antibody MPDL3280A in cancer patients. Nature. 2014;515:563–7.
43. Tumeh PC, Harview CL, Yearley JH, Shintaku IP, Taylor EJ, Robert L, Chmielowski B, Spasic M, Henry G, Ciobanu V, West AN, Carmona M, Kivork C, Seja E, Cherry G, Gutierrez AJ, Grogan TR, Mateus C, Tomasic G, Glaspy JA, Emerson RO, Robins H, Pierce RH, Elashoff DA, Robert C, Ribas A. PD-1 blockade induces responses by inhibiting adaptive immune resistance. Nature. 2014;515:568–71.
44. Robert C, Thomas L, Bondarenko I, O'Day S, Weber J, Garbe C, Lebbe C, Baurain JF, Testori A, Grob JJ, Davidson N, Richards J, Maio M, Hauschild A, Miller WH, Gascon P, Lotem M, Harmankaya K, Ibrahim R, Francis S, Chen TT, Humphrey R, Hoos A, Wolchok JD. Ipilimumab plus dacarbazine for previously untreated metastatic melanoma. N Engl J Med. 2011;364:2517–26.
45. Munn DH, Mellor AL. IDO in the tumor microenvironment: inflammation, counter-regulation, and tolerance. Trends Immunol. 2016;37:193–207.
46. Munn DH, Zhou M, Attwood JT, Bondarev I, Conway SJ, Marshall B, Brown C, Mellor AL. Prevention of allogeneic fetal rejection by tryptophan catabolism. Science. 1998;281:1191–3.
47. Muller AJ, Duhadaway JB, Donover PS, Sutanto-Ward E, Prendergast GC. Inhibition of indoleamine 2,3-dioxygenase, an immunoregulatory target of the cancer suppression gene Bin1, potentiates cancer chemotherapy. Nat Med. 2005;11:312–9.
48. Mellor AL, Sivakumar J, Chandler P, Smith K, Molina H, Mao D, Munn DH. Prevention of T cell-driven complement activation and inflammation by tryptophan catabolism during pregnancy. Nat Immunol. 2001;2:64–8.
49. Matteoli G, Mazzini E, Iliev ID, Mileti E, Fallarino F, Puccetti P, Chieppa M, Rescigno M. Gut CD103+ dendritic cells express indoleamine 2,3-dioxygenase which influences T regulatory/T effector cell balance and oral tolerance induction. Gut. 2010;59:595–604.
50. van der Marel AP, Samsom JN, Greuter M, van Berkel LA, O'Toole T, Kraal G, Mebius RE. Blockade of IDO inhibits nasal tolerance induction. J Immunol. 2007;179:894–900.
51. Sucher R, Fischler K, Oberhuber R, Kronberger I, Margreiter C, Ollinger R, Schneeberger S, Fuchs D, Werner ER, Watschinger K, Zelger B, Tellides G, Pilat N, Pratschke J, Margreiter

R, Wekerle T, Brandacher G. IDO and regulatory T cell support are critical for cytotoxic T lymphocyte-associated Ag-4 Ig-mediated long-term solid organ allograft survival. J Immunol. 2012;188:37–46.
52. Grohmann U, Orabona C, Fallarino F, Vacca C, Calcinaro F, Falorni A, Candeloro P, Belladonna ML, Bianchi R, Fioretti MC, Puccetti P. CTLA-4-Ig regulates tryptophan catabolism in vivo. Nat Immunol. 2002;3:1097–101.
53. Mellor AL, Baban B, Chandler P, Marshall B, Jhaver K, Hansen A, Koni PA, Iwashima M, Munn DH. Cutting edge: induced indoleamine 2,3 dioxygenase expression in dendritic cell subsets suppresses T cell clonal expansion. J Immunol. 2003;171:1652–5.
54. Guillonneau C, Hill M, Hubert FX, Chiffoleau E, Herve C, Li XL, Heslan M, Usal C, Tesson L, Menoret S, Saoudi A, Le Mauff B, Josien R, Cuturi MC, Anegon I. CD40Ig treatment results in allograft acceptance mediated by CD8CD45RC T cells, IFN-gamma, and indoleamine 2,3-dioxygenase. J Clin Invest. 2007;117:1096–106.
55. Tsai S, Shameli A, Yamanouchi J, Clemente-Casares X, Wang J, Serra P, Yang Y, Medarova Z, Moore A, Santamaria P. Reversal of autoimmunity by boosting memory-like autoregulatory T cells. Immunity. 2010;32:568–80.
56. Lan Z, Ge W, Arp J, Jiang J, Liu W, Gordon D, Healey D, DeBenedette M, Nicolette C, Garcia B, Wang H. Induction of kidney allograft tolerance by soluble CD83 associated with prevalence of tolerogenic dendritic cells and indoleamine 2,3-dioxygenase. Transplantation. 2010;90:1286–93.
57. Swanson KA, Zheng Y, Heidler KM, Mizobuchi T, Wilkes DS. CDllc+ cells modulate pulmonary immune responses by production of indoleamine 2,3-dioxygenase. Am J Respir Cell Mol Biol. 2004;30:311–8.
58. Matino D, Gargaro M, Santagostino E, Di Minno MN, Castaman G, Morfini M, Rocino A, Mancuso ME, Di Minno G, Coppola A, Talesa VN, Volpi C, Vacca C, Orabona C, Iannitti R, Mazzucconi MG, Santoro C, Tosti A, Chiappalupi S, Sorci G, Tagariello G, Belvini D, Radossi P, Landolfi R, Fuchs D, Boon L, Pirro M, Marchesini E, Grohmann U, Puccetti P, Iorio A, Fallarino F. IDO1 suppresses inhibitor development in hemophilia A treated with factor VIII. J Clin Invest. 2015;125:3766–81.
59. Jasperson LK, Bucher C, Panoskaltsis-Mortari A, Taylor PA, Mellor AL, Munn DH, Blazar BR. Indoleamine 2,3-dioxygenase is a critical regulator of acute GVHD lethality. Blood. 2008;111:3257–65.
60. Lu Y, Giver CR, Sharma A, Li JM, Darlak KA, Owens LM, Roback JD, Galipeau J, Waller EK. IFN-gamma and indoleamine 2,3-dioxygenase signaling between donor dendritic cells and T cells regulates graft versus host and graft versus leukemia activity. Blood. 2012;119:1075–85.
61. Gurtner GJ, Newberry RD, Schloemann SR, McDonald KG, Stenson WF. Inhibition of indoleamine 2,3-dioxygenase augments trinitrobenzene sulfonic acid colitis in mice. Gastroenterology. 2003;125:1762–73.
62. Szanto S, Koreny T, Mikecz K, Glant TT, Szekanecz Z, Varga J. Inhibition of indoleamine 2,3-dioxygenase-mediated tryptophan catabolism accelerates collagen-induced arthritis in mice. Arthritis Res Ther. 2007;9:R50.
63. Yan Y, Zhang GX, Gran B, Fallarino F, Yu S, Li H, Cullimore ML, Rostami A, Xu H. IDO upregulates regulatory T cells via tryptophan catabolite and suppresses encephalitogenic T cell responses in experimental autoimmune encephalomyelitis. J Immunol. 2010;185:5953–61.
64. Fallarino F, Volpi C, Zelante T, Vacca C, Calvitti M, Fioretti MC, Puccetti P, Romani L, Grohmann U. IDO mediates TLR9-driven protection from experimental autoimmune diabetes. J Immunol. 2009;183:6303–12.
65. Romani L, Fallarino F, De Luca A, Montagnoli C, D'Angelo C, Zelante T, Vacca C, Bistoni F, Fioretti MC, Grohmann U, Segal BH, Puccetti P. Defective tryptophan catabolism underlies inflammation in mouse chronic granulomatous disease. Nature. 2008;451:211–5.
66. Grohmann U, Volpi C, Fallarino F, Bozza S, Bianchi R, Vacca C, Orabona C, Belladonna ML, Ayroldi E, Nocentini G, Boon L, Bistoni F, Fioretti MC, Romani L, Riccardi C, Puccetti

P. Reverse signaling through GITR ligand enables dexamethasone to activate IDO in allergy. Nat Med. 2007;13:579–86.
67. Metz R, Duhadaway JB, Kamasani U, Laury-Kleintop L, Muller AJ, Prendergast GC. Novel tryptophan catabolic enzyme IDO2 is the preferred biochemical target of the antitumor indoleamine 2,3-dioxygenase inhibitory compound D-1-methyl-tryptophan. Cancer Res. 2007;67:7082–7.
68. Ball HJ, Yuasa HJ, Austin CJ, Weiser S, Hunt NH. Indoleamine 2,3-dioxygenase-2; a new enzyme in the kynurenine pathway. Int J Biochem Cell Biol. 2009;41:467–71.
69. Fatokun AA, Hunt NH, Ball HJ. Indoleamine 2,3-dioxygenase 2 (IDO2) and the kynurenine pathway: characteristics and potential roles in health and disease. Amino Acids. 2013;45:1319–29.
70. Munn DH, Sharma MD, Baban B, Harding HP, Zhang Y, Ron D, Mellor AL. GCN2 kinase in T cells mediates proliferative arrest and anergy induction in response to indoleamine 2,3-dioxygenase. Immunity. 2005;22:633–42.
71. Rodriguez PC, Quiceno DG, Ochoa AC. L-arginine availability regulates T-lymphocyte cell-cycle progression. Blood. 2007;109:1568–73.
72. Fallarino F, Grohmann U, You S, McGrath BC, Cavener DR, Vacca C, Orabona C, Bianchi R, Belladonna ML, Volpi C, Santamaria P, Fioretti MC, Puccetti P. The combined effects of tryptophan starvation and tryptophan catabolites down-regulate T cell receptor zeta-chain and induce a regulatory phenotype in naive T cells. J Immunol. 2006;176:6752–61.
73. Ravindran R, Loebbermann J, Nakaya HI, Khan N, Ma H, Gama L, Machiah DK, Lawson B, Hakimpour P, Wang YC, Li S, Sharma P, Kaufman RJ, Martinez J, Pulendran B. The amino acid sensor GCN2 controls gut inflammation by inhibiting inflammasome activation. Nature. 2016;531:523–7.
74. Mezrich JD, Fechner JH, Zhang X, Johnson BP, Burlingham WJ, Bradfield CA. An interaction between kynurenine and the aryl hydrocarbon receptor can generate regulatory T cells. J Immunol. 2010;185:3190–8.
75. Liu H, Huang L, Bradley J, Liu K, Bardhan K, Ron D, Mellor AL, Munn DH, McGaha TL. GCN2-dependent metabolic stress is essential for endotoxemic cytokine induction and pathology. Mol Cell Biol. 2014;34:428–38.
76. Quintana FJ, Murugaiyan G, Farez MF, Mitsdoerffer M, Tukpah AM, Burns EJ, Weiner HL. An endogenous aryl hydrocarbon receptor ligand acts on dendritic cells and T cells to suppress experimental autoimmune encephalomyelitis. Proc Natl Acad Sci U S A. 2010;107:20768–73.
77. Jaronen M, Quintana FJ. Immunological relevance of the coevolution of IDO1 and AHR. Front Immunol. 2014;5:521.
78. Manlapat AK, Kahler DJ, Chandler PR, Munn DH, Mellor AL. Cell-autonomous control of interferon type I expression by indoleamine 2,3-dioxygenase in regulatory CD19(+) dendritic cells. Eur J Immunol. 2007;37:1064–71.
79. Mellor AL, Baban B, Chandler PR, Manlapat A, Kahler DJ, Munn DH. Cutting edge: CpG oligonucleotides induce splenic CD19+ dendritic cells to acquire potent indoleamine 2,3-dioxygenase-dependent T cell regulatory functions via IFN type 1 signaling. J Immunol. 2005;175:5601–5.
80. Sharma MD, Huang L, Choi JH, Lee EJ, Wilson JM, Lemos H, Pan F, Blazar BR, Pardoll DM, Mellor AL, Shi H, Munn DH. An inherently bifunctional subset of Foxp3 T helper cells is controlled by the transcription factor Eos. Immunity. 2013;38:998–1012.
81. Huang L, Li L, Lemos H, Chandler PR, Pacholczyk G, Baban B, Barber GN, Hayakawa Y, McGaha TL, Ravishankar B, Munn DH, Mellor AL. Cutting edge: DNA sensing via the STING adaptor in myeloid dendritic cells induces potent tolerogenic responses. J Immunol. 2013;191:3509–13.
82. Thornton AM, Piccirillo CA, Shevach EM. Activation requirements for the induction of CD4+CD25+ T cell suppressor function. Eur J Immunol. 2004;34:366–76.
83. Levine AG, Arvey A, Jin W, Rudensky AY. Continuous requirement for the TCR in regulatory T cell function. Nat Immunol. 2014;15:1070–8.

84. Chaudhry A, Rudensky AY. Control of inflammation by integration of environmental cues by regulatory T cells. J Clin Invest. 2013;123:939–44.
85. Hou DY, Muller AJ, Sharma MD, Duhadaway JB, Banerjee T, Johnson M, Mellor AL, Prendergast GC, Munn DH. Inhibition of IDO in dendritic cells by stereoisomers of 1-methyl-tryptophan correlates with anti-tumor responses. Cancer Res. 2007;67:792–801.
86. Holmgaard RB, Zamarin D, Li Y, Gasmi B, Munn DH, Allison JP, Merghoub T, Wolchok JD. Tumor-expressed IDO recruits and activates MDSCs in a Treg-dependent manner. Cell Rep. 2015;13:412–24.
87. Holmgaard RB, Zamarin D, Munn DH, Wolchok JD, Allison JP. Indoleamine 2,3-dioxygenase is a critical resistance mechanism in antitumor T cell immunotherapy targeting CTLA-4. J Exp Med. 2013;210:1389–402.
88. Wainwright DA, Chang AL, Dey M, Balyasnikova IV, Kim CK, Tobias A, Cheng Y, Kim JW, Qiao J, Zhang L, Han Y, Lesniak MS. Durable therapeutic efficacy utilizing combinatorial blockade against IDO, CTLA-4, and PD-L1 in mice with brain tumors. Clin Cancer Res. 2014;20:5290–301.
89. Spranger S, Koblish HK, Horton B, Scherle PA, Newton R, Gajewski TF. Mechanism of tumor rejection with doublets of CTLA-4, PD-1/PD-L1, or IDO blockade involves restored IL-2 production and proliferation of CD8(+) T cells directly within the tumor microenvironment. J Immunother Cancer. 2014;2:3.
90. Liu X, Shin N, Koblish HK, Yang G, Wang Q, Wang K, Leffet L, Hansbury MJ, Thomas B, Rupar M, Waeltz P, Bowman KJ, Polam P, Sparks RB, Yue EW, Li Y, Wynn R, Fridman JS, Burn TC, Combs AP, Newton RC, Scherle PA. Selective inhibition of indoleamine 2,3-dioxygenase (IDO1) effectively regulates mediators of anti-tumor immunity. Blood. 2010;115:3520–30.
91. Koblish HK, Hansbury MJ, Bowman KJ, Yang G, Neilan CL, Haley PJ, Burn TC, Waeltz P, Sparks RB, Yue EW, Combs AP, Scherle PA, Vaddi K, Fridman JS. Hydroxyamidine inhibitors of indoleamine-2,3-dioxygenase potently suppress systemic tryptophan catabolism and the growth of IDO-expressing tumors. Mol Cancer Ther. 2010;9:489–98.
92. Bakmiwewa SM, Fatokun AA, Tran A, Payne RJ, Hunt NH, Ball HJ. Identification of selective inhibitors of indoleamine 2,3-dioxygenase 2. Bioorg Med Chem Lett. 2012;22:7641–6.
93. Opitz CA, Litzenburger UM, Sahm F, Ott M, Tritschler I, Trump S, Schumacher T, Jestaedt L, Schrenk D, Weller M, Jugold M, Guillemin GJ, Miller CL, Lutz C, Radlwimmer B, Lehmann I, von Deimling A, Wick W, Platten M. An endogenous tumour-promoting ligand of the human aryl hydrocarbon receptor. Nature. 2011;478:197–203.
94. Pilotte L, Larrieu P, Stroobant V, Colau D, Dolusic E, Frederick R, De Plaen E, Uyttenhove C, Wouters J, Masereel B, Van den Eynde BJ. Reversal of tumoral immune resistance by inhibition of tryptophan 2,3-dioxygenase. Proc Natl Acad Sci U S A. 2012;109:2497–502.
95. Ball HJ, Jusof FF, Bakmiwewa SM, Hunt NH, Yuasa HJ. Tryptophan-catabolizing enzymes—party of three. Front Immunol. 2014;5:485.
96. Ugel S, De Sanctis F, Mandruzzato S, Bronte V. Tumor-induced myeloid deviation: when myeloid-derived suppressor cells meet tumor-associated macrophages. J Clin Invest. 2015;125:3365–76.
97. Franklin RA, Liao W, Sarkar A, Kim MV, Bivona MR, Liu K, Pamer EG, Li MO. The cellular and molecular origin of tumor-associated macrophages. Science. 2014;344:921–5.
98. Rybinski B, Franco-Barraza J, Cukierman E. The wound healing, chronic fibrosis, and cancer progression triad. Physiol Genomics. 2014;46:223–44.
99. Balkwill F, Mantovani A. Inflammation and cancer: back to Virchow? Lancet. 2001;357:539–45.
100. Colegio OR, Chu NQ, Szabo AL, Chu T, Rhebergen AM, Jairam V, Cyrus N, Brokowski CE, Eisenbarth SC, Phillips GM, Cline GW, Phillips AJ, Medzhitov R. Functional polarization of tumour-associated macrophages by tumour-derived lactic acid. Nature. 2014;513:559–63.
101. Mitchem JB, Brennan DJ, Knolhoff BL, Belt BA, Zhu Y, Sanford DE, Belaygorod L, Carpenter D, Collins L, Piwnica-Worms D, Hewitt S, Udupi GM, Gallagher WM, Wegner

C, West BL, Wang-Gillam A, Goedegebuure P, Linehan DC, DeNardo DG. Targeting tumor-infiltrating macrophages decreases tumor-initiating cells, relieves immunosuppression, and improves chemotherapeutic responses. Cancer Res. 2013;73:1128–41.
102. Ries CH, Cannarile MA, Hoves S, Benz J, Wartha K, Runza V, Rey-Giraud F, Pradel LP, Feuerhake F, Klaman I, Jones T, Jucknischke U, Scheiblich S, Kaluza K, Gorr IH, Walz A, Abiraj K, Cassier PA, Sica A, Gomez-Roca C, de Visser KE, Italiano A, Le Tourneau C, Delord JP, Levitsky H, Blay JY, Ruttinger D. Targeting tumor-associated macrophages with anti-CSF-1R antibody reveals a strategy for cancer therapy. Cancer Cell. 2014;25:846–59.
103. Kumar V, Patel S, Tcyganov E, Gabrilovich DI. The nature of myeloid-derived suppressor cells in the tumor microenvironment. Trends Immunol. 2016;37:208–20.
104. Trinchieri G. Cancer immunity: lessons from infectious diseases. J Infect Dis. 2015;212(Suppl 1):S67–73.
105. Goldszmid RS, Dzutsev A, Trinchieri G. Host immune response to infection and cancer: unexpected commonalities. Cell Host Microbe. 2014;15:295–305.
106. Thevenot PT, Sierra RA, Raber PL, Al-Khami AA, Trillo-Tinoco J, Zarreii P, Ochoa AC, Cui Y, Del Valle L, Rodriguez PC. The stress-response sensor CHOP regulates the function and accumulation of myeloid-derived suppressor cells in tumors. Immunity. 2014;41:389–401.
107. Marvel D, Gabrilovich DI. Myeloid-derived suppressor cells in the tumor microenvironment: expect the unexpected. J Clin Invest. 2015;125:3356–64.
108. Solito S, Marigo I, Pinton L, Damuzzo V, Mandruzzato S, Bronte V. Myeloid-derived suppressor cell heterogeneity in human cancers. Ann N Y Acad Sci. 2014;1319:47–65.
109. Draghiciu O, Lubbers J, Nijman HW, Daemen T. Myeloid derived suppressor cells-an overview of combat strategies to increase immunotherapy efficacy. Oncoimmunology. 2015;4:e954829.
110. Ding ZC, Lu X, Yu M, Lemos H, Huang L, Chandler P, Liu K, Walters M, Krasinski A, Mack M, Blazar BR, Mellor AL, Munn DH, Zhou G. Immunosuppressive myeloid cells induced by chemotherapy attenuate antitumor CD4+ T-cell responses through the PD-1-PD-L1 axis. Cancer Res. 2014;74:3441–53.
111. Spranger S, Spaapen RM, Zha Y, Williams J, Meng Y, Ha TT, Gajewski TF. Up-regulation of PD-L1, IDO, and Tregs in the melanoma tumor microenvironment is driven by CD8+ T cells. Sci Transl Med. 2013;5:200ra116.
112. Liu Z, Gerner MY, Van Panhuys N, Levine AG, Rudensky AY, Germain RN. Immune homeostasis enforced by co-localized effector and regulatory T cells. Nature. 2015;528:225–30.
113. Zitvogel L, Apetoh L, Ghiringhelli F, Andre F, Tesniere A, Kroemer G. The anticancer immune response: indispensable for therapeutic success? J Clin Invest. 2008;118:1991–2001.
114. Ciampricotti M, Hau CS, Doornebal CW, Jonkers J, de Visser KE. Chemotherapy response of spontaneous mammary tumors is independent of the adaptive immune system. Nat Med. 2012;18:344–6; author reply 6
115. Li M, Bolduc AR, Hoda MN, Gamble DN, Dolisca SB, Bolduc AK, Hoang K, Ashley C, McCall D, Rojiani AM, Maria BL, Rixe O, MacDonald TJ, Heeger PS, Mellor AL, Munn DH, Johnson TS. The indoleamine 2,3-dioxygenase pathway controls complement-dependent enhancement of chemo-radiation therapy against murine glioblastoma. J Immunother Cancer. 2014;2:21.
116. Zakharia Y, Colman H, Mott F, Lukas R, Vahanian N, Link C, Kennedy E, Sadek R, Munn D, Rixe O. Updates on phase 1B/2 combination study of the IDO pathway inhibitor indoximod with temozolomide for adult patients with temozolomide-refractory primary malignant brain tumors. Neuro-Oncology. 2015;17:v112.
117. Bahary N, Garrido-Laguna I, Wang-Gillam A, Nyak-Kapoor A, Kennedy E, Vahanian NN, Link CJ, editors. Results of the phase Ib portion of a phase I/II trial of the indoleamine 2,3-dioxygenase pathway (IDO) inhibitor indoximod plus gemcitabine/nab-paclitaxel for the treatment of metastatic pancreatic cancer. ASCO Annual Meeting Proceedings; 2016.
118. Müller P, Kreuzaler M, Khan T, Thommen DS, Martin K, Glatz K, Savic S, Harbeck N, Nitz U, Gluz O, von Bergwelt-Baildon M, Kreipe H, Reddy S, Christgen M, Zippelius

A. Trastuzumab emtansine (T-DM1) renders HER2+ breast cancer highly susceptible to CTLA-4/PD-1 blockade. Sci Transl Med. 2015;7:315ra188.

119. Ercolini AM, Ladle BH, Manning EA, Pfannenstiel LW, Armstrong TD, Machiels JP, Bieler JG, Emens LA, Reilly RT, Jaffee EM. Recruitment of latent pools of high-avidity CD8(+) T cells to the antitumor immune response. J Exp Med. 2005;201:1591–602.
120. Emens LA, Asquith JM, Leatherman JM, Kobrin BJ, Petrik S, Laiko M, Levi J, Daphtary MM, Biedrzycki B, Wolff AC, Stearns V, Disis ML, Ye X, Piantadosi S, Fetting JH, Davidson NE, Jaffee EM. Timed sequential treatment with cyclophosphamide, doxorubicin, and an allogeneic granulocyte-macrophage colony-stimulating factor-secreting breast tumor vaccine: a chemotherapy dose-ranging factorial study of safety and immune activation. J Clin Oncol. 2009;27:5911–8.
121. Brandsma D, Stalpers L, Taal W, Sminia P, van den Bent MJ. Clinical features, mechanisms, and management of pseudoprogression in malignant gliomas. Lancet Oncol. 2008;9:453–61.
122. Mittal D, Gubin MM, Schreiber RD, Smyth MJ. New insights into cancer immunoediting and its three component phases—elimination, equilibrium and escape. Curr Opin Immunol. 2014;27:16–25.
123. Wolchok JD, Hoos A, O'Day S, Weber JS, Hamid O, Lebbe C, Maio M, Binder M, Bohnsack O, Nichol G, Humphrey R, Hodi FS. Guidelines for the evaluation of immune therapy activity in solid tumors: immune-related response criteria. Clin Cancer Res. 2009;15:7412–20.
124. Golden EB, Apetoh L. Radiotherapy and immunogenic cell death. Semin Radiat Oncol. 2015;25:11–7.
125. Burnette B, Weichselbaum RR. The immunology of ablative radiation. Semin Radiat Oncol. 2015;25:40–5.
126. Pilones KA, Vanpouille-Box C, Demaria S. Combination of radiotherapy and immune checkpoint inhibitors. Semin Radiat Oncol. 2015;25:28–33.
127. Postow MA, Callahan MK, Barker CA, Yamada Y, Yuan J, Kitano S, Mu Z, Rasalan T, Adamow M, Ritter E, Sedrak C, Jungbluth AA, Chua R, Yang AS, Roman RA, Rosner S, Benson B, Allison JP, Lesokhin AM, Gnjatic S, Wolchok JD. Immunologic correlates of the abscopal effect in a patient with melanoma. N Engl J Med. 2012;366:925–31.
128. Bloy N, Pol J, Manic G, Vitale I, Eggermont A, Galon J, Tartour E, Zitvogel L, Kroemer G, Galluzzi L. Trial watch: radioimmunotherapy for oncological indications. Oncoimmunology. 2014;3:e954929.
129. Brody JD, Ai WZ, Czerwinski DK, Torchia JA, Levy M, Advani RH, Kim YH, Hoppe RT, Knox SJ, Shin LK, Wapnir I, Tibshirani RJ, Levy R. In situ vaccination with a TLR9 agonist induces systemic lymphoma regression: a phase I/II study. J Clin Oncol. 2010;28:4324–32.

Chapter 3
Allogeneic Stem Cell Transplantation

Patrick Schlegel, Christian Seitz, Peter Lang, and Rupert Handgretinger

Abstract Allogeneic stem cell transplantation in malignant diseases has evolved as a treatment option for patients with otherwise incurable diseases. The principle of this treatment is a significant tumor reduction by pretransplant chemotherapy or irradiation and immunological consolidation by various effector cells of the adaptive as well as of the innate immune system. The role of Graft versus Host disease (GvHD) and the concomitant Graft versus Tumor (GvT) effects is discussed and therapeutic approaches exploiting alloreactive T cell responses and ways to separate GvHD from GvT are shown. Antitumor response mechanisms that are also induced by alloreactive Natural Killer (NK) cells and γδ + T-cells belonging to the innate immune system are described. The innate donor-derived immune system might significantly contribute to the anti-tumor effects of allogeneic transplantation and the selection of donors will extend beyond classical high resolution typing of HLA alleles and finding the best matched HLA identical donor. The Killer Inhibitory Immunoglobuline-like Receptor (KIR) system is almost as polymorphic but independent from the HLA system and allows the selection of the optimal donor for certain malignant diseases. Especially in haploidentical transplantion, the KIR system plays an important role and new donor selection strategies might also apply in the future for the treatment of refractory solid tumors.

Keywords Allogeneic hematopoietic stem cell transplantation • Graft-versus-leukemia effect • Graft-versus-tumor effect • Graft manipulation • Haploidentical stem cell transplantation

Allogeneic haematological stem cell transplantation (HSCT) was one of the first forms of immunotherapy demonstrated to have clinical benefit in cancer, and is now widely used as an established therapy, largely in patients with relapsed or refractory haematological malignancies and in patients with otherwise incurable non-malignant hematological diseases. In contrast to autologous stem transplantation, allogeneic HSCT has the potential for additional immunological benefit, including

P. Schlegel, M.D. • C. Seitz, M.D. • P. Lang, M.D. • R. Handgretinger, M.D. (✉)
Hematology/Oncology, University Children's Hospital Tübingen, Tübingen, Germany
e-mail: rupert.handgretinger@med.uni-tuebingen.de

J.C. Gray, A. Marabelle (eds.), *Immunotherapy for Pediatric Malignancies*,
https://doi.org/10.1007/978-3-319-43486-5_3

a 'graft versus leukaemia' (GvL) or 'graft versus tumor' (GvT) effect. In this chapter, we discuss the indications for allogeneic transplant in children, the choice of donor stem cells, and how the graft may be manipulated to maximize the GvL effect, whilst minimizing graft versus host disease (GvHD) and other transplant related morbidity. The potential role of allogeneic HSCT in solid tumours is also reviewed.

3.1 Indications for Allogeneic HSCT in Children

Allogeneic HSCT has been most widely used in patients with haematological malignancies. Long-term survival in paediatric acute lymphoblastic leukaemia is now in the order of 85%–90%, and HSCT is generally reserved for children with refractory and relapsed disease [1, 2]. For those children with early disease relapse (e.g. within 6 months of achieving complete remission) allogeneic HSCT has been demonstrated to significantly improve leukemia-free and overall survival [3]. Allogeneic HSCT is also considered in later relapses in those patients who fail to clear minimal residual disease (MRD) after initial relapse chemotherapy [4, 5]. To date, few patients with relapsed ALL who fail to achieve remission with relapse protocols are cured by allogeneic transplant [6]. However, the rapidly evolving field of immunotherapy might offer new strategies to improve the outcome of these patients [7, 8]. Patients with less common forms of ALL, including Philadelphia chromosome positive ALL t(9;22), MLL-AF4 t(4;11) rearrangements, T lineage leukaemias, patients with poor response to initial treatment and patients with persistent MRD may also benefit from HSCT in first remission (CR1) [3, 9–11].

Despite intensive chemotherapy, survival of children with AML remains in the order of 60%–65%, and as the management of transplant-associated toxicity, transplant-related mortality (TRM) and post-transplant complications have improved, allogeneic transplant is more and more considered for these patients [12–14]. Allogeneic transplant in children with AML is recommended in CR1 in patients with high risk cytogenetics, such as t(10;11)(p12;q23)/MLLT10-MLL, t(6;9)(p23;q34)/DEK-NUP214, inv.(3)(q21q26.2 or t(3;3)(q21;q26.2)/RPN1-EVI1 [15], in patients who are slow to achieve remission and have persistent MRD status at the end of induction, and in patients with molecular mutations such as FLT3 mutations with high allelic ratios [16]. In patients with relapsed AML, the indication for transplant is clearer, and is generally considered a standard of care in most patients who achieve a second remission (CR2), provided a suitable donor is available [17–19]. An important adverse prognostic factor is the leukemic load at the time of transplantation [20–22], although transplant is still sometimes considered in children who fail to achieve a complete morphological remission.

Allogeneic transplantation may also offer the best chance for cure for patients with less frequent types of childhood leukemia, such as juvenile myelomonocytic leukemia (JMML) and chronic myelogenous leukemia (CML), achieving survival rates of more than 50% for both JMML and CML patients, dependent on the time point of HSCT [23, 24]. However, for CML, newer targeted therapies with tyrosine kinase inhibitors (TKIs) such as imatinib or new generation TKIs such as dasatinib and nilotinib, are now recommended as first line treatment for most children and allotransplant should generally be postponed until CML becomes refractory to imatinib [25, 26].

3.2 Graft Versus Leukemia Response and the Use of Donor Lymphocyte Infusion

Allogeneic HSCT in leukemia aims to provide a new healthy immune system that reconstitutes in the 'foreign' recipient bone marrow niche and lymphatic tissues. The most important prerequisite for successful HSCT is to consider Human Leucocyte Antigen (HLA) matching of donor and recipient, however other genetic differences such as minor histocompatibility antigens, killer immunoglobulin-like receptor (KIR) genes and variations in cytokine-, innate immunity- and pharmacological relevant polymorphisms as well as structural variations such as single nucleotide polymorphisms (SNPs) might also play a role [27]. HLA-based immune interaction is key for controlling highly individualized physiological intracellular protein processing by presentation of diverse oligopeptides for major histocompatibiltiy (MHC) class I and polypeptides for MHC II and for recognition of polymorphic fragments of foreign HLA molecules to distinguish between self- and foreign invaders such as viruses, bacteria but also aberrant cells in tumorigenesis [28] and allotransplantation [27]. State of the art HLA typing comprises typing at HLA-A, -B, -C, -DRB1 and -DQB1 genetic loci. The role of HLA-DPB1 for donor-recipient matching remains unclear [27]. HLA mismatch accounts for increased risk of graft rejection and graft versus host disease (GvHD) [29]. Nonetheless there seems to be a hierarchy in HLA disparities, accordingly grouped into permissive and non-permissive HLA mismatches that correlate with clinical features like GvHD [30]. In order to facilitate allogeneic HSCT, it is necessary to use a sufficient preparative regimen. The intensity of conditioning regimens can vary substantially, and when selecting the optimal conditioning regimen for any given patient, disease-related factors such as diagnosis and remission status, as well as patient-related factors including age, donor availability, and presence of co-morbidities, need to be considered. In children with severe combined immunodeficiency or patients with severe aplastic anemia who have syngeneic donors, HCT can be performed without the administration of a preparative regimen [31]. The most intensive high-dose conditioning regimens, namely total body irradiation (TBI), usually applied as fractionated therapy and intensified by additional chemotherapy, is especially used in haematological malignancies. Radiotherapy penetrates all immunologically and pharmaceutically hidden tumour sites and an increased TBI dose is associated with increased tumour control but is also associated with high rate of TRM [32].

Alternatively, non-TBI based conditioning regimens are also used, including busulphan plus cyclophosphamide or fludarabine, as well as melphalan based condition regimens with fludarabine, thiotepa and others [31]. Moreover, treosulfan-based conditioning regimens have been used with fludarabine for autologous and allogeneic transplant in childhood hematological malignancies, with favorable toxicity profile especially for second allo-HSCT [33, 34].

The concept of reduced intensity non-myeloablative conditioning regimens arose from the observation that patients had a benefit from robust immune reconstitution not only for protection from infectious complications, but also for the induction of an anti-tumour response. The observation of enhanced tumour control was linked to the development of acute and chronic GvHD [35, 36] after allotransplantation as well as clarified by the comparison of un-modified allogeneic grafts to autologous [37], syngeneic [38] and T cell depleted grafts [39]. Graft versus tumour or graft versus leukaemia effects contributed to improved relapse-free survival and opened the therapeutic window for patients in reduced general condition to undergo allogeneic HSCT, who were otherwise ineligible to receive myeloablative conditioning regimens [31]. *In vivo* depletion of host and allogeneic T cells has markedly reduced the rate of graft rejection, however at the price of delayed immune reconstitution. Its use is commonly integrated in preparative regimens and plays also a role in T cell depleted transplant [40]. The timing and dosing of in vivo T-cell depleting agents such as anti-thymocyte globulines (ATG) or alemtuzumab is crucial and due to the different composition and biological origins (horse, rabbit) and different mode of actions, it is difficult to directly compare these in vivo-T-cell depletion approaches [41, 42].

After allogeneic HSCT, the reconstitution of the donor immune system is crucial for immunological control of the primary disease to maintain complete remission in hematologic malignancies [43]. Individual pattern of short tandem repeats can be measured by Polymerase Chain Reaction (PCR) and can be reliably quantified to monitor the origin of the reconstituting cells [44]. Full donor chimerism and increasing donor chimerism post-transplant is associated with prolonged survival and lower risk of relapse [43], whereas mixed chimerism and decreasing donor chimerism is associated with an increase of recipient chimerism and results in significantly higher rate for relapse in myeloid and lymphoid malignancies [45]. To overcome mixed chimerism and to prevent leukaemia recurrence or to treat leukemic relapse, donor lymphocyte infusion (DLI) can successfully be used as a therapeutic tool in some patients. In this approach, donor lymphocytes are isolated from the peripheral blood and applied at defined escalating doses until response is observed while GvHD, the principal complication of DLI, is carefully balanced [46].

In general, HSCT provides the opportunity to regenerate a life-long healthy immune system, with the aim of potentially reducing MRD and maintaining remission by the development of a GvL effect. It does, however, involve considerable risks, including acute and chronic GvHD, which can be a severe or even lethal complication of HSCT [47, 48]. HLA matching between donors and recipients is the most important factor associated with acute graft-versus-host disease (GVHD) following allogeneic hematopoietic stem cell transplantation [49] and the underlying principle of GvHD is a complex alloimmune response, that requires the interaction of a variety of immune cells, mainly antigen presenting cells and T cells that in most cases recognize host-specific MHC presented peptides. The pathogenesis of GvHD is not completely understood, but naïve CD45RA$^+$ T cells are most likely responsible for alloreactive, host-attacking T cells in the highly inflammatory milieu posttransplant. There are different mechanisms in acute and chronic GvHD [48]. In matched transplant, GvHD is still a major complication, however it appears more often in HLA-mismatched transplants [49]. Single nucleotide polymorphisms can also account for the induction of GvHD and they can be stratified as organ-specific risk profiles [50, 51].

Graft versus Leukemia effects have been demonstrated to correlate with chronic GvHD, and there is some evidence that patients with well-controlled chronic GvHD are more likely to have concurrent GvL and a reduced incidence of leukemia recurrence and prolonged survival [52, 53]. However, GvHD is not a pre-requisite for a beneficial GvL effect.

The importance of T cells in the GvL effect was further demonstrated when ex vivo T cell depletion was introduced into clinical practice with the aim of prevention of GVHD. In CML, the beneficial effect of T-cell depletion on GVHD was negated because of an increased relapse rate. Increased relapse after T-cell depletion was most pronounced in CML, less in AML, and lowest in ALL [39], suggesting the relative importance of a GvL in these different leukaemias. In CML, T cells appear to induce the most potent and durable GvL with DLI-mediated complete response rates of 70%–80% in patients treated for hematologic and cytogenetic relapse. GvL can be induced post-transplant by DLI, and several reports have demonstrated long-term survival with this approach [39, 54]. DLI can augment GvL significantly and clear molecular relapses in 80% of CML patients [54]. In AML, only 15% of the patients respond to DLI and in ALL the benefit for DLI is even lower and remains controversial [39, 54]. However, a risk-adapted strategy involving pre-emptive DLI in paediatric patients who had undergone allogeneic HSCT for ALL, AML or CML, and who had mixed chimerism has been shown to reduce the risk of leukaemia recurrence with acceptable rates of GvHD. DLI was given at a small starting dose dependent on the donor, and dose-escalation guided by monitoring of chimerism and withholding further DLI once patients achieved full donor chimerism. Full donor chimerism was achieved in around 80% of the patients, in whom there was a significantly lower relapse rates and improved survival compared to those patients with persistent mixed chimerism [55].

Although the role of GvL in paediatric ALL appears to be less than in AML and CML, there is nevertheless evidence that allogeneic HSCT can also induce immunological anti-leukemic control in these patients and patients can benefit from HSCT [2, 56] independent of the donor source [3, 57–59] and there is clear evidence that the repopulating lymphocytes post allotransplant play a vital role in the early post-transplantation period by destroying residual tumor cells, reducing the relapse rate [60]. Previous studies have shown that delayed lymphocyte recovery post-

HSCT is associated with an increased risk of relapse in AML and ALL in adults. A clear indication for the critical role of GvL in childhood ALL in the context of allotransplantation is that low absolute lymphocyte count (ALC) in the early post-transplant phase is associated with an increased leukemia recurrence and reduced long-term event-free survival. Interestingly, increasing ALC is not associated with increased incidence of acute or chronic GVHD or TRM. Thus, early lymphocyte recovery post-HSCT appears to allow significant GvL without increase of GVHD [61].

The question which donor source is best able to induce GvL is still unanswered. The ALL-SCT-BFM-2003 trial demonstrated excellent EFS and OS in children with high-risk ALL conditioned with TBI and etoposide with HLA-matched siblings or well-matched unrelated (MUD) donors. MUD-HSCT is therefore generally considered a standard of care for patients with ALL who have a high risk of relapse and who lack a matched related donor [62]. However, improvement in transplant management and risk-adjustment has led to a similar outcome of MUD, matched related (MSD), umbilical cord blood (UCB) and haploidentical allotransplants [63]. Donor selection algorithms are primarily based on donor availability. In general, UCB and haploidentical donors currently are considered if there is no matched related or unrelated donor within an appropriate time frame. Retrospective studies have shown no substantial differences in outcomes and the transplant center's experience and donor availability currently determines the choice of donor [64]. However, in adult AML, unmanipulated haploidentical HSCT was superior to UCB and comparable to MSD, MUD and mismatched-UD HSCT, with lower incidence of acute and chronic GvHD, TRM and by tendency increased overall survival [65]. In future prospective randomized trials, donor origin might be determined for malignant diseases in favor of new alloreactivity aspects and potential post-transplant donor availability for the generation of supportive cell products including DLI, virus-specific T cells, tumor-antigen-specific T cells and genetically engineered T cells with TcR and CAR modified effector functional T cells [26, 58, 59, 66–70].

Minor histocompatibility antigens (mHAs) expressed on hematopoietic cells can also be targets for donor T cells to exert GvL by CD8+ as well as CD4+ T cells [71], but can also cause GvHD, since mHAs are also commonly expressed in non-hematopoietic tissues [72]. Sex restricted antigens, due to Y-chromosome encoding, has led to the identification of GvHD responsible genes recognized by female donors only [73] and differential expression of mHAs due to homozygous deletion of genes [74] and the recognition of mHAs by alloreactive T cells expressed on other organs than bone marrow, such as skin, gastrointestinal tract, liver or even brain can induce GvHD. If the mHAs are exclusively expressed on haematopoietic tissue, GvL effects might result in control of the leukemic cells [75]. Further strategies might exploit T cells targeting tumor associated antigens such as the non-polymorphic protein Wilms tumor 1 (WT1), proteinase 3, survivin, telomerase reverse transcriptase, CYPB1 and immature laminin receptor [75, 76]. The adoptive transfer of WT1-specific T cells and WT1 vaccination trials have been taken into clinical application and to date, more than 200 trials are registered at https://clinicaltrials.gov/, most of them for the treatment of AML. In order to retain the alloreactive potential of allogeneic grafts, selective T-cell depletion methods are under development with the limitation so far that the GvL and GvHD is closely linked to each other with T cells exerting the main effector function and the best clinical strategies with respect to patient-donor individual HLA-constellation including minor histocompatibility antigens or genetic HLA-relevant polymorphisms have yet to be explored [75, 77–79].

3.3 The Role of the Innate Immunity

In contrast to conventional (TCRαβ⁺) T-lymphocytes, NK cells and gamma delta (TCRγδ⁺) T cells can exert HLA-non-restricted anti-leukaemic functions [80–82] and thus can provide anti-leukaemic response in the early post-transplant phase, especially in haploidentical HSCT [83]. While conventional T-cells recognize individual peptides presented by HLA molecules, NK and γδ T cells play an important role in the initiation of an innate immune response. However, also more and more adaptive aspects of immune response of NK and γδ T cells are being discovered [84–86]. The activation state of NK and γδ T cells is regulated by activatory, inhibitory, and costimulatory receptors; and their migration is regulated by specific chemokines which are partially shared with αβ T cells. A specific feature of γδ T cells is that antigen-specificity can occur in a MHC-dependent and independent manner [87, 88]. Especially after haploidentical HSCT, TcR αβ T cells are lacking in the early post-transplant phase and NK and γδ T-cells protect the recipient from infectious complications. For controlling of cytomegalovirus (CMV) reactivation, the Vδ1 subset of γδ T-cells expand significantly and show anti-viral activity [83]. Moreover, γδ T-cells cross-talk with NK cells and enhance antitumor effector function [89]. In the context of HSCT, NK cell reconstitution and activity is critical to control malignancy in haploidentical and matched donor transplantation [90] and NK as well γδ T-cells exert Antibody-Dependent CellularCytotoxicity (ADCC) via the FcγIIIa receptor [91, 92]. In haploidentical HSCT using ex vivo depletion of TCRαβ T-cells, γδ T lymphocytes are very important effector cells especially in the early post-transplant phase, in which the function of adaptive immunity is still impaired and the expansion of anti-CMV γδ T cells in patients who reactivated CMV might contribute to control of leukaemia due to the anti-leukaemic activity of this lymphocyte subset [83].

HLA class I molecules are the main inhibitory ligands for NK cells and their corresponding receptors are the KIRs [93–96]. NK cells circulate in a pre-activated state and are continuously inhibited, primarily by HLA class I interaction. The missing-self recognition hypothesis which describes the loss of HLA antigens during viral infection or malignant transformation is a major mode of action of NK cells and the lack of inhibitory signaling (i.e. loss or reduction of HLA class I antigen expression) leads to target cytolysis and release of pro-inflammatory cytokines such as IFNγ and IL2 [97–99]. Another mode of action is the induced-self mechanism. Induced-self ligands are molecules that are not expressed or only expressed at low levels on most normal cells, but upregulated on unhealthy cells due to the activation of pathways associated with malignancy, infection or stress [100]. The NKG2D-receptor-ligand axis is an example of induced-self recognition wherein NK cells recognize self-ligands via the NKG2D receptor. NKG2D ligands (NKG2D-L) are upregulated on unhealthy cells and NKG2D recognition of target cells results in killing of tumor cells. Other receptors on NK cells, such as DNAM-1, recognize self-molecules that are widely expressed by healthy cells but can be further upregulated under conditions of stress. DNAM-1 interacts with the adhesion receptor LFA-1 on the surface of NK cells and may therefore play a role in regulating adhesion [101, 102]. In pediatric ALL, DNAM-1 ligand nectin-2 (PRR2/CD112) and NKG2D ligands ULBP-1 and ULBP3 are higher expressed compared to adult ALL and have been identified to play a key role in NK mediated cytolysis. Interestingly, increased NKG2D-ligand (NKG2DL) expression has been described in BCR/ABL-positive high risk ALL and tyrosine kinase inhibitors (TKIs) have been shown to induce enhanced NK mobilization, activation and proliferation *in vivo* and could therefore increase the recognition of ALL blasts by NK cells [103]. In adult leukemias, NKG2D-L has been shown to be higher expressed in chronic compared to acute leukemias. Moreover, leukemic blasts shed NKG2D-L, resulting in reduced NKG2D-L expression which might result in immune escape [104]. Moreover, in childhood ALL, reduced expression of HLA I was demonstrated in childhood ALL to be inversely correlated with NK cytolysis [105, 106], whereas in AML NKG2D-L signaling was identified as an important factor for NK cytotoxicity [107].

3.4 The Basis of NK Alloreactivity

Alloreactive NK cells are thought to be one of the most important anti-leukemic effector cells in allogeneic transplantation [108]. As early as day 14 post-transplant, NK cells start to reconstitute in number and maturation to fully immune competent NK cells begins. The same is observed for $TcR\gamma\delta^+$ T cells in $TcR\alpha\beta^+/CD19^+$ depleted transplants, whereas reconstitution of $TcR\alpha\beta^+$ T cells start to reconstitute only late, after many weeks or months, depending on the mode of transplant [109–111]. It is not clear at what time the NK cell gain complete function to eradicate leukemic blasts and whether alloreactive NK cells persist and contribute to long-term leukemia control. As already described, NK activity is controlled by a balance of inhibitory and activatory signals, of which the KIRs are the best characterized. KIRs are a family of type I transmembrane glycoproteins expressed on the plasma membrane of natural killer NK and a minority of T cells. They have two or three extracellular immunglobulin domains that are designated KIR2D and KIR3D, respectively [81].

The KIR family is polymorphic and the genetic variation determines NK mediated GvL reactions [112, 113]. The alloreactive potential of NK cells was first seen in haploidentical HSCT [114]. The mechanism became clearer with better understanding of KIR gene variability and interaction with HLA molecules. KIR2D family members recognize HLA-C alleles with Lys80 (C2 epitope) or Asn80 (C1 epitope) residues), whereas KIR3D family members recognize HLA-B alleles with a Bw4 supertypic specifity. In Fig. 3.1, possible constellations of NK alloreactivity based on the interaction of inhibitory KIRs with their respective ligands are depicted.

Based on the 17 KIR genes and two pseudogens, two donor haplotypes can be distinguished; KIR haplotype A donors express mainly inhibitory receptors, whereas haplotype B donors additionally express various numbers of activatory receptors.

Patients who received a transplant from MUD donors who had KIR B haplotypes had a better survival compared to patient who received grafts from haplotype A donors [113]. Pediatric patients who received T-cell depleted grafts had also a better outcome when donors had KIR B haplotypes compared to those with KIR A haplotype donors [115]. Similar results were seen in adult patients with AML who received an ex vivo T-cell depleted graft [116]. Further subgrouping of KIR B genotypes into centromeric and telomeric KIR B genes showed the importance of the centromeric located KIR genes, which mainly encode for the inhibitory KIRs

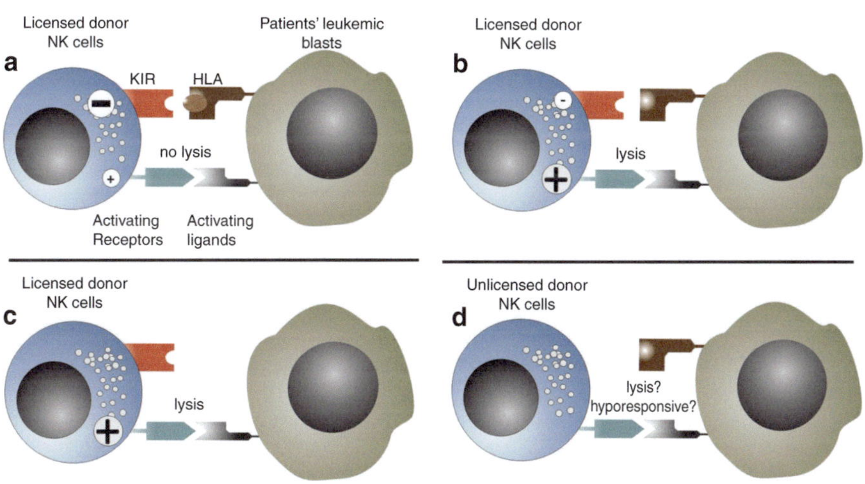

Fig. 3.1 Possible constellations of NK alloreactivity are shown. In (**a**) licensed donor NK cells (i.e. NK cells that have inhibitory KIRs for self-HLA class I) are inhibited by the recipients HLA class I antigens (inhibitory KIR ligands) and this presents a NK non-alloreactive situation. In (**b**) licensed NK cells are not inhibited since the recipient expresses HLA class I antigens which are not recognized by donor KIRs. This results in NK alloreactivity. In (**c**) HLA class I antigens are not expressed on the recipients blasts and the donor NK cells are therefore not inhibited, resulting in NK alloreactivity. In (**d**) NK cells do not express KIRs and therefore are not licensed. They are hypo responsive, but might become responsive upon cytokine stimulation

interacting with HLA-C alleles [113, 117]. In Fig. 3.2, strategies for defining the optimal donor based on the donor KIR genotype are shown. It has also been shown that the relapse protection with donor KIR B grafts is enhanced in recipients who have one or two C1-bearing HLA-C allotypes, compared to C2 homozygous recipients. In C1 recipients, mismatch at HLA-C was protective in patients who received grafts with ≥2 KIR B motifs, irrespective of the KIR ligand match/mismatch constellation and the survival advantage in C1/x recipients compared with homozygous C2 recipients was similar irrespective of the particular donor KIR B genes [117]. In contrast, in pediatric haploidentical CD3/CD19 depleted transplantation, a lower survival was demonstrated for recipients homozygous for C1 compared to non-homozygous recipients [118]. The prediction of NK alloreactivity evolves to be more and more complex, due to variable distribution of single KIR positive NK cells and inconsistent KIR avidity to HLA class I molecules. Further NK education or 'licensing' resulting in responsiveness is altered hereby and leads to a complex network of interaction [119, 120]. Nevertheless, alloreactivity models will help to improved donor selection algorithm which can be used as "donor of choice" as well as "donor of avoidance" [113, 117]. This might initiate a new era of donor selection

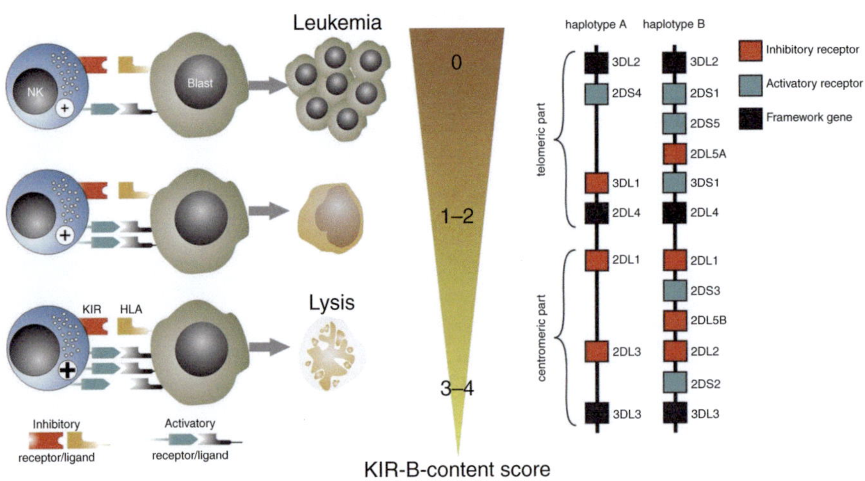

Fig. 3.2 Defining the optimal donor according to KIR haplotypes. According to the haplotype A which has a fixed gene content of 6 inhibitory KIRs and 1 activatory KIRs (aKIRs) and haplotype B with variable gene content with up to 5 aKIRs, donors can be assigned either to KIR genotype A/A (i.e. homozygous for A haplotypes) or to genotype B/x (i.e. having 1 or 2 B haplotypes). The centromeric (Cen) and telomeric (Tel) regions can reassemble to recombinant haplotypes. Genetic association studies showed that an optimal alloreactive donor will have a mismatch of his KIRs with the recipients KIR ligands and have multiple aKIRs (haplotype B). The KIR B content score reflects the number of activatory KIRs and the highest score is assocated with the highest number of aKIRs. NK cells from haplotype B donors with a high KIR B content score should exert a strong antileukemic NK—mediated response. It has also been shown that transplantation with donors homozygous for Cen KIR B haplotpyes is associated with the lowest risk of relapse and highest overall survival. Note that the majority of haplotype B donors do not express all genes shown in the figure

strategy in ALL and AML with focus on alloreactive potential of donors rather than preferring a matched donor [63, 113, 115, 116]. Since the recipients' genetic features are given [121], the best donor providing excellent alloreactive features need to be chosen [113, 115–117].

Along with the discovery of KIR alloreactivity and the introduction of models of recipient-donor interaction such as the KIR ligand-ligand model (LL) [114], the receptor-ligand model (RL) [122], the KIR genotyping model [123], the understanding of NK licensing (education) [124, 125] and the observation of the homozygosity model [118, 121], KIR immunology could bring allotransplant to a new level based on the KIR immunogenetic system independent of the HLA system. The impact of KIR genetics on clinical outcome in terms of leukemia-free survival and overall survival was demonstrated in T cell replete MUD transplant for adult AML, and in childhood ALL for haploidentical T cell depleted transplant [126]. In donor selection via KIR genotyping, the KIR receptor/ligand mismatch in GvL direction has been demonstrated to increase NK alloreactivity significantly in childhood ALL and AML, if the donor encoded for the polymorphism containing the functionally stronger KIR2DL1 allele with arginine at amino acid position 245 (KIR2DL1-R^{245}) instead of cysteine. Thus, donor KIR2DL1 allelic polymorphism might be incorporated into donor selection algorithms, even if the frequency of KIR2DL1-R^{245} polymorphism is low [127, 128]. In a pilot study in childhood AML, patients who completed primary therapy, safety, feasibility and engraftment of haploidentical adoptively transferred KIR-mismatched NK cells and subsequent interleukin-2 application after an immunosuppressive regimen with cyclophosphamide and fludarabine was demonstrated. Toxicity was acceptably low and results indicate that the adoptive transfer of haploidentical NK cells is a promising therapy for patients with AML in remission [129]. No influence of KIR receptor-ligand match versus mismatch was observed in adult patients who received $CD34^+$ enriched grafts [130] or in children with ALL, AML and advanced myelodysplastic syndrome who received a CD3/CD19 depleted allotransplant from a haploidentical family donor [118].

3.5 Haploidentical Transplantation

Major risks of allotransplantation in leukemia are relapse and post-transplant complications, including severe bacterial, viral and fungal infections as well as the development of acute and chronic GvHD [63, 131]. Thus the challenges for allotransplant is to reduce leukemic relapse by improved immunological control of leukemia, rapid immune reconstitution of innate and adaptive immune responses to avert lethal infections and at the same time to prevent GvHD while retaining an intensive GvL response [63, 131, 132].

Several strategies to meet these needs have evolved over time to rebuild the immune system post-transplant. Haploidentical HSCT especially, has improved tremendously and has become a therapeutic option, potentially broadening the indications for allotransplant [64]. Although the risk for GvHD clearly depends on the degree of HLA disparity, haploidentical HSCT has paved the way for previously unexpected immune tolerance [114, 133]. Alloreactive T cells have been identified to be responsible for the induction of GvHD, thus the balance of T cell immunity for leukemic control as well as the prevention of severe infections and GvHD are the critical point in the cure of leukemia by transplant [48, 131].

In the case of related HLA-mismatched donors, unmanipulated marrow grafts induce high grade acute GvHD in almost every patient [133]. Therefore, ex-vivo depletion strategies have been established which can very efficiently decrease the number of T cells in the graft. These strategies have facilitated allotransplantion from full haplotype mismatched donors, since the number of residual T cells in the graft is the most critical factor associated with GvHD [134]. Profound T cell depletion in the range of 4–5 log-fold is required to significantly reduce the risk of GvHD [109, 135]. Even very low numbers of T cells, as low as 3×10^4 T cells per kg bodyweight, are capable of inducing severe GvHD if no post-transplant immunosuppressive treatment is applied [136]. Most children who receive haploidentical HSCT grafts containing T cell doses below 5×10^4/kg do not develop higher grade GvHD [137, 138]. Children receiving less than 2.5×10^4 T cells per Kg can be considered to have a very low risk of developing GvHD. With higher T cell doses, calcineurin antagonists such as cyclosporine A (CSA), tacrolimus or mycophenolate mofetil (MMF) are recommended to reduce the risk of GvHD [118].

Less intensive ex vivo T-cell depletion resulted in a higher incidence of GvHD [139]. However methods for the clinical isolation of mobilised peripheral CD34+ stem cells facilitated haploidentical transplants with low or even no risk of GvHD [109, 140, 141]. However, CD34+ positive selection was associated with a delayed immune recovery and a high incidence of infections. Therefore, other ex vivo T-cell depletion techniques were introduced aiming to accelerate the immune recovery [142]. Additional in vivo or ex vivo B-cell depletion was used to prevent post-transplant lymphoproliferative disease (PLTD) of B cells [40]. The crucial advantage of T and B cell depleted grafts is the high number of effector cells retained in the graft that can potentially improve immune reconstitution by co-stimulation, antigen presentation, and innate immune effector functions [81, 143, 144]. Besides $CD34^+$ hematopoietic progenitors, CD3/CD19 depleted grafts comprise large numbers of NK cells which might prevent infections and result in antitumor responses [64, 90, 114–116, 118]. The preparative regimen has also to be taken into account since TRM, leukemic relapse, immune reconstitution, lymphoreconstitution and engraftment failure is determined hereby [145]. While myeloablative TBI-based conditioning and non-TBI myeloablative conditioning both provide the maximum of tolerable anti-leukemic effects, TRM is increased compared to reduced intensity conditioning regimens which facilitate a more rapid immune reconstitution [142, 145, 146]. In extensively pre-treated patients, non-TBI based conditioning regimens with fludarabine, thiotepa, melphalan, and anti-CD3 antibody OKT-3 have been demonstrated to be feasible with excellent outcome and acceptable GvHD rates. The cumulative incidence of acute GvHD grade III-IV was below 10% and chronic GvHD was observed in only a few patients. Non-TBI based conditioning might reduce the risk of infectious complications with less frequent transmission of bacteria and rapid immune reconstitution [146]. In subsequent trials, promising results were observed in children [147] but also adults [148, 149]. However, a delayed immune reconstitution was still observed in the adult patients, whereas NK reconstitution was rapid with physiological NK cell counts as early as day 20 post-transplant and a TRM of 7% and 39% was observed at day +100 and day +200, respectively [148]. In pediatric patients transplanted with CD3/CD19 depleted haploidentical grafts, TRM and infectious complications seemed to be more favourable [150, 151].

γδ T-cells have been of interest in antitumor response and their role in allotransplant in terms of engraftment, infectious immunological support, crosstalk with NK cells, the linkage to adaptive immune responses, GvT and GvL response as well as GvHD has been investigated [88, 89, 152]. After successful introduction of CD3/CD19 depleted grafts, the next step in graft manipulation was to retain γδ T cells in the graft to further enhance engraftment especially in reduced-intensity conditioning preparative regimens and to facilitate a more rapid T cell reconstitution to prevent severe viral infections and induce strong antitumor and antileukemic response [153, 154]. γδ T cells share in part receptors of NK cells including the natural cytotoxicity receptors (NCR) and KIRs, enabling them to recognize and kill tumor cells (e.g. leukemic AML blasts) [155] independent from the HLA presentation, and they interact with the tumor environment and influence immune responses [88, 156]. Thus, γδ T cells are able to mediate GvL without an allogeneic response. An overall favourable effect of rapid γδ T cell immune reconstitution after HSCT has been connected to a significantly higher overall survival rate and a decreased rate of acute GvHD in patients with elevated numbers of γδ T cells compared to patients with low or normal γδ T cell counts [157, 158]. The depletion of αβ TcR positive cells by anti-TcRαβ coated microbeads results in a profound depletion of TcRαβ T-cells of 4–5 logs. The TcRαβ/CD19 depleted grafts include γδ T cells in addition to effector cells present in CD3/CD19 depleted grafts [118, 154]. The first experience in haploidentical TcRαβ/CD19 depleted grafts were promising and a more rapid immune recovery compared to the CD34+ selection or CD3/CD19 depletion was observed [111, 154, 159]. In pediatric AML, patients receiving TcRαβ/CD19 depleted grafts from haploidentical and matched unrelated donors after a treosulfan-based conditioning regimen had a high engraftment rate, low incidence of acute GvHD and the cumulative incidence of chronic GvHD was 30% using various GvHD prophylaxis regimens, suggesting no advantage of MUD compared to haploidentical donor HSCT [160]. The clinical impact of this accelerated immune recovery is currently being evaluated in a multi-center phase I/II safety and feasibility study using CliniMACS TCRα/β/CD19 depleted stem cell grafts from haploidentical donors children and adults (EudraCT Number: 2011-005562-38). Currently, there are no prospective comparative studies of $CD34^+$ enriched and CD3/CD19 depleted grafts, but both are encouraging and have been reported to cure very high-risk leukemia [111, 161]. Only historical controls can be used for comparing the different graft manipulation procedures. However, the strongest prognostic factors of leukemia-free survival and outcome might still be leukemic load prior to transplant and the time interval of primary treatment and leukemia recurrence [3, 162].

The depletion of naïve, potentially alloreactive CD45RA⁺ T-cells might be able to retain a broad spectrum of both effector memory T cells (T_{EM}) and central memory T cells (T_{CM}) in the graft [163]. T_{EM} and T_{CM} cells could provide protection against infections before stem cell-derived thymopoiesis is initiated, as there is clear evidence that insufficient recovery of thymopoiesis is associated with opportunistic infections in allogeneic hematopoietic stem cell transplant recipients [164–166]. The disadvantage of CD45RA depletion could be that the depletion of alloreactive T cells, especially of the $CD4^+$ T cell subset, might be insufficient [163]. In a cohort of 17 patients with hematologic malignancies who received a conditioning regimen based on total nodal irradiation (TNI), fludarabine, cyclophosphamide, thiotepa and melphalan without serotherapy, patients received a haploidentical $CD34^+$ enriched graft with $CD45RA^-$ T cell-and $CD56^+CD3^-$ enriched NK cell add backs. Surprisingly, high numbers of regulatory T cells expanded early while naïve T cells remained absent and allowed discontinuation of GvHD prophylaxis without significant development of acute or chronic GvHD. Moreover, Vβ spectratyping showed diversity in predominantly $CD45RO^+$ T cells responsive to antigen stimulation, indicating the successful adoptive transfer of broad T cell specificity [167]. Eight pediatric patients with lymphoma or sarcoma conditioned with alemtuzumab, fludarabine, busulfan and melphalan and who received a $CD45RA^-$ depleted haploidentical graft also showed rapid immune reconstitution without induction of GvHD [168]. In 5 patients with primary combined immunodeficiency transplanted after busulfan-based conditioning and serotherapy with ATG who received CD45RA-depleted bone marrow grafts from 1-2/10 HLA loci mismatched donors, antiviral response was documented for CMV in 2/5 patients and no severe GvHD was observed after pharmacologic posttransplant GvHD prophylaxis with CsA and MMF [169].

However, the results are difficult to compare with studies due to the novel conditioning regimen and the use of CD34+ and CD56+ cells. Further clinical data are necessary to evaluate the risk of GvHD after infusion of CD45RA-depleted T-cells.

3.6 Post-transplant Allodepletion by Cyclophosphamide

The counterpart of *ex vivo* T cell depletion is *in vivo* T cell depletion, taking advantage of the time-dependent priming and expansion of alloreactive T cells [170]. *In vivo* T cell depletion can be done by application of high dose (50 mg/kg) cyclophosphamide on day 3 and 4 post-transplant (PTCy) to induce specific allodepletion of preactivated and proliferating T cells, while resting lymphocytes are spared [171]. Only limited data are available in pediatric HSCT with PTCy. In children with advanced leukemia, PTCy has been shown to facilitate stable neutrophil and platelet engraftment after fludarabine-, busulfan- and melphalan-based conditioning with medium-term immunosuppression with CSA (6 months) and MMF (3 weeks). The cumulative incidence of acute GvHD grade II-IV and chronic GVHD was 35% and 5% respectively. TRM at 1 year post transplant was 20% [172]. In adults, the outcome of T-Cell replete haploidentical HSCT with PTCy for hematologic malignancies (ALL, AML, NHL and others) is equivalent to matched related donor and MUD transplantation [173, 174] and a low cumulative incidence of acute and chronic GvHD was found in sirolimus treated patients after treosulfan-based myeloablative conditioning and peripheral blood stem cell grafts [175]. Similar results were obtained after nonmyeloablative conditioning in adults with hematologic malignancies with low rate of graft failure of 13% and with a cumulative incidence of high grade acute GvHD of 34% and chronic GvHD of 22% [171]. Given the low toxicity profile in adults, this approach might also be applicable to pediatric patients, especially in countries with limited resources or lack of donor registries [172]. However, it is still not clear whether this approach is associated with an increased risk of relapse due to the intensive immune suppression by PTCy [176–178].

3.7 Allogeneic Stem Cell Transplantation for Solid Tumors

In leukemias, which are basically fluid tumors, allotransplant has tremendously increased leukemia-free survival and overall survival [6, 9, 179–181]. The experience in allotransplant for solid tumors of childhood is very limited. Nevertheless, allotransplantation is an evolving field and besides other immunotherapeutical strategies, HSCT has become safer and might deserve broader clinical evaluation while embedding new strategies to multimodal individualized approaches [182, 183]. Allotransplantation in solid tumors has been used to induce an immunological response and tumor control [184]. The better understanding of tumor biology, particularly of the tumor microenvironment [185], tumor infiltrating lymphocytes [186], mechanisms of tumor associated antigen specific T cell recognition [66], CAR T cells [187], immune checkpoint inhibition [188], vaccination approaches [189, 190] as well as targeting antibodies [191] and NK-based tumor therapies [192] are setting set the basis for using allogeneic transplantation as a platform to treat solid tumors by combining several post-transplant antitumor strategies.

Patients with higher stage solid tumors such as Ewing's sarcoma, neuroblastoma, renal cell carcinoma, melanoma and others might benefit from allotransplantation [183, 184, 193, 194]. However, the responsible mode of action is not always clear and thus the transfer of case reports into systematic clinical application is difficult and larger clinical studies will be necessary. Furthermore, it is currently not possible to predict which patient will develop clinically relevant anti-tumor response which would allow a better selection of patients for allotransplantation [195].

In renal cell carcinoma, allotransplantation led to the cure of an incurable patient after nonmyeloablative fludarabine and cyclophosphamide-based preparative regimen, and tumor regression was associated with acute and chronic GvHD [196]. Several other transplant trials in renal cell carcinoma showed some encouraging results with response rates between 0% and 57%. Strategies to increase the GvT response are to leave high numbers of T cells in the graft with rapid withdrawal of pharmacologic GvHD prophylaxis, and rigorously treating mixed chimerism or using DLI and lymphokines to increase GvT effects with the risk of induction of severe GvHD [194]. There is a close connection between survival in renal cell carcinoma patients, the application of DLIs and the development of chronic GvHD and the clinical relevant GvT response [197]. Besides renal cell carcinoma, melanoma is one of the most immunogenic tumors, but still hard to treat in a metastasized stage even by HSCT [198]. However, the concept of adoptively transfering tumor infiltrating lymphocytes (TILs) was introduced by Rosenberg et al. in metastatic melanoma with an objective response rate in 50% of the patients [199].

Children with metastasized soft tissue sarcomas, neuroblastoma and other solid tumors have still a very poor outcome despite intensive chemotherapy [191, 200, 201]. In a haploidentical transplanted patient with Ewing's sarcoma, an impressive tumor regression was observed even of cerebral metastasis, which was associated with the development of GvHD [184]. In addition, haploidentical HSCT has shown anti-tumor response in rhabdomyosarcoma, nasopharyngeal carcinoma, desmoplastic tumor, Ewing's sarcoma and neuroblastoma [183]. Thus, multimodal treatment of primary metastatic and relapsed soft tissue sarcomas including haploidentical HSCT could facilitate long-term remission and survival and there is evidence that patients with partial remission prior to transplant might also benefit from the establishment of a new immune system [202].

In neuroblastoma, immunotherapy with anti-GD2 antibodies improved survival after autologous SCT [191, 203–205]. Prior to antibody therapy, allogeneic transplantation has been investigated for advanced neuroblastoma using a multimodality treatment with local irradiation, high dose chemotherapy and TBI. However, the TRM was unacceptably high (>50%) mainly due to infectious complications [206]. Another cohort of patients with refractory neuroblastoma and Ewing's sarcoma who failed conventional therapy experienced transplant-related complications including prolonged hospitalization, pancytopenia, sepsis and gastrointestinal toxicity. While treatment toxicity was prominent, efficacy was moderate with only partial or transient response in the majority of patients and no sustained remissions were observed [207]. Since the risk of allogeneic HSCT was estimated higher than in autologous HSCT, it was used primarily for patients who failed to harvest substantial amounts of autologous stem cells for hematopoietic reconstitution. It was observed that the outcome after auto- or allotransplantation was similar for high-risk neuroblastoma patients with acceptable low rates of GvHD [208]. Over the years, supportive care strategies improved and allogeneic transplantation should be reconsidered in the treatment of non-haematological malignancies exploiting potential graft-versus-solid tumor effects [13, 182]. More recent evidence suggest a potential clinical efficacy of allogeneic transplantation in neuroblastoma [209, 210].

The introduction of reduced intensity conditioning regimens led to significant reduction of TRM and other complications using either umbilical cord blood or T-cell depleted haploidentical grafts [193, 211]. A clinical study for the treatment of relapsed neuroblastoma has been initiated using haploidentical transplantation followed by immunotherapy with anti-GD2 antibodies and Interleukin-2 (ClinicalTrials.gov Identifier: NCT02258815). This study is still ongoing and preliminary analyses have shown encouraging survival rates [212]. In summary, allotransplantation has become safer in terms of rapid hematopoietic engraftment and with a very low TRM even in heavily pretreated patients. As in hematological malignancies, the tumor burden at time of transplantation seems to be of prognostic importance [213]. More prospective clinical trials are necessary to demonstrate the benefit of allotransplantation in pediatric solid tumors and to further identify risk-adaptive strategies to apply allotransplantation in very high risk patients at earlier stages of treatment or even as a frontline therapy for patients with an otherwise very poor prognosis.

References

1. Pieters R, et al. Successful therapy reduction and intensification for childhood acute lymphoblastic leukemia based on minimal residual disease monitoring: study ALL10 from the Dutch Childhood Oncology Group. J Clin Oncol. 2016;34(22):2591–601.
2. Horowitz M, et al. Graft-versus-leukemia reactions after bone marrow transplantation. Blood. 1990;75(3):555–62.
3. Pulsipher MA, Peters C, Pui C-H. High risk pediatric acute lymphoblastic leukemia: to transplant or not to transplant? Biol Blood Marrow Transplant. 2011;17(1 Suppl):S137–48.
4. Boulad F, et al. Allogeneic bone marrow transplantation versus chemotherapy for the treatment of childhood acute lymphoblastic leukemia in second remission: a single-institution study. J Clin Oncol. 1999;17(1):197.
5. Tallen G, et al. Long-term outcome in children with relapsed acute lymphoblastic leukemia after time-point and site-of-relapse stratification and intensified short-course multidrug chemotherapy: results of trial ALL-REZ BFM 90. J Clin Oncol. 2010;28(14):2339–47.
6. von Stackelberg A, et al. Outcome of children and adolescents with relapsed acute lymphoblastic leukaemia and non-response to salvage protocol therapy: a retrospective analysis of the ALL-REZ BFM Study Group. Eur J Cancer. 2011;47(1):90–7.
7. Schlegel P, et al. Pediatric posttransplant relapsed/refractory B-precursor acute lymphoblastic leukemia shows durable remission by therapy with the T-cell engaging bispecific antibody blinatumomab. Haematologica. 2014;99(7):1212–9.
8. Maude SL, et al. Chimeric antigen receptor T cells for sustained remissions in leukemia. N Engl J Med. 2014;371(16):1507–17.
9. Schrauder A, et al. Allogeneic hematopoietic SCT in children with ALL: current concepts of ongoing prospective SCT trials. Bone Marrow Transplant. 2008;41(Suppl 2):S71–4.
10. Bader P, et al. Prognostic value of minimal residual disease quantification before allogeneic stem-cell transplantation in relapsed childhood acute lymphoblastic leukemia: the ALL-REZ BFM Study Group. J Clin Oncol. 2009;27(3):377–84.
11. Bader P, et al. Minimal residual disease (MRD) status prior to allogeneic stem cell transplantation is a powerful predictor for post-transplant outcome in children with ALL. Leukemia. 2002;16(9):1668–72.
12. Tomas F, et al. Autologous or allogeneic bone marrow transplantation for acute myeloblastic leukemia in second complete remission. Importance of duration of first complete remission in final outcome. Bone Marrow Transplant. 1996;17(6):979–84.
13. Mateos MK, et al. Transplant-related mortality following allogeneic hematopoeitic stem cell transplantation for pediatric acute lymphoblastic leukemia: 25-year retrospective review. Pediatr Blood Cancer. 2013;60(9):1520–7.
14. Horan JT, et al. Reducing the risk for transplantation-related mortality after allogeneic hematopoietic cell transplantation: how much progress has been made? J Clin Oncol. 2011;29(7):805–13.
15. Creutzig U, et al. Diagnosis and management of acute myeloid leukemia in children and adolescents: recommendations from an international expert panel. Blood. 2012;120(16):3187–205.

16. Kelly MJ, et al. Comparable survival for pediatric acute myeloid leukemia with poor-risk cytogenetics following chemotherapy, matched related donor, or unrelated donor transplantation. Pediatr Blood Cancer. 2014;61(2):269–75.
17. Woods WG, et al. A comparison of allogeneic bone marrow transplantation, autologous bone marrow transplantation, and aggressive chemotherapy in children with acute myeloid leukemia in remission: a report from the Children's Cancer Group. Blood. 2001;97(1):56–62.
18. Godder K, et al. Autologous hematopoietic stem-cell transplantation for children with acute myeloid leukemia in first or second complete remission: a prognostic factor analysis. J Clin Oncol. 2004;22(18):3798–804.
19. Thol F, et al. How I treat refractory and early relapsed acute myeloid leukemia. Blood. 2015;126(3):319–27.
20. Kaspers GJL, et al. Improved outcome in pediatric relapsed acute myeloid leukemia: results of a randomized trial on liposomal daunorubicin by the International BFM Study Group. J Clin Oncol. 2013;31(5):599–607.
21. Bitan M, et al. Transplantation for children with acute myeloid leukemia: a comparison of outcomes with reduced intensity and myeloablative regimens. Blood. 2014;123(10):1615–20.
22. Sander A, et al. Consequent and intensified relapse therapy improved survival in pediatric AML: results of relapse treatment in 379 patients of three consecutive AML-BFM trials. Leukemia. 2010;24(8):1422–8.
23. Locatelli F, Niemeyer CM. How I treat juvenile myelomonocytic leukemia. Blood. 2015;125(7):1083–90.
24. Cwynarski K, et al. Stem cell transplantation for chronic myeloid leukemia in children. Blood. 2003;102(4):1224–31.
25. Suttorp M, Millot F. Treatment of pediatric chronic myeloid leukemia in the year 2010: use of tyrosine kinase inhibitors and stem-cell transplantation. Hematology Am Soc Hematol Educ Program. 2010;2010:368–76.
26. Andolina JR, Neudorf SM, Corey SJ. How I treat childhood CML. Blood. 2012;119(8):1821–30.
27. Nowak J. Role of HLA in hematopoietic SCT. Bone Marrow Transplant. 2008;42(S2):S71–6.
28. Schultz ES, et al. A MAGE-A3 peptide presented by HLA-DP4 is recognized on tumor cells by $CD4^{+}$ cytolytic T lymphocytes. Cancer Res. 2000;60(22):6272–5.
29. Lee SJ, et al. High-resolution donor-recipient HLA matching contributes to the success of unrelated donor marrow transplantation. Blood. 2007;110(13):4576–83.
30. Passweg JR, et al. High-resolution HLA matching in unrelated donor transplantation in Switzerland: differential impact of class I and class II mismatches may reflect selection of nonimmunogenic or weakly immunogenic DRB1/DQB1 disparities. Bone Marrow Transplant. 2015;50(9):1201–5.
31. Gyurkocza B, Sandmaier BM. Conditioning regimens for hematopoietic cell transplantation: one size does not fit all. Blood. 2014;124(3):344–53.
32. Clift R, et al. Allogeneic marrow transplantation in patients with acute myeloid leukemia in first remission: a randomized trial of two irradiation regimens [see comments]. Blood. 1990;76(9):1867–71.
33. Scheulen ME, et al. Clinical phase I dose escalation and pharmacokinetic study of high-dose chemotherapy with treosulfan and autologous peripheral blood stem cell transplantation in patients with advanced malignancies. Clin Cancer Res. 2000;6(11):4209–16.
34. Wachowiak J, et al. Treosulfan-based preparative regimens for allo-HSCT in childhood hematological malignancies: a retrospective study on behalf of the EBMT pediatric diseases working party. Bone Marrow Transplant. 2011;46(12):1510–8.
35. Sullivan K, et al. Influence of acute and chronic graft-versus-host disease on relapse and survival after bone marrow transplantation from HLA-identical siblings as treatment of acute and chronic leukemia [published erratum appears in Blood 1989 Aug 15;74(3):1180]. Blood. 1989;73(6):1720–8.
36. Weiden PL, et al. Antileukemic effect of chronic graft-versus-host disease: contribution to improved survival after allogeneic marrow transplantation. N Engl J Med. 1981;304(25):1529–33.

37. Gorin NC, et al. Retrospective evaluation of autologous bone marrow transplantation vs. allogeneic bone marrow transplantation from an HLA identical related donor in acute myelocytic leukemia. A study of the European Cooperative Group for Blood and Marrow Transplantation (EBMT). Bone Marrow Transplant. 1996;18(1):111–7.
38. Fefer A, et al. Graft versus leukemia effect in man: the relapse rate of acute leukemia is lower after allogeneic than after syngeneic marrow transplantation. Prog Clin Biol Res. 1987;244:401–8.
39. Kolb H-J. Graft-versus-leukemia effects of transplantation and donor lymphocytes. Blood. 2008;112(12):4371–83.
40. Lang P, et al. A comparison between three graft manipulation methods for haploidentical stem cell transplantation in pediatric patients: preliminary results of a pilot study. Klin Padiatr. 2005;217(6):334–8.
41. Pérez-Simón JA, et al. Nonmyeloablative transplantation with or without alemtuzumab: comparison between 2 prospective studies in patients with lymphoproliferative disorders. Blood. 2002;100(9):3121–7.
42. Kumar A, et al. Antithymocyte globulin for acute-graft-versus-host-disease prophylaxis in patients undergoing allogeneic hematopoietic cell transplantation: a systematic review. Leukemia. 2012;26(4):582–8.
43. Tang X, et al. Increasing chimerism after allogeneic stem cell transplantation is associated with longer survival time. Biol Blood Marrow Transplant. 2014;20(8):1139–44.
44. Quantitative analysis of chimerism after allogeneic stem cell transplantation using multiplex PCR amplification of short tandem repeat markers and fluorescence detection. Leukemia. 2001;15(2):303–6.
45. Barrios M, et al. Chimerism status is a useful predictor of relapse after allogeneic stem cell transplantation for acute leukemia. Haematologica. 2003;88(7):801–10.
46. Nikiforow S, Alyea EP. Maximizing GVL in allogeneic transplantation: role of donor lymphocyte infusions. Hematology Am Soc Hematol Educ Program. 2014;2014(1):570–5.
47. Bleakley M, Riddell SR. Molecules and mechanisms of the graft-versus-leukaemia effect. Nat Rev Cancer. 2004;4(5):371–80.
48. Blazar BR, Murphy WJ, Abedi M. Advances in graft-versus-host disease biology and therapy. Nat Rev Immunol. 2012;12(6):443–58.
49. Kanda J. Effect of HLA mismatch on acute graft-versus-host disease. Int J Hematol. 2013;98(3):300–8.
50. Dickinson AM. SNPs and GVHD prediction: where to next? Blood. 2012;119(22):5066–8.
51. Kim D, et al. Risk stratification of organ-specific GVHD can be improved by single-nucleotide polymorphism-based risk models. Bone Marrow Transplant. 2014;49(5):649–56.
52. Ringdén O, et al. Is there a graft-versus-leukaemia effect in the absence of graft-versus-host disease in patients undergoing bone marrow transplantation for acute leukaemia? Br J Haematol. 2000;111(4):1130–7.
53. Jernberg Gustafsson A, et al. Graft-versus-leukaemia effect in children: chronic GVHD has a significant impact on relapse and survival. Bone Marrow Transplant. 2003;31(3):175–81.
54. Kolb H, et al. Graft-versus-leukemia effect of donor lymphocyte transfusions in marrow grafted patients. European Group for blood and marrow transplantation working party chronic leukemia [see comments]. Blood. 1995;86(5):2041–50.
55. Rujkijyanont P, et al. Risk-adapted donor lymphocyte infusion based on chimerism and donor source in pediatric leukemia. Blood Cancer J. 2013;3:e137.
56. Gaynon PS, et al. Bone marrow transplantation versus prolonged intensive chemotherapy for children with acute lymphoblastic leukemia and an initial bone marrow relapse within 12 months of the completion of primary therapy: Children's Oncology Group Study CCG-1941. J Clin Oncol. 2006;24(19):3150–6.
57. Rocha V, et al. Comparison of outcomes of unrelated bone marrow and umbilical cord blood transplants in children with acute leukemia. Blood. 2001;97(10):2962–71.
58. Oevermann L, et al. Immune reconstitution and strategies for rebuilding the immune system after haploidentical stem cell transplantation. Ann N Y Acad Sci. 2012;1266:161–70.

59. Oevermann L, Handgretinger R. New strategies for haploidentical transplantation. Pediatr Res. 2012;71(4 Pt 2):418–26.
60. Cornelissen JJ, et al. Unrelated marrow transplantation for adult patients with poor-risk acute lymphoblastic leukemia: strong graft-versus-leukemia effect and risk factors determining outcome. Blood. 2001;97(6):1572–7.
61. Ishaqi MK, et al. Early lymphocyte recovery post-allogeneic hematopoietic stem cell transplantation is associated with significant graft-versus-leukemia effect without increase in graft-versus-host disease in pediatric acute lymphoblastic leukemia. Bone Marrow Transplant. 2008;41(3):245–52.
62. Peters C, et al. Stem-cell transplantation in children with acute lymphoblastic leukemia: a prospective international multicenter trial comparing sibling donors with matched unrelated donors-the ALL-SCT-BFM-2003 trial. J Clin Oncol. 2015;33(11):1265–74.
63. Weisdorf D. Which donor or graft source should you choose for the strongest GVL? Is there really any difference. Best Pract Res Clin Haematol. 2013;26(3):293–6.
64. Velardi A. Haplo-BMT: which approach? Blood. 2013;121(5):719–20.
65. Raiola AM, et al. Unmanipulated haploidentical transplants compared with other alternative donors and matched sibling grafts. Biol Blood Marrow Transplant. 2014;20(10):1573–9.
66. van den Ancker W, et al. Priming of PRAME- and WT1-specific CD8(+) T cells in healthy donors but not in AML patients in complete remission: implications for immunotherapy. Oncoimmunology. 2013;2(4):e23971.
67. Saglio F, Hanley PJ, Bollard CM. The time is now: moving toward virus-specific T cells after allogeneic hematopoietic stem cell transplantation as the standard of care. Cytotherapy. 2014;16(2):149–59.
68. Leen A, et al. Multi-virus-specific T-cell therapy for patients after hematopoietic stem cell and cord blood transplantation. Blood. 2013;122(21):140.
69. Feuchtinger T, et al. Clinical grade generation of hexon-specific T cells for adoptive T-cell transfer as a treatment of adenovirus infection after allogeneic stem cell transplantation. J Immunother. 2008;31(2):199–206.
70. Icheva V, et al. Adoptive transfer of epstein-barr virus (EBV) nuclear antigen 1–specific T cells as treatment for EBV reactivation and lymphoproliferative disorders after allogeneic stem-cell transplantation. J Clin Oncol. 2013;31(1):39–48.
71. Fontaine P, et al. Adoptive transfer of minor histocompatibility antigen-specific T lymphocytes eradicates leukemia cells without causing graft-versus-host disease. Nat Med. 2001;7(7):789–94.
72. Akatsuka Y, et al. Disparity for a newly identified minor histocompatibility antigen, HA-8, correlates with acute graft-versus-host disease after haematopoietic stem cell transplantation from an HLA-identical sibling. Br J Haematol. 2003;123(4):671–5.
73. Wang W, et al. Human H-Y: a male-specific histocompatibility antigen derived from the SMCY protein. Science. 1995;269(5230):1588–90.
74. Murata M, Warren EH, Riddell SR. A human minor histocompatibility antigen resulting from differential expression due to a gene deletion. J Exp Med. 2003;197(10):1279–89.
75. Bleakley M, Riddell SR. Exploiting T cells specific for human minor histocompatibility antigens for therapy of leukemia. Immunol Cell Biol. 2011;89(3):396–407.
76. Anguille S, Van Tendeloo VF, Berneman ZN. Leukemia-associated antigens and their relevance to the immunotherapy of acute myeloid leukemia. Leukemia. 2012;26(10):2186–96.
77. Stuehler C, et al. Selective depletion of alloreactive T cells by targeted therapy of heat shock protein 90: a novel strategy for control of graft-versus-host disease. Blood. 2009;114(13):2829–36.
78. Hartwig UF, et al. Depletion of alloreactive T cells via CD69: implications on antiviral, antileukemic and immunoregulatory T lymphocytes. Bone Marrow Transplant. 2005;37(3):297–305.
79. Amrolia PJ, et al. Selective depletion of donor alloreactive T cells without loss of antiviral or antileukemic responses. Blood. 2003;102(6):2292–9.
80. Kruse PH, et al. Natural cytotoxicity receptors and their ligands. Immunol Cell Biol. 2014;92(3):221–9.
81. Vivier E, et al. Functions of natural killer cells. Nat Immunol. 2008;9(5):503–10.

82. Takada K, Jameson SC. Naive T cell homeostasis: from awareness of space to a sense of place. Nat Rev Immunol. 2009;9(12):823–32.
83. Airoldi I, et al. γδ T-cell reconstitution after HLA-haploidentical hematopoietic transplantation depleted of TCR-αβ+/CD19+ lymphocytes. Blood. 2015;125(15):2349–58.
84. Vantourout P, Hayday A. Six-of-the-best: unique contributions of [gamma][delta] T cells to immunology. Nat Rev Immunol. 2013;13(2):88–100.
85. Paust S, von Andrian UH. Natural killer cell memory. Nat Immunol. 2011;12(6):500–8.
86. Felix NJ, Allen PM. Specificity of T-cell alloreactivity. Nat Rev Immunol. 2007;7(12):942–53.
87. Zheng J, et al. [ggr][dgr]-T cells: an unpolished sword in human anti-infection immunity. Cell Mol Immunol. 2013;10(1):50–7.
88. Carding SR, Egan PJ. Gammadelta T cells: functional plasticity and heterogeneity. Nat Rev Immunol. 2002;2(5):336–45.
89. Maniar A, et al. Human gammadelta T lymphocytes induce robust NK cell-mediated antitumor cytotoxicity through CD137 engagement. Blood. 2010;116(10):1726–33.
90. Lang P, et al. Natural killer cell activity influences outcome after T cell depleted stem cell transplantation from matched unrelated and haploidentical donors. Best Pract Res Clin Haematol. 2011;24(3):403–11.
91. Seidel UJE, et al. Reduction of minimal residual disease in pediatric B-lineage acute lymphoblastic leukemia by an Fc-optimized CD19 antibody. Mol Ther. 2016;24(9):1634–43.
92. Seidel UJ, et al. gammadelta T cell-mediated antibody-dependent cellular cytotoxicity with CD19 antibodies assessed by an impedance-based label-free real-time cytotoxicity assay. Front Immunol. 2014;5:618.
93. Vivier E, et al. Innate or adaptive immunity? The example of natural killer cells. Science. 2011;331(6013):44–9.
94. Leung W. Use of NK cell activity in cure by transplant. Br J Haematol. 2011;155(1):14–29.
95. Colonna M, et al. A high-resolution view of NK-cell receptors: structure and function. Immunol Today. 2000;21(9):428–31.
96. Yokoyama WM, Plougastel BFM. Immune functions encoded by the natural killer gene complex. Nat Rev Immunol. 2003;3(4):304–16.
97. Raulet DH, Vance RE. Self-tolerance of natural killer cells. Nat Rev Immunol. 2006;6(7):520–31.
98. Kumar V, McNerney ME. A new self: MHC-class-I-independent Natural-killer-cell self-tolerance. Nat Rev Immunol. 2005;5(5):363–74.
99. Borrego F. The first molecular basis of the "missing self" hypothesis. J Immunol. 2006;177(9):5759–60.
100. Raulet DH. Roles of the NKG2D immunoreceptor and its ligands. Nat Rev Immunol. 2003;3(10):781–90.
101. Jaeger BN, Vivier E. Natural killer cell tolerance: control by self or self-control? Cold Spring Harb Perspect Biol. 2012;4(3):a007229.
102. Shifrin N, Raulet DH, Ardolino M. NK cell self tolerance, responsiveness and missing self recognition. Semin Immunol. 2014;26(2):138–44.
103. Torelli GF, et al. Recognition of adult and pediatric acute lymphoblastic leukemia blasts by natural killer cells. Haematologica. 2014;99(7):1248–54.
104. Hilpert J, et al. Comprehensive analysis of NKG2D ligand expression and release in leukemia: implications for NKG2D-mediated NK cell responses. J Immunol. 2012;189(3):1360–71.
105. Feuchtinger T, et al. Cytolytic activity of NK cell clones against acute childhood precursor-B-cell leukaemia is influenced by HLA class I expression on blasts and the differential KIR phenotype of NK clones. Bone Marrow Transplant. 2009;43(11):875–81.
106. Pfeiffer M, et al. Intensity of HLA class I expression and KIR-mismatch determine NK-cell mediated lysis of leukaemic blasts from children with acute lymphatic leukaemia. Br J Haematol. 2007;138(1):97–100.
107. Schlegel P, et al. NKG2D signaling leads to NK cell mediated lysis of childhood AML. J Immunol Res. 2015;2015:10.
108. Locatelli F, Bertaina A. Reconstitution of repertoire of natural killer cell receptors after transplantation: just a question of time[quest]. Bone Marrow Transplant. 2010;45(6):968–9.

109. Handgretinger R, et al. Megadose transplantation of purified peripheral blood CD34(+) progenitor cells from HLA-mismatched parental donors in children. Bone Marrow Transplant. 2001;27(8):777–83.
110. Seggewiss R, Einsele H. Immune reconstitution after allogeneic transplantation and expanding options for immunomodulation: an update. Blood. 2010;115(19):3861–8.
111. Lang P, et al. Improved immune recovery after transplantation of TCRalphabeta/CD19-depleted allografts from haploidentical donors in pediatric patients. Bone Marrow Transplant. 2015;50(Suppl 2):S6–10.
112. Uhrberg M. The KIR gene family: life in the fast lane of evolution. Eur J Immunol. 2005;35(1):10–5.
113. Cooley S, et al. Donor selection for natural killer cell receptor genes leads to superior survival after unrelated transplantation for acute myelogenous leukemia. Blood. 2010;116(14):2411–9.
114. Ruggeri L, et al. Effectiveness of donor natural killer cell alloreactivity in mismatched hematopoietic transplants. Science. 2002;295(5562):2097–100.
115. Oevermann L, et al. KIR B haplotype donors confer a reduced risk for relapse after haploidentical transplantation in children with ALL. Blood. 2014;124(17):2744–7.
116. Michaelis SU, et al. KIR haplotype B donors but not KIR-ligand mismatch result in a reduced incidence of relapse after haploidentical transplantation using reduced intensity conditioning and CD3/CD19-depleted grafts. Ann Hematol. 2014;93(9):1579–86.
117. Cooley S, et al. Donor killer cell Ig-like receptor B haplotypes, recipient HLA-C1, and HLA-C mismatch enhance the clinical benefit of unrelated transplantation for acute myelogenous leukemia. J Immunol. 2014;192(10):4592–600.
118. Lang P, et al. Transplantation of CD3/CD19 depleted allografts from haploidentical family donors in paediatric leukaemia. Br J Haematol. 2014;165(5):688–98.
119. Moretta A, et al. Activating and inhibitory killer immunoglobulin-like receptors (KIR) in haploidentical haemopoietic stem cell transplantation to cure high-risk leukaemias. Clin Exp Immunol. 2009;157(3):325–31.
120. Pende D, et al. Anti-leukemia activity of alloreactive NK cells in KIR ligand-mismatched haploidentical HSCT for pediatric patients: evaluation of the functional role of activating KIR and redefinition of inhibitory KIR specificity. Blood. 2009;113(13):3119–29.
121. Pfeiffer MM, et al. Reconstitution of natural killer cell receptors influences natural killer activity and relapse rate after haploidentical transplantation of T- and B-cell depleted grafts in children. Haematologica. 2010;95(8):1381–8.
122. Leung W, et al. Determinants of antileukemia effects of allogeneic NK cells. J Immunol. 2004;172(1):644–50.
123. McQueen KL, et al. Donor-recipient combinations of group A and B KIR haplotypes and HLA class I ligand affect the outcome of HLA-matched, sibling donor hematopoietic cell transplantation. Hum Immunol. 2007;68(5):309–23.
124. Huntington ND, Vosshenrich CA, Di Santo JP. Developmental pathways that generate natural-killer-cell diversity in mice and humans. Nat Rev Immunol. 2007;7(9):703–14.
125. Tarek N, et al. Unlicensed NK cells target neuroblastoma following anti-GD2 antibody treatment. J Clin Invest. 2012;122(9):3260–70.
126. Handgretinger R. Donor selection for AML: do the KIR. Blood. 2010;116(14):2407–9.
127. Bari R, et al. Effect of donor KIR2DL1 allelic polymorphism on the outcome of pediatric allogeneic hematopoietic stem-cell transplantation. J Clin Oncol. 2013;31(30):3782–90.
128. O'Reilly RJ. Allelic polymorphisms of inhibitory killer immunoglobulin-like receptor natural killer cell function can also influence the graft-versus-leukemia response. J Clin Oncol. 2013;31(30):3742–5.
129. Rubnitz JE, et al. NKAML: a pilot study to determine the safety and feasibility of haploidentical natural killer cell transplantation in childhood acute myeloid leukemia. J Clin Oncol. 2010;28(6):955–9.
130. Weisdorf D, et al. T cell-depleted partial matched unrelated donor transplant for advanced myeloid malignancy: KIR ligand mismatch and outcome. Biol Blood Marrow Transplant. 2012;18(6):937–43.

131. Ringden O, et al. Is there a stronger graft-versus-leukemia effect using HLA-haploidentical donors compared with HLA-identical siblings[quest]. Leukemia. 2016;30(2):447–55.
132. Verneris MR. NK Cell—KIR-TREGs: how to manipulate a graft for optimal GVL. ASH Education Book. 2013;2013:335–41.
133. Anasetti C, Hansen JA. Effect of HLA incompatibility in marrow transplantation from unrelated and HLA-mismatched related donors. Transfus Sci. 1994;15(3):221–30.
134. Lang P, Handgretinger R. Haploidentical SCT in children: an update and future perspectives. Bone Marrow Transplant. 2008;42(S2):S54–9.
135. Reisner Y, Martelli MF. Tolerance induction by 'megadose' transplants of CD34+ stem cells: a new option for leukemia patients without an HLA-matched donor. Curr Opin Immunol. 2000;12(5):536–41.
136. Aversa F, et al. Mismatched T cell-depleted hematopoietic stem cell transplantation for children with high-risk acute leukemia. Bone Marrow Transplant. 1998;22(Suppl 5):S29–32.
137. Lang P, et al. Long-term outcome after haploidentical stem cell transplantation in children. Blood Cells Mol Dis. 2004;33(3):281–7.
138. Marks DI, et al. Haploidentical stem cell transplantation for children with acute leukaemia. Br J Haematol. 2006;134(2):196–201.
139. Henslee-Downey PJ, et al. Use of partially mismatched related donors extends access to allogeneic marrow transplant. Blood. 1997;89(10):3864–72.
140. Lang P, et al. Transplantation of a combination of CD133+ and CD34+ selected progenitor cells from alternative donors. Br J Haematol. 2004;124(1):72–9.
141. Peters C, et al. Transplantation of highly purified peripheral blood CD34+ cells from HLA-mismatched parental donors in 14 children: evaluation of early monitoring of engraftment. Leukemia. 1999;13(12):2070–8.
142. Chen X, et al. Rapid immune reconstitution after a reduced-intensity conditioning regimen and a CD3-depleted haploidentical stem cell graft for paediatric refractory haematological malignancies. Br J Haematol. 2006;135(4):524–32.
143. Foley B, et al. The biology of NK cells and their receptors affects clinical outcomes after hematopoietic cell transplantation (HCT). Immunol Rev. 2014;258(1):45–63.
144. Velardi A, Ruggeri L, Mancusi A. Killer-cell immunoglobulin-like receptors reactivity and outcome of stem cell transplant. Curr Opin Hematol. 2012;19(4):319–23.
145. Hale GA, et al. Haploidentical stem cell transplantation with CD3 depleted mobilized peripheral blood stem cell grafts for children with hematologic malignancies. Blood. 2005;106(11):2910.
146. Hale GA, et al. Mismatched family member donor transplantation for patients with refractory hematologic malignancies: long-term followup of a prospective clinical trial. Blood. 2006;108(11):3137.
147. Handgretinger R, et al. Feasibility and outcome of reduced-intensity conditioning in haploidentical transplantation. Ann N Y Acad Sci. 2007;1106(1):279–89.
148. Federmann B, et al. Immune reconstitution after haploidentical hematopoietic cell transplantation: impact of reduced intensity conditioning and CD3/CD19 depleted grafts. Leukemia. 2011;25(1):121–9.
149. Bethge WA, et al. Haploidentical allogeneic hematopoietic cell transplantation in adults with reduced-intensity conditioning and CD3/CD19 depletion: fast engraftment and low toxicity. Exp Hematol. 2006;34(12):1746–52.
150. Dufort G, et al. Feasibility and outcome of haploidentical SCT in pediatric high-risk hematologic malignancies and Fanconi anemia in Uruguay. Bone Marrow Transplant. 2012;47(5):663–8.
151. Palma J, et al. Haploidentical stem cell transplantation for children with high-risk leukemia. Pediatr Blood Cancer. 2012;59(5):895–901.
152. Drobyski WR, Majewski D, Hanson G. Graft-facilitating doses of ex vivo activated gammadelta T cells do not cause lethal murine graft-vs.-host disease. Biol Blood Marrow Transplant. 1999;5(4):222–30.

153. Halary F, et al. Shared reactivity of Vδ2(neg) γδ T cells against cytomegalovirus-infected cells and tumor intestinal epithelial cells. J Exp Med. 2005;201(10):1567–78.
154. Handgretinger R, et al. Transplantation of TcRαβ/CD19 depleted stem cells from haploidentical donors: robust engraftment and rapid immune reconstitution in children with high risk leukemia. Blood. 2011;118(21):1005.
155. Dolstra H, et al. TCR gamma delta cytotoxic T lymphocytes expressing the killer cell-inhibitory receptor p58.2 (CD158b) selectively lyse acute myeloid leukemia cells. Bone Marrow Transplant. 2001;27(10):1087–93.
156. Gajewski TF, Schreiber H, Fu Y-X. Innate and adaptive immune cells in the tumor microenvironment. Nat Immunol. 2013;14(10):1014–22.
157. Minculescu L, Sengeløv H. The role of gamma delta T cells in haematopoietic stem cell transplantation. Scand J Immunol. 2015;81(6):459–68.
158. Godder KT, et al. Long term disease-free survival in acute leukemia patients recovering with increased [gamma][delta] T cells after partially mismatched related donor bone marrow transplantation. Bone Marrow Transplant. 2007;39(12):751–7.
159. Handgretinger R. Negative depletion of CD3(+) and TcRalphabeta(+) T cells. Curr Opin Hematol. 2012;19(6):434–9.
160. Maschan M, et al. TCR-alpha/beta and CD19 depletion and treosulfan-based conditioning regimen in unrelated and haploidentical transplantation in children with acute myeloid leukemia. Bone Marrow Transplant. 2016;51(5):668–74.
161. Leung W, et al. High success rate of hematopoietic cell transplantation regardless of donor source in children with very high-risk leukemia. Blood. 2011;118(2):223–30.
162. Eckert C, et al. Use of allogeneic hematopoietic stem-cell transplantation based on minimal residual disease response improves outcomes for children with relapsed acute lymphoblastic leukemia in the intermediate-risk group. J Clin Oncol. 2013;31(21):2736–42.
163. Teschner D, et al. Depletion of naive T cells using clinical grade magnetic CD45RA beads: a new approach for GVHD prophylaxis. Bone Marrow Transplant. 2014;49(1):138–44.
164. Mackay CR. Dual personality of memory T cells. Nature. 1999;401(6754):659–60.
165. Chang JT, Wherry EJ, Goldrath AW. Molecular regulation of effector and memory T cell differentiation. Nat Immunol. 2014;15(12):1104–15.
166. Wils E-J, et al. Insufficient recovery of thymopoiesis predicts for opportunistic infections in allogeneic hematopoietic stem cell transplant recipients. Haematologica. 2011;96(12):1846–54.
167. Triplett BM, et al. Rapid memory T-cell reconstitution recapitulating CD45RA-depleted haploidentical transplant graft content in patients with hematologic malignancies. Bone Marrow Transplant. 2015;50(7):968–77.
168. Shook DR, et al. Haploidentical stem cell transplantation augmented by CD45RA negative lymphocytes provides rapid engraftment and excellent tolerability. Pediatr Blood Cancer. 2015;62(4):666–73.
169. Touzot F, et al. CD45RA depletion in HLA-mismatched allogeneic hematopoietic stem cell transplantation for primary combined immunodeficiency: a preliminary study. J Allergy Clin Immunol. 2015;135(5):1303.e3–9.e3.
170. Luznik L, et al. Posttransplantation cyclophosphamide facilitates engraftment of major histocompatibility complex-identical allogeneic marrow in mice conditioned with low-dose total body irradiation. Biol Blood Marrow Transplant. 2002;8(3):131–8.
171. Luznik L, et al. HLA-haploidentical bone marrow transplantation for hematologic malignancies using nonmyeloablative conditioning and high-dose, posttransplantation cyclophosphamide. Biol Blood Marrow Transplant. 2008;14(6):641–50.
172. Jaiswal SR, et al. Haploidentical peripheral blood stem cell transplantation with post-transplantation cyclophosphamide in children with advanced acute leukemia with fludarabine-, busulfan-, and melphalan-based conditioning. Biol Blood Marrow Transplant. 2016;22(3):499–504.
173. Bashey A, et al. T-cell-replete HLA-haploidentical hematopoietic transplantation for hematologic malignancies using post-transplantation cyclophosphamide results in outcomes equivalent to those of contemporaneous HLA-matched related and unrelated donor transplantation. J Clin Oncol. 2013;31(10):1310–6.

174. Ciurea SO, et al. Haploidentical transplant with posttransplant cyclophosphamide vs. matched unrelated donor transplant for acute myeloid leukemia. Blood. 2015;126(8):1033–40.
175. Cieri N, et al. Post-transplantation cyclophosphamide and sirolimus after haploidentical hematopoietic stem cell transplantation using a treosulfan-based myeloablative conditioning and peripheral blood stem cells. Biol Blood Marrow Transplant. 2015;21(8):1506–14.
176. Bacigalupo A, et al. Unmanipulated haploidentical bone marrow transplantation and post-transplant cyclophosphamide for hematologic malignanices following a myeloablative conditioning: an update. Bone Marrow Transplant. 2015;50(S2):S37–9.
177. Fuchs EJ. HLA-haploidentical blood or marrow transplantation with high-dose, post-transplantation cyclophosphamide. Bone Marrow Transplant. 2015;50(S2):S31–6.
178. Kasamon YL, et al. Nonmyeloablative HLA-haploidentical bone marrow transplantation with high-dose posttransplantation cyclophosphamide: effect of HLA disparity on outcome. Biol Blood Marrow Transplant. 2010;16(4):482–9.
179. Schrappe M, et al. Key treatment questions in childhood acute lymphoblastic leukemia: results in 5 consecutive trials performed by the ALL-BFM study group from 1981 to 2000. Klin Padiatr. 2013;225(Suppl 1):S62–72.
180. Schrauder A, et al. Superiority of allogeneic hematopoietic stem-cell transplantation compared with chemotherapy alone in high-risk childhood T-cell acute lymphoblastic leukemia: results from ALL-BFM 90 and 95. J Clin Oncol. 2006;24(36):5742–9.
181. Peters C, et al. Allogeneic haematopoietic stem cell transplantation in children with acute lymphoblastic leukaemia: the BFM/IBFM/EBMT concepts. Bone Marrow Transplant. 2005;35(Suppl 1):S9–11.
182. Barrett D, Fish JD, Grupp SA. Autologous and allogeneic cellular therapies for high-risk pediatric solid tumors. Pediatr Clin N Am. 2010;57(1):47–66.
183. Perez-Martinez A, et al. Natural killer cells can exert a graft-vs-tumor effect in haploidentical stem cell transplantation for pediatric solid tumors. Exp Hematol. 2012;40(11):882.e1–91.e1.
184. Koscielniak E, et al. Graft-versus-Ewing sarcoma effect and long-term remission induced by haploidentical stem-cell transplantation in a patient with relapse of metastatic disease. J Clin Oncol. 2005;23(1):242–4.
185. Albini A, Sporn MB. The tumour microenvironment as a target for chemoprevention. Nat Rev Cancer. 2007;7(2):139–47.
186. Baldan V, et al. Efficient and reproducible generation of tumour-infiltrating lymphocytes for renal cell carcinoma. Br J Cancer. 2015;112(9):1510–8.
187. Singh N, et al. Nature of tumor control by permanently and transiently modified GD2 chimeric antigen receptor T cells in xenograft models of neuroblastoma. Cancer Immunol Res. 2014;2(11):1059–70.
188. Topalian SL, et al. Mechanism-driven biomarkers to guide immune checkpoint blockade in cancer therapy. Nat Rev Cancer. 2016;16(5):275–87.
189. Rammensee H-G. Some considerations on the use of peptides and mRNA for therapeutic vaccination against cancer. Immunol Cell Biol. 2006;84(3):290–4.
190. Walter S, et al. Multipeptide immune response to cancer vaccine IMA901 after single-dose cyclophosphamide associates with longer patient survival. Nat Med. 2012;18:1254–61.
191. Navid F, et al. Phase I trial of a novel anti-GD2 monoclonal antibody, Hu14.18K322A, designed to decrease toxicity in children with refractory or recurrent neuroblastoma. J Clin Oncol. 2014;32(14):1445–52.
192. Pfeiffer MM, et al. IL-15-stimulated CD3/CD19-depleted stem-cell boosts in relapsed pediatric patients after haploidentical SCT. Leukemia. 2012;26(11):2435–9.
193. Lang P, et al. Haploidentical stem cell transplantation in patients with pediatric solid tumors: preliminary results of a pilot study and analysis of graft versus tumor effects. Klin Padiatr. 2006;218(6):321–6.
194. Yang JC, Childs R. Immunotherapy for renal cell cancer. J Clin Oncol. 2006;24(35):5576–83.
195. Ringdén O, et al. The allogeneic graft-versus-cancer effect. Br J Haematol. 2009;147(5):614–33.
196. Childs RW, et al. Successful treatment of metastatic renal cell carcinoma with a nonmyeloablative allogeneic peripheral-blood progenitor-cell transplant: evidence for a graft-versus-tumor effect. J Clin Oncol. 1999;17(7):2044.

197. Barkholt L, et al. Allogeneic haematopoietic stem cell transplantation for metastatic renal carcinoma in Europe. Ann Oncol. 2006;17(7):1134–40.
198. Childs R, Srinivasan R. Advances in allogeneic stem cell transplantation: directing graft-versus-leukemia at solid tumors. Cancer J. 2002;8(1):2–11.
199. Rosenberg SA, et al. Adoptive cell transfer: a clinical path to effective cancer immunotherapy. Nat Rev Cancer. 2008;8(4):299–308.
200. Carli M, et al. High-dose melphalan with autologous stem-cell rescue in metastatic rhabdomyosarcoma. J Clin Oncol. 1999;17(9):2796–803.
201. Koscielniak E, et al. Do patients with metastatic and recurrent rhabdomyosarcoma benefit from high-dose therapy with hematopoietic rescue? Report of the German/Austrian Pediatric Bone Marrow Transplantation Group. Bone Marrow Transplant. 1997;19(3):227–31.
202. Schlegel P, et al. Favorable NK cell activity after haploidentical hematopoietic stem cell transplantation in stage IV relapsed Ewing's sarcoma patients. Bone Marrow Transplant. 2015;50(Suppl 2):S72–6.
203. Simon T, et al. Long term outcome of high-risk neuroblastoma patients after immunotherapy with antibody ch14.18 or oral metronomic chemotherapy. BMC Cancer. 2011;11:21.
204. Handgretinger R, et al. A phase I study of human/mouse chimeric antiganglioside GD2 antibody ch14.18 in patients with neuroblastoma. Eur J Cancer. 1995;31A(2):261–7.
205. Ozkaynak MF, et al. Phase I study of chimeric human/murine anti-ganglioside G(D2) monoclonal antibody (ch14.18) with granulocyte-macrophage colony-stimulating factor in children with neuroblastoma immediately after hematopoietic stem-cell transplantation: a Children's Cancer Group Study. J Clin Oncol. 2000;18(24):4077–85.
206. August CS, et al. Treatment of advanced neuroblastoma with supralethal chemotherapy, radiation, and allogeneic or autologous marrow reconstitution. J Clin Oncol. 1984;2(6):609–16.
207. Graham-Pole J, et al. High-dose melphalan therapy for the treatment of children with refractory neuroblastoma and Ewing's sarcoma. Am J Pediatr Hematol Oncol. 1984;6(1):17–26.
208. Matthay KK, et al. Allogeneic versus autologous purged bone marrow transplantation for neuroblastoma: a report from the Childrens Cancer Group. J Clin Oncol. 1994;12(11):2382–9.
209. Rousseau RF, et al. Local and systemic effects of an allogeneic tumor cell vaccine combining transgenic human lymphotactin with interleukin-2 in patients with advanced or refractory neuroblastoma. Blood. 2003;101(5):1718–26.
210. Marabelle A, et al. Graft-versus-tumour effect in refractory metastatic neuroblastoma. Bone Marrow Transplant. 2007;39(12):809–10.
211. Del Toro G, et al. Reduced intensity (RI) allogeneic cord blood hematopoietic cell transplantation (Allo CBHCT) in pediatric patients with malignant and non-malignant diseases. Blood. 2005;106(11):5463.
212. Lang P, et al. Haploidentical stem cell transplantation and subsequent immunotherapy with antiGD2 antibody for patients with relapsed metastatic neuroblastoma. J Clin Oncol. 2015;33(suppl; abstr 10056.)
213. Kanold J, et al. Allogeneic or haploidentical HSCT for refractory or relapsed solid tumors in children: toward a neuroblastoma model. Bone Marrow Transplant. 2008;42(S2):S25–30.

Chapter 4
Overview of Monoclonal Antibody Therapies

Juliet C. Gray and Paul M. Sondel

Abstract The advent of monoclonal antibody technology in the 1970s brought with it the possibility of generating virtually unlimited amounts of pure antibody targeting almost any antigen of choice, opening the door to widespread application. Since the first monoclonal antibody was licensed for clinical use 30 years ago, there has been an exponential growth in our knowledge of how they may be used therapeutically, particularly in the treatment to cancer. The attraction of antibodies as therapeutics lies in part in their exquisite specificity, with little off target binding, but also in their relative ease of production and storage (as compared to cellular immunotherapies) and their long in vivo half-life (as compared to small molecules). Although the development of monoclonal antibodies for paediatric cancers has lagged behind their use for adult malignancies, there are increasing numbers of antibodies in paediatric clinical trials, and in 2015, dinutuximab, the first monoclonal antibody specifically for a paediatric malignancy (neuroblastoma), was approved.

Keywords Monoclonal antibody • Chimeric • Antibody Dependent Cellular Cytotoxicity (ADCC) • Dinutuximab • Rituximab

The concept of using antibodies as therapeutics dates back over 100 years, to when Emil Adolf von Behring demonstrated that immunity to diphtheria and tetanus could be transferred between mice, by the transfer of small amounts of serum from one animal to another [1]. At around the same time, Paul Ehrlich suggested the idea of a 'magic bullet'; a perfect therapeutic, which was highly specific for the molecules or pathogens responsible for disease but spared healthy tissues [2]. However, attempts

J.C. Gray, M.A., FRCPCH, Ph.D. (✉)
Cancer Sciences Unit, University of Southampton, Southampton, UK
e-mail: j.c.gray@soton.ac.uk

P.M. Sondel, M.D., Ph.D.
Departments of Pediatrics, Human Oncology, and Genetics, University of Wisconsin, American Family Children's Hospital, Madison, WI, USA
e-mail: pmsondel@humonc.wisc.edu

J.C. Gray, A. Marabelle (eds.), *Immunotherapy for Pediatric Malignancies*,
https://doi.org/10.1007/978-3-319-43486-5_4

at early antibody therapies were dependent on polyclonal antibodies generated by immunising large animals, which significantly limited any clinical development. The advent of monoclonal antibody technology offered the prospect of generating virtually unlimited amounts of pure, monoclonal antibody (mAb) targeting virtually any antigen of choice, and the door was opened to their widespread application to patients. Since the first monoclonal antibody was licensed for clinical use 30 years ago, there has been an exponential growth in our knowledge of how they may be used therapeutically in many different areas of medicine, but it is perhaps their contribution to the treatment to cancer that has been most successful. In 2016, the monoclonal antibody industry is worth over $60 billion dollars a year, there are 24 monoclonal antibodies licensed by the FDA for the treatment of cancer, and over 500 other antibodies in development. The attraction of antibodies as therapeutics lies in part in their exquisite specificity, with little off target binding, but also in their relative ease of production and storage (as compared to cellular immunotherapies) and their long in vivo half-life (as compared to small molecules). Although the development of monoclonal antibodies for paediatric cancers has lagged behind their use for adult malignancies, there are increasing numbers of antibodies in paediatric clinical trials, and in 2015, dinutuximab, the first monoclonal antibody specifically for a paediatric malignancy (neuroblastoma), was approved.

4.1 Monoclonal Antibody Production

The generation of the first monoclonal antibodies, described by Köhler and Milstein in 1975, involved the hybridoma technique [3]. This entailed vaccinating rodents with a specific epitope or antigen and obtaining the B-lymphocytes from the spleen of the immunized animal. The B-lymphocytes were then fused (by chemical means) with an immortal myeloma cell line. These cells were then cultured *in vitro* in a selection medium which only allowed survival of 'hybridoma' cells, which were the product of the fusion between a primary B-lymphocyte and a myeloma cell. The initial culture contains a mixture of hybridoma cells derived from many different primary B-lymphocyte clones, each secreting its own specific antibody. The next step in the process, in order to make the antibody 'monoclonal' was therefore to separate secreting hybridoma cells out into individual culture wells, and then screen for those wells containing the desired antibody. All the hybridoma cells within the well are derived from the same original single B-lymphocyte clone, and the antibody produced will therefore be monoclonal, with specificity for the same epitope. The positive hybridoma identified can then be expanded in culture, and antibody purified from the culture medium. The immortal nature of the myeloma component of the hybridoma allows the culture to be continued indefinitely, while retaining the specificity of the B cell clone.

Since this original technique was described, a number of other methodologies have been developed, generally with the aim of improving the efficiency of the fusion and selection processes, the range of target epitopes to which antibodies can be generated against or the affinity of the antibodies produced [4]. Of these, phage display technology has been widely used, whereby antibodies are displayed on the surface of phage by fusing the coding sequence of the antibody variable regions to the phage coat protein [5]. Large libraries of antibodies are created, and can be rapidly screened for target antigen binding. As the antibody genes are cloned at the same time as selection they can be further engineered to potentially increase their affinity, modulating their specificity or effector function.

4.1.1 Reducing the Immunogenicity of Monoclonal Antibodies

Rodent-derived antibodies are recognised as foreign by the human immune system and will usually provoke a human anti-mouse antibody (HAMA) response when used repeatedly in immunocompetent patients [6]. This anti-globulin response is usually detectable within 8–12 days of receiving the mAb and reaches a peak between 20–30 days. In early clinical trials of murine mAbs, HAMA responses were reported in over 50% of patients [7]. Such responses not only increase the clearance rate of the mAb from the serum thus reducing efficacy, but can also result in serious allergic responses precluding the long term, repeated use of that same mAb or of other murine mAbs. This limited the clinical use of early monoclonal antibodies, and only four rodent antibodies have been successfully licensed for use in patients. A number of strategies have been used to reduce the immunogenicity of rodent mAbs. The first technology to be widely used was chimerisation, in which the antibody was genetically engineered, to retain the variable components of the parent rodent mAb for the immunoglobulin heavy and light chains that comprise the antigen binding end of the antibody's Fab region, thereby retaining the antigen binding specificity of the initial rodent mAb. These were then genetically fused to human constant regions for the light and heavy immunoglobulin chains, comprising the constant part of the Fab region and the Fc region [8, 9] (see Fig. 4.1). This was found to be an effective way of preserving the specificity and affinity of the antibody whilst reducing its immunogenicity to immunocompetent patients [10, 11]. A more elaborate technique is to further "humanise" the antibody by grafting human

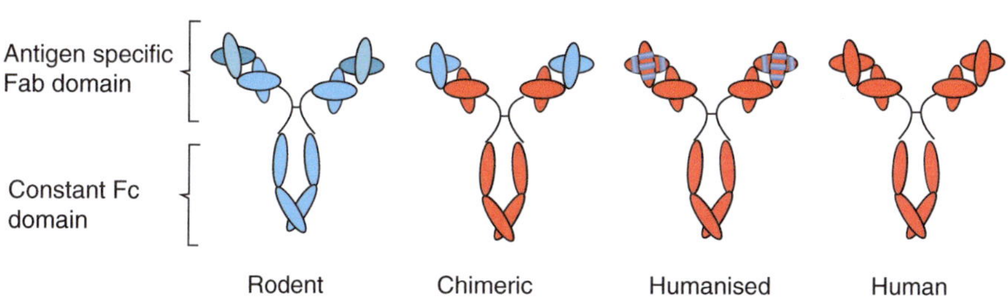

Fig. 4.1 Schematic representation of monoclonal antibody structure. *Blue areas* represent parent murine protein, and *red areas* represent human antibody sequences introduced by either chimerisation or humanisation

framework regions into the variable region, in order to retain only the murine complementarity-determining regions (CDRs) that control the original antigen binding specificity, thereby removing most murine-derived amino acid sequences from the entire mAb [12]. More recently, transgenic mice with human immunoglobulin genes have been engineered [13]; these produce fully human antibodies when immunised. Although fully humanised antibodies may have the advantage of reducing immunogenicity as compared to chimeric antibodies, they are potentially more difficult and expensive to produce, and have been associated with reduced affinity [12]. In addition, extensive humanisation may in itself not always be necessary. The anti-CD20 mAb, Rituximab, is a chimeric mouse/ human antibody and has been used extensively in over 300,000 patients, with human anti-chimeric antibody (HACA) responses reported in only approximately 1% of patients [14]. This low immunogenicity for the chimeric Rituximab reflects, at least in part, that its functional target is the elimination of mature B lymphocytes, thereby effectively blocking the induction of an antibody response against its rodent derived components. In the case of the mouse/human chimeric anti-GD2 antibody, ch14.18/CHO, HACA are reported in 21% of neuroblastoma patients, but only in 7.5% of neuroblastoma patients are the levels high (≥10 μg/mL), and capable of neutralising circulating ch14.18 [15]. In contrast, when the chimeric ch14.18 mAb has been given to adult patients with melanoma, strong HACA responses are seen more frequently [16, 17]. This likely reflects the potent immunosuppressive effects of the chemotherapy regimens received by the neuroblastoma patients vs. the relative absence of immunosuppressive chemotherapy used for treatment of melanoma. Currently, the majority of new monoclonal antibodies in development are fully human.

4.2 Mechanisms of Action of Monoclonal Antibodies

With the advent of monoclonal antibody technology, it was envisaged that antibodies recognising tumour antigens would be able to bind to malignant cells and that such 'opsonised' cells would be destroyed by complement and effector cells of the host immune system. There was early optimism that this would be therapeutically beneficial and this was supported by success with mAbs directed against lymphoma surface immunoglobulin (anti-idiotype mAbs), with long-term complete remission in some patients [18]. However these anti-idiotype monoclonal antibodies had to be custom made for each lymphoma patient, limiting their general use. In general, antibodies raised against other identified tumour antigens met with less success, with therapeutic effect being limited by failure to effectively recruit immune effectors, down-regulation of targeted antigens, difficulty in the penetration of mAbs (due to their large size of ~150 kD) into the interstitial spaces of large solid tumors or immunogenicity of the antibodies [10, 19, 20]. Despite these difficulties, there are several mAbs that directly target tumour antigens that have proved to be clinically beneficial and have been granted FDA approval for therapeutic use (Table 4.1), with many more experimental tumor reactive mAbs in preclinical and clinical

Table 4.1 Monoclonal antibodies with FDA approval for use in cancer patients

Monoclonal antibody	Target antigen target	Form	Disease indication	Year of FDA approval
Antibodies targeting hematopoietic differentiation antigens				
Rituximab	CD20	Chimeric	NHL	1997
Gemtuzumab ozogamicin	CD33	Humanized, conjugated	AML	2000
Alemtuzumab	CD52	Humanized	CLL	2001
Ibritumomab tiuxetan	CD20	Mouse, conjugated to radioisotope	NHL	2002
Tositumomab	CD20	Mouse, conjugated to radioisotope	NHL	2002
Ofatumumab	CD20	Human	CLL	2009
Brentuximab vedotoxin	CD30	Chimeric, conjugated to toxin	HL	2012
Obinutuzumab	CD20	Humanised, gylcoengineered	Follicular lymphoma	2013
Blinatumomab	CD19/CD3	Bi-specific T cell engager (BiTE)	ALL	2014
Daratumomab	CD38	Human	Myeloma	2015
Elotuzuamab	CD319	Humanised	Myeloma	2015
Antibodies targeting growth and differentiation signals				
Trastuzumab	HER2/neu	Humanized	Breast cancer	1998
Cetuximab	EGFR	Chimeric	CRC	2004
Panitumomab	EGFR	Human	CRC	2006
Pertuzumab	HER2	Humanized	Breast	2012
Trastuzumab emtansine	HER2/neu	Humanized, conjugated to drug	Breast	2013
Denosumab	RANK Ligand	Human	Giant cell bone tumours	2013
Necitumumab	EGFR	Human	Lung	2015
Antibodies target tumor vasculature				
Bevacizumab	VEGF	Humanized	CRC	2004
Ramucirumab	VEGFR2	Human	CRC	2014
Antibodies targeting the immune system				
Iplimumab	CTLA-4	Human	Melanoma	2011
Nivolumab	PD-1	Human	Renal, Lung	2014
Pembrolizumab	PD-1	Humaized	Lung	2014
Siltuxiamab	IL-6	Chimeric	Castleman's disease	2014
Antibodies targeting gangliosides				
Dinutuximab	GD2	Chimeric	Neuroblastoma	2015

Abbreviations: *NHL* non-Hodgkin's lymphoma, *HL* Hodgkin's lymphoma, *AML* acute myeloid leukaemia, *CLL* chronic lymphocytic leukaemia, *EDGF* epidermal growth factor receptor, *VEGF* vascular endothelial growth factor, *CRC* colorectal carcinoma development. In addition, over the last 5 years, a separate class of mAbs has proven to be very useful in clinical cancer therapy; rather than targeting antigens on the tumor, these are immunomodulatory mAbs that directly target the immune system and thereby can augment endogenous anti-tumor immune reactions.

4.2.1 Antibodies Directly Targeting Tumour Antigens

The potential mechanisms by which antibodies directly targeting an antigen on tumor cells make evoke cell death are illustrated in Fig. 4.2.

4.2.1.1 Antibody Dependent Cellular Cytotoxicity (ADCC)

Immune-mediated destruction of cancer cells that are coated or opsonized by antibody may be carried out by a number of immune effector cells, including Natural Killer cells, neutrophils and macrophages. The process is initiated by, and

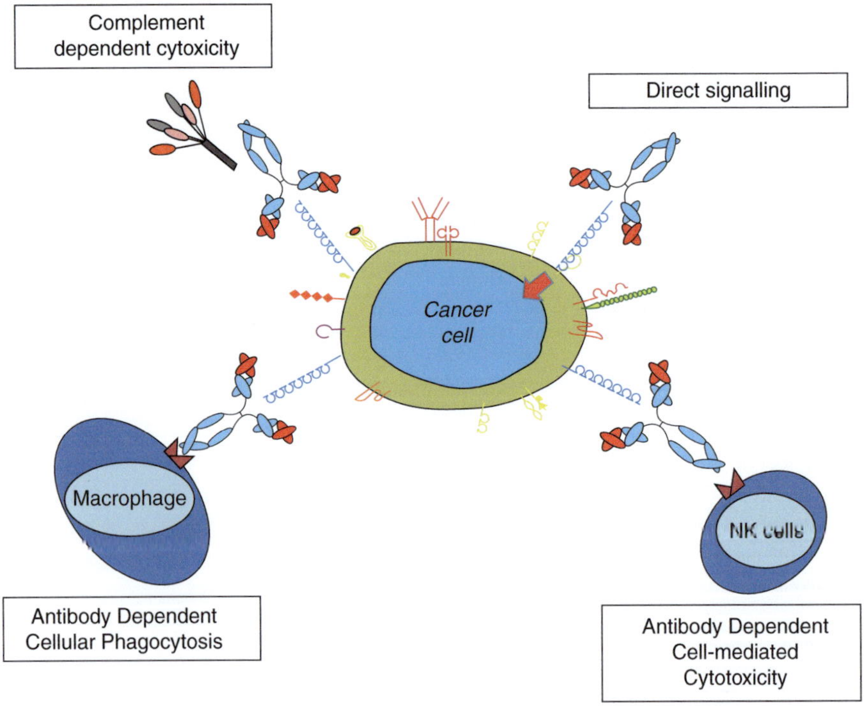

Fig. 4.2 Schematic representation of mechanisms of immune mediated cell death triggered by monoclonal antibodies directly targeting tumour antigens. The relative importance of these mechanisms varies between antibodies, and may be influenced by antibody isotype, affinity and glycosylation, and by tumour antigen density and proximity to the cell surface

dependent upon, the binding of the constant domain (Fc) of the antibody to an Fc gamma receptor (FcγR) on an effector cell. There are several human FcγR, differing in their ability to either enhance (e.g. FcγRIIA, FcγRIIIA) or inhibit (FcγRIIB) the effect of the antibody on the immune system [21]. The overall effector response triggered is determined by the relative interaction with activatory/inhibitory receptors. The engagement of activating FcγR by antibody triggers recruitment of adapter proteins and activation of the effector cell, resulting in the release of lytic enzymes such as perforin and granzymes, as well as production of interferon gamma (IFN-γ). The latter has a number of potential effects, including inhibition of target cell proliferation, up-regulation of MHC surface expression, inhibition of angiogenesis, as well as potentially fueling a secondary T cell mediated immune response. In addition, NK cells can also initiate the transduction of death signals to the tumour cell through death receptor/ligand (e.g Fas/FasL) signaling. Therapeutic efficacy will be achieved if the combined effects of these mechanisms results in immune-mediated destruction of the adjacent tumour cell.

Early *in vitro* work and murine models suggested ADCC as the key effector mechanism responsible for the therapeutic effect of mAb targeting tumour antigens. However, as discussed below, additional mechanisms, separate from ADCC, also appear to influence the activity of tumor-reactive mAbs [22].

4.2.1.2 Antibody Dependent Cellular Phagocytosis (ADCP)

Macrophages are increasingly recognized to play a key role in the mechanism of action of therapeutic anti-cancer mAbs. They are innate immune cells, derived from circulating monocytes, and are the dominant leukocyte population found within the tumor microenvironment of most cancers. Tumor associated macrophages (TAMs) express Fcγ receptors that can bind to the Fc fragment of antibodies and enable them to engage in mAb-dependent phagocytosis, with engulfment of the opsonized target tumor cell. There is now strong pre-clinical evidence to support that this is an important therapeutic mechanism for antibodies such as Trastuzumab (anti-HER2) and Rituximab (anti-CD20), and increasing evidence of the clinical importance of this mechanism. Similar to ADCP, which can cause direct cell death of tumors, is the process of antibody-facilitated antigen uptake and presentation by antigen presenting cells, particularly dendritic cells and macrophages. Here, antibody binding to apoptotic cells or their membrane fragments is recognized via Fc receptors on the antigen-presenting cell, augmenting antigen uptake, presentation and subsequent induction of adaptive immunity [23].

Although TAMs are potentially potent immune effector cells they can also actively promote tumor growth, development and immune evasion. They display heterogeneity of expression of FcγR and cytokine secretion, with distinct pro-inflammatory (M1) and pro-tumour (M2) phenotypes recognized [24]. The relative expression of activatory FcγR (e.g FcγRIIA and FcγR IIIA) as compared to inhibitory FcγR (e.g FcγRIIB), is higher on 'M1' macrophages than on their pro-tumour 'M2' counterparts. It is therefore likely that the phenotype of resident TAMs will influence the efficacy of ADCP, and that therapeutic mAbs may be more effective in tumors where there is a predominance of M1 TAMs. Polarisation of TAM towards an M2 phenotype may thus not only promote tumour growth, but also limit the efficacy of monoclonal antibody therapies.

4.2.1.3 Complement Dependent Cytotoxicity (CDC)

The complement cascade is mediated by a series of complement proteins found in serum, and can be triggered by the binding of the complement protein C1q to the Fc region of antibody bound to a target tumour cell. The degree to which CDC is triggered by antibody binding is dependent on a number of factors including the level of antigen expression and antibody binding, as well as expression of complement-regulatory proteins (e.g. CD46, CD55, and CD59), which may be found on the tumour surface and negatively regulate complement activation [25]. Although high levels of CDC may be observed in vitro, this does not necessarily correlate with importance in vivo. Indeed, in some instances CDC has been associated with toxicity rather than therapeutic efficacy, and some antibodies have been specifically engineered to try to prevent complement activation [26].

4.2.1.4 Altering Signal Transduction in Downstream Intracellular Pathways

Cancer cells, by definition, exhibit dysregulation of growth signals that control cell proliferation and survival. If such signaling molecules are expressed on the cell surface, then targeting with monoclonal antibody may inhibit proliferation and promote cell death. Such mechanisms probably play a significant contribution to the efficacy of anti-EGFR and anti-HER-2 mAbs [27]. Direct signally and induction of programmed cell death is also thought to have a role in the mechanism of anti-CD20 mAbs, despite the fact that the CD20 molecule itself does not have a clearly identified role in controlling cell proliferation or survival [28]. The role of direct signaling mechanisms in other mAbs is less clear. For example, induction of apoptosis in neuroblastoma cell lines after *in vitro* incubation with anti-GD2 has been reported, but only at relatively high concentrations of antibody [29].

In most cases, the relative contributions of each of the above mechanisms of action in patients are unclear. In vitro studies, demonstrating cytotoxicity in the absence of immune effector cells, may give some indication of direct (signaling) effects of an antibody, which may be clinically relevant if the effects are seen at concentrations of antibody achieved in patients. Immune mediated killing observed in *in vitro* or *in vivo* models may not necessarily be extrapolated to patients. Equally, immune effects observed in peripheral blood of patients do not necessarily reflect intratumoral activity. The existence of polymorphisms in Fcγ receptors, with identified low and higher affinity alleles for the different classes of Fcγ receptors, provides some evidence of clinical importance of different mechanisms. For instance polymorphisms of the activatory FcγRIIA have been shown to predict clinical response to 3F8 (anti-GD2) in patients with neuroblastoma [30], as well as predict clinical responses for the therapeutic use of Rituximab, Trastuzumab and Cetuximab, in appropriate clinical settings [31, 32]. As FcγRIIA is not expressed on NK cells, this suggests that macrophages (or other myeloid cells) also play a key role in this antibody therapy. Identifying and understanding such *in vivo* mechanisms is important in order to improve antibody function, for instance in selection of optimal antibody isotype or in choosing immune adjuvants for combinational therapies.

4.2.2 Immunomodulatory Monoclonal Antibodies

In the last decade, a group of monoclonal antibodies have emerged which, rather than recognising the tumour itself, target key receptors in the immune system. The aim of such antibodies is to boost weak, ineffective endogenous anti-tumour immune responses, to a level that is therapeutic and capable of providing effective tumour immunity [27]. Agonistic antibodies have been used as surrogate ligands, mimicking costimulatory molecules in order to optimise antigen presentation and T cell activation. Blocking antibodies have been used to counteract inhibitory signals and immunoregulatory cells [33–36]. Attractive aspects of this strategy is that the immune response generated should be directed against multiple epitopes, reducing the chances of tumour escape variants and that the targeted antigens need not be identified. Furthermore, because this class of antibodies recognise receptors expressed by all patients, they are a potentially 'off the shelf' and 'universal' therapy; they are not dependent on identification of individuals of a certain HLA type or whose tumour expresses a particular antigen of interest. In animal tumour models, antibodies against a number of target molecules on immune cells have been shown to provoke powerful tumour specific T cell responses capable of eradicating established tumour and, in some instances, leaving the animal immune to re-challenge with the same tumour, indicating long term tumour immunity. Several of these have now shown considerable clinical success, particular those targeting the checkpoint blockade molecules PD-1, PD-L1 and CTLA-4. These antibodies are being widely explored in adult malignancies, and are already of proven success in a number of cancer types. Experience in children is more limited, but the first early phase trials of these agents in the paediatric population are now in progress.

4.2.3 Antibodies Targeting the Tumour Vasculature

Tumour growth is dependent on new blood vessel growth in order to maintain supply of nutrition and oxygen to the tumour. Such angiogenesis is driven by release of Vascular Endothelial Growth Factor (VEGF) and other vascular growth factors by the tumour. These pathways can potentially be blocked by either small molecular agents or by monoclonal antibodies. The latter may have the advantage that, in general, antibodies have much longer serum half-life, as compared to small molecule drugs. In some adult malignancies, synergy between anti-VEGF mAb and conventional chemotherapy agents is reported, with normalization of blood vessels and (paradoxically) improved drug delivery. The anti-VEGF mAb, bevacizumab, is the mAb in this class that has been most widely used clinically, and has FDA approval in colorectal, breast, renal, cervical, ovarian and non-small cell lung cancer [37, 38]. Bevacizumab is being investigated in the paediatric population in a number of tumour types (including neuroblastoma, rhabdomyosarcoma and high grade glioma), but there is as yet no established benefit in any paediatric malignancy.

4.3 Improving the Efficacy of Monoclonal Antibodies

A number of different strategies have been employed to optimize and improve the function of monoclonal antibody therapies.

4.3.1 Conjugation to Toxin, Drug or Radioisotope

Monoclonal antibodies potentially provide a highly specific mechanism for delivering drug or toxin to the site of antigen expression (the tumour), without high systemic exposure. Toxins, enzymes, radionuclides and cytotoxic drugs can all be potentially chemical coupled to an antibody, usually via a thiol, amine groups or carbohydrates [27, 39]. This combines the specificity of the antibody with the cytotoxicity of the toxin, and removes the need to engage the patient's immune effector mechanisms. Several conjugated antibodies have proven therapeutic success, and have approval for use in specific malignancies (Table 4.1). Despite the attractive nature of this approach, it does have limitations, and success in solid malignancies has been limited, perhaps because of challenges of achieving adequate delivery of the conjugate to solid tumors. Heterogeneity of antigen expression on the tumor surface, and expression of the antigen by normal tissues may also limit success. These challenges may be easier to overcome in patients with leukemia and lymphoma, where delivery of the antibody conjugate to all malignant cells may be more achievable.

4.3.2 Fc Engineering to Modify Effector Function

The majority of early clinical therapeutic antibodies directly targeting tumour antigens were designed to have a human IgG1 isotype, based on pre-clinical evidence that this isotype would best promote ADCC and immune effector engagement [40]. More recently, as understanding of effector mechanisms has grown, more sophisticated antibodies have been engineered to optimize effector function. This is perhaps best exemplified by the development of the anti-CD20 mAbs. After the original first generation, chimeric anti-CD20 mAb rituximab, a number of second generation, fully humanized antibodies were developed. These had similar potency and efficacy to rituximab, but had the advantage of reduced immunogenicity. Most recently, third generation anti-CD20 antibodies have been genetically engineered either by amino-acid substitution or glycoengineering to promote interaction with FcR, particularly FcRIIIa, based on clinical data suggesting favorable outcome in patients with lymphoma with the high affinity FcγRIIIa allele [28]. Other antibodies have been glycoengineered to promote FcγRIIa binding, with the aim of optimizing macrophage interaction and ADCP [41].

In the case of neuroblastoma, an anti-GD2 mAb has been engineered to modify effector function with the aim of reducing toxicity, rather than directly improving efficacy; a specific point mutation K332A in the Fc region of hu14.18 has been introduced to prevent complement activation. This K332A mutant demonstrated a significant reduction in antibody induced pain (thought to be complement mediated) in a rat model, and has shown activity in a completed Phase I trial in patients with relapsed neuroblastoma [42].

Isotype selection is also, perhaps unexpectedly, important in order to optimise the efficacy of immunomodulatory antibodies [43]. Although such mAbs were initially thought to function primarily by either blocking key inhibitory pathways (checkpoint blockade) or by agonistically binding costimulatory receptors, recent preclinical data suggest that some such antibodies (anti-OX40, anti-CTLA-4, anti-PD-L1) actually deliver much of their therapeutic effect through deletion of intratumoral T regulatory (Treg) cells [44]. The effectiveness of this, at least in pre-clinical models, appears to be heavily isotype dependent, requiring activatory FcγR engagement on effector cells in the tumor microenvironment. Paradoxically, other agonistic immunomodulatory mAb (e.g. anti-CD40) appear to be dependent on engagement of the inhibitory FcγRIIb for their immunostimulatory effects [45]. It is likely that the relative contribution of blockade/agonistic signalling and Treg depletion is different for individual mAbs, and may even vary for the same mAb used in different cancers, depending on the tumour microenvironment. Further work is needed to better elucidate the mechanisms involved in order to fully optimize individual antibodies to maximize clinical benefit.

4.3.3 Combining with Other Therapies

It is likely that the ultimate success of most mAb therapies will be in combination with other therapeutic agents. The potential for combining different modalities of treatment and different immunotherapies is vast, and only a fraction of possible combinational therapies have been explored clinically. Understanding mechanisms of action is key to rationally designing combinational studies, especially in paediatric populations where limited patient numbers restricts the number of different studies that can be undertaken. For instance if the key mechanism of action of a mAb is thought to be Natural Killer cell mediated ADCC, then there may be value in administering concurrent immune adjuvants (e.g. IL-2 and/or GM-CSF) to activate this effector population [46]. The choice of adjuvant will be different if macrophages or other immune effectors are believed to the key effectors. Interestingly in paediatric oncology, the approach, until recently, has been to combine anti-GD2 mAb with different adjuvants, whereas in adult oncology directly targeting mAbs (e.g rituximab and trastuzumab) have been routinely given with conventional chemotherapy, and there has been relative little attention given to combining with other immune agents. Recently, however pilot data has been reported by the US Children's Oncology Group, suggesting high response rates in patients with relapsed/refractory neuroblastoma that received anti-GD2 (ch14.18/SP2/0) in combination with temozolamide and irinotecan [47]. On the basis of this very encouraging early data, it is likely that other similar combinations will be explored.

There is good rationale, and increasing preclinical data to suggest that there will be value in combining immunomodulatory mAbs with other agents, whether it be other immunotherapies, chemotherapy of radiotherapy [48]. Other therapies (e.g. chemotherapy) which induce cell death can potentially provide tumour antigen to initiate an immune response fueled by the immunomodulatory mAb. Specific chemotherapy agents, and indeed radiotherapy, may also have beneficial immune effects (e.g Treg depletion) which synergize with the effects of immunomodulatroy mAbs. The selection of chemotherapy agent, as well as dose and timing, is likely to be important. Testing this in pre-clinical models is not necessarily straightforward, but may provide proof of principle of synergy between modalities of treatment.

References

1. Winau F, Winau R. Emil von Behring and serum therapy. Microbes Infect. 2002;4(2):185–8.
2. Strebhardt K, Ullrich A. Paul Ehrlich's magic bullet concept: 100 years of progress. Nat Rev Cancer. 2008;8(6):473–80.
3. Kohler G, Milstein C. Continuous cultures of fused cells secreting antibody of predefined specificity. Nature. 1975;256(5517):495–7.
4. Liu JK. The history of monoclonal antibody development—progress, remaining challenges and future innovations. Ann Med Surg (Lond). 2014;3(4):113–6.
5. Winter G, Griffiths AD, Hawkins RE, Hoogenboom HR. Making antibodies by phage display technology. Annu Rev Immunol. 1994;12:433–55.
6. Schroff RW, Foon KA, Beatty SM, Oldham RK, Morgan AC Jr. Human anti-murine immunoglobulin responses in patients receiving monoclonal antibody therapy. Cancer Res. 1985;45(2):879–85.
7. Shawler DL, Bartholomew RM, Smith LM, Dillman RO. Human immune response to multiple injections of murine monoclonal IgG. J Immunol. 1985;135(2):1530–5.
8. Boulianne GL, Hozumi N, Shulman MJ. Production of functional chimaeric mouse/human antibody. Nature. 1984;312(5995):643–6.
9. Morrison SL, Johnson MJ, Herzenberg LA, Oi VT. Chimeric human antibody molecules: mouse antigen-binding domains with human constant region domains. Proc Natl Acad Sci U S A. 1984;81(21):6851–5.
10. Glennie MJ, Johnson PW. Clinical trials of antibody therapy. Immunol Today 2000;21(8):403–10.

11. Pavlinkova G, Colcher D, Booth BJ, Goel A, Wittel UA, Batra SK. Effects of humanization and gene shuffling on immunogenicity and antigen binding of anti-TAG-72 single-chain Fvs. Int J Cancer. 2001;94(5):717–26.
12. Clark M. Antibody humanization: a case of the 'Emperor's new clothes'? Immunol Today. 2000;21(8):397–402.
13. Bruggemann M, Spicer C, Buluwela L, Rosewell I, Barton S, Surani MA, et al. Human antibody production in transgenic mice: expression from 100 kb of the human IgH locus. Eur J Immunol. 1991;21(5):1323–6.
14. Cragg MS, Walshe CA, Ivanov AO, Glennie MJ. The biology of CD20 and its potential as a target for mAb therapy. Curr Dir Autoimmun. 2005;8:140–74.
15. Siebert N, Eger C, Seidel D, Juttner M, Zumpe M, Wegner D, et al. Pharmacokinetics and pharmacodynamics of ch14.18/CHO in relapsed/refractory high-risk neuroblastoma patients treated by long-term infusion in combination with IL-2. MAbs. 2016;8(3):604–16.
16. Albertini MR, Gan J, Jaeger P, Hank JA, Storer B, Schell K, et al. Systemic interleukin-2 modulates the anti-idiotypic response to chimeric anti-GD2 antibody in patients with melanoma. J Immunother Emphasis Tumor Immunol. 1996;19(4):278–95.
17. Albertini MR, Hank JA, Schiller JH, Khorsand M, Borchert AA, Gan J, et al. Phase IB trial of chimeric antidisialoganglioside antibody plus interleukin 2 for melanoma patients. Clin Cancer Res. 1997;3(8):1277–88.
18. Davis TA, Maloney DG, Czerwinski DK, Liles TM, Levy R. Anti-idiotype antibodies can induce long-term complete remissions in non-Hodgkin's lymphoma without eradicating the malignant clone. Blood. 1998;92(4):1184–90.
19. Pesando JM, Hoffman P, Abed M. Antibody-induced antigenic modulation is antigen dependent: characterization of 22 proteins on a malignant human B cell line. J Immunol. 1986;137(11):3689–95.
20. Glennie MJ, van de Winkel JG. Renaissance of cancer therapeutic antibodies. Drug Discov Today. 2003;8(11):503–10.
21. Nimmerjahn F, Ravetch JV. Fcgamma receptors as regulators of immune responses. Nat Rev Immunol. 2008;8(1):34–47.
22. Seidel UJ, Schlegel P, Lang P. Natural killer cell mediated antibody-dependent cellular cytotoxicity in tumor immunotherapy with therapeutic antibodies. Front Immunol. 2013;4:76.
23. Rafiq K, Bergtold A, Clynes R. Immune complex-mediated antigen presentation induces tumor immunity. J Clin Invest. 2002;110(1):71–9.
24. Chanmee T, Ontong P, Konno K, Itano N. Tumor-associated macrophages as major players in the tumor microenvironment. Cancers (Basel). 2014;6(3):1670–90.
25. Rogers LM, Veeramani S, Weiner GJ. Complement in monoclonal antibody therapy of cancer. Immunol Res. 2014;59(1–3):203–10.
26. Sorkin LS, Otto M, Baldwin WM 3rd, Vail E, Gillies SD, Handgretinger R, et al. Anti-GD(2) with an FC point mutation reduces complement fixation and decreases antibody-induced allodynia. Pain. 2010;149(1):135–42.
27. Scott AM, Wolchok JD, Old LJ. Antibody therapy of cancer. Nat Rev Cancer. 2012;12(4):278–87.
28. Lim SH, Beers SA, French RR, Johnson PW, Glennie MJ, Cragg MS. Anti-CD20 monoclonal antibodies: historical and future perspectives. Haematologica. 2010;95(1):135–43.
29. Alvarez-Rueda N, Desselle A, Cochonneau D, Chaumette T, Clemenceau B, Leprieur S, et al. A monoclonal antibody to O-acetyl-GD2 ganglioside and not to GD2 shows potent anti-tumor activity without peripheral nervous system cross-reactivity. PLoS One. 2011;6(9):e25220.
30. Cheung NK, Sowers R, Vickers AJ, Cheung IY, Kushner BH, Gorlick R. FCGR2A polymorphism is correlated with clinical outcome after immunotherapy of neuroblastoma with anti-GD2 antibody and granulocyte macrophage colony-stimulating factor. J Clin Oncol. 2006;24(18):2885–90.
31. Musolino A, Naldi N, Bortesi B, Pezzuolo D, Capelletti M, Missale G, et al. Immunoglobulin G fragment C receptor polymorphisms and clinical efficacy of trastuzumab-based therapy in patients with HER-2/neu-positive metastatic breast cancer. J Clin Oncol. 2008;26(11):1789–96.

32. Weng WK, Levy R. Genetic polymorphism of the inhibitory IgG Fc receptor FcgammaRIIb is not associated with clinical outcome in patients with follicular lymphoma treated with rituximab. Leuk Lymphoma. 2009;50(5):723–7.
33. Pardoll DM. The blockade of immune checkpoints in cancer immunotherapy. Nat Rev Cancer. 2012;12(4):252–64.
34. Homet Moreno B, Ribas A. Anti-programmed cell death protein-1/ligand-1 therapy in different cancers. Br J Cancer. 2015;112(9):1421–7.
35. Lee CS, Cragg M, Glennie M, Johnson P. Novel antibodies targeting immune regulatory checkpoints for cancer therapy. Br J Clin Pharmacol. 2013;76(2):233–47.
36. Marabelle A, Gray J. Tumor-targeted and immune-targeted monoclonal antibodies: going from passive to active immunotherapy. Pediatr Blood Cancer. 2015;62(8):1317–25.
37. Ferrara N, Adamis AP. Ten years of anti-vascular endothelial growth factor therapy. Nat Rev Drug Discov. 2016;15(6):385–403.
38. Sullivan LA, Brekken RA. The VEGF family in cancer and antibody-based strategies for their inhibition. MAbs. 2010;2(2):165–75.
39. de Goeij BE, Lambert JM. New developments for antibody-drug conjugate-based therapeutic approaches. Curr Opin Immunol. 2016;40:14–23.
40. Isaacs JD, Greenwood J, Waldmann H. Therapy with monoclonal antibodies. II. The contribution of Fc gamma receptor binding and the influence of C(H)1 and C(H)3 domains on in vivo effector function. J Immunol. 1998;161(8):3862–9.
41. Herter S, Birk MC, Klein C, Gerdes C, Umana P, Bacac M. Glycoengineering of therapeutic antibodies enhances monocyte/macrophage-mediated phagocytosis and cytotoxicity. J Immunol. 2014;192(5):2252–60.
42. Navid F, Sondel PM, Barfield R, Shulkin BL, Kaufman RA, Allay JA, et al. Phase I trial of a novel anti-GD2 monoclonal antibody, Hu14.18K322A, designed to decrease toxicity in children with refractory or recurrent neuroblastoma. J Clin Oncol. 2014;32(14):1445–52.
43. DiLillo DJ, Ravetch JV. Fc-receptor interactions regulate both cytotoxic and immunomodulatory therapeutic antibody effector functions. Cancer Immunol Res. 2015;3(7):704–13.
44. Beers SA, Glennie MJ, White AL. Influence of immunoglobulin isotype on therapeutic antibody function. Blood. 2016;127(9):1097–101.
45. White AL, Dou L, Chan HT, Field VL, Mockridge CI, Moss K, et al. Fcgamma receptor dependency of agonistic CD40 antibody in lymphoma therapy can be overcome through antibody multimerization. J Immunol. 2014;193(4):1828–35.
46. Yu AL, Gilman AL, Ozkaynak MF, London WB, Kreissman SG, Chen HX, et al. Anti-GD2 antibody with GM-CSF, interleukin-2, and isotretinoin for neuroblastoma. N Engl J Med. 2010;363(14):1324–34.
47. Mody R, Naranjo A, Van Ryn C, Yu AL, London WB, Shulkin BL, Parisi MT, Servaes SE, Diccianni MB, Sondel PM, Bender JG, Maris JM, Park JR, Bagatell R. Irinotecan-temozolomide with temsirolimus or dinutuximab in children with refractory or relapsed neuroblastoma (COGANBL1221): an open-label, randomised, phase 2 trial. Lancet Oncol. 2017;18(7):946–957. doi: 10.1016/S1470-2045(17)30355-8. Epub 2017 May 23.
48. Morris ZS, Guy EI, Francis DM, Gressett MM, Werner LR, Carmichael LL, et al. In situ tumor vaccination by combining local radiation and tumor-specific antibody or immunocytokine treatments. Cancer Res. 2016;76(13):3929–41.

Chapter 5
Monoclonal Antibodies Targeting Hematological Malignancies

Matthew J. Barth, Jessica Hochberg, Nader Kim El-Mallawany, and Mitchell S. Cairo

Abstract The current prognosis is excellent for children with Acute Lymphoblastic Leukemia (ALL), Non-Hodgkin's Lymphoma (NHL) and Hodgkin's Lymphoma (HL). However, patients who relapse or progress can have a dismal prognosis. Further, children with Acute Myeloid Leukemia (AML) have a good, but not excellent, prognosis with upfront therapy. Furthermore, despite these advances in outcome, children still suffer acute and long-term morbidity and mortality from upfront and re-induction chemotherapy. Surface targets have been identified in ALL, AML, NHL and HL and concomitant monoclonal antibodies have been developed to these surface targets and many have been recently approved by regulatory authorities. In this review, we summarize the safety and clinical application of therapeutic monoclonal antibodies in the treatment of paediatric haematological malignancies and discuss the future direction of this new targeted therapy approach.

Keywords Hematological malignancy • Children • Antibody • Non-Hodgkin lymphoma • Acute lymphoblastic leukaemia • Acute myeloid leukaemia • Hodgkin lymphoma • Immune therapy

---

Supported in part by grants from the Pediatric Cancer Research Foundation and the St. Baldrick's Foundation.

M.J. Barth, M.D.
Pediatric Hematology and Oncology, Women and Children's Hospital of Buffalo/Roswell Park Cancer Institute, Buffalo, NY, USA

J. Hochberg, M.D.
Division Pediatric Hematology, Oncology and Stem Cell Transplant, Westchester Medical Center, Valhalla, NY, USA

N.K. El-Mallawany, M.D.
Pediatric Hematology, Oncology, and Stem Cell Transplantation, Maria Fareri Children's Hospital, New York Medical College, Valhalla, NY, USA

M.S. Cairo, M.D. (✉)
Department of Pediatrics, New York Medical College, Valhalla, NY, USA
e-mail: Mitchell_cairo@nymc.edu

J.C. Gray, A. Marabelle (eds.), *Immunotherapy for Pediatric Malignancies*,
https://doi.org/10.1007/978-3-319-43486-5_5

5.1 Introduction

While the use of current combination chemotherapy and radiation approaches has resulted in overall improved cure rates, especially in paediatric hematological malignancies, there has been a relative plateau over the past decade and cancer remains the most common cause of disease-related mortality in the United States. In addition, patients with relapsed or refractory cancer have limited treatment options which often require further intensification of chemotherapy or radiation.

As we have developed a better understanding of the immune mechanisms involved in the regulation of various malignancies, the area of targeted cancer immunotherapy has rapidly emerged as an example of how we can utilise the patient's own immune system alone or in combination with more traditional chemotherapy strategies to further improve overall outcomes with less toxicities. Both cellular and humoral immunotherapy approaches have been investigated in hematological malignancies with varying success (Fig. 5.1) [1]. Newer cellular therapy approaches such as chimeric antigen receptor modified T or natural killer (NK) cells or vaccine trials have been promising. In addition, there are several monoclonal antibodies that have now been FDA approved or under investigation. In this chapter, we will focus on those monoclonal antibodies that have shown the most success in treating paediatric hematological malignancies.

5.2 B-Cell Non-Hodgkin Lymphoma

5.2.1 Monoclonal Antibodies Targeting CD20

Treatment of B-cell non-Hodgkin lymphoma (B-NHL) has been significantly enhanced by the addition of monoclonal antibody therapy in recent decades (Table 5.1). A number of surface targets or receptors are expressed on B-cell malignancies (Fig. 5.2). Rituximab, a chimeric monoclonal antibody targeting the B-cell associated antigen CD20, has exhibited significant activity in adults with B-NHL. As a single agent, rituximab led to responses in nearly half of adults with follicular lymphoma (FL); and when added to the chemotherapy regimen incorporating cyclophosphamide, doxorubicin, vincristine and prednisone (CHOP) led to an improvement in response rates and survival compared to CHOP alone in adults with both indolent and aggressive forms of B-NHL [2–5]. While data is more limited and results mixed in the setting of adult Burkitt lymphoma (BL), recent data suggests that there is in fact a survival benefit to adding rituximab to chemotherapy for BL [6, 7]. With these findings, rituximab is currently standard of care for treatment of B-NHL in adults.

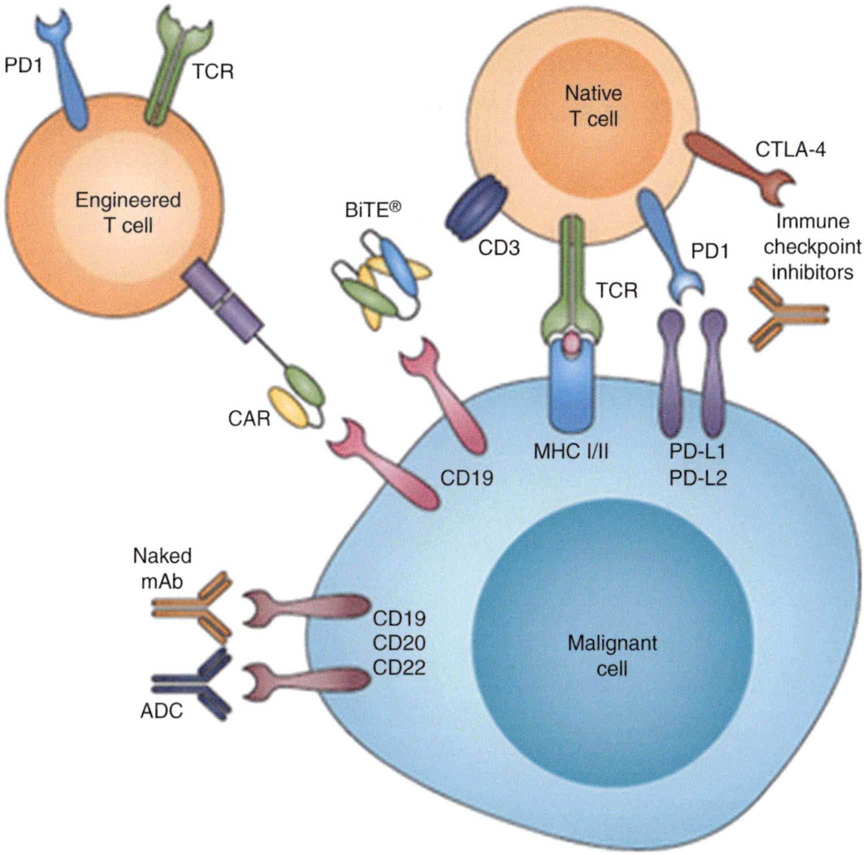

Fig. 5.1 Mechanisms of action of immunotherapy modalities. Native T cells can recognise tumour-specific antigens in an MHC-dependent manner. The T cells also require co-stimulation for activation. Upon antigen recognition, without co-stimulatory signal, or with the stimulation of inhibitory molecules, such as through the PD-1–PD-L1 axis, the T cells can be induced to anergy or become exhausted. Immune-checkpoint inhibitors can block the inhibitory signal of T cells to avert T cells from anergy. BiTE® antibodies bring T cells and malignant cells into close proximity through dual antigen binding, and can induce T-cell activation without co-stimulatory signals. T-cells can also be engineered to express CARs to recognize cell-surface molecules independent of MHC. Later-generation CARs have both TCR and co-stimulatory signalling components, thereby activating the T cells without additional co-stimulatory signal. Abbreviations: ADC, antibody–drug conjugate; BiTE®, bispecific T-cell engager antibody; CAR, chimeric antigen receptor; CTLA-4, cytotoxic T-lymphocyte-associated protein 4; mAb, monoclonal antibody; MHC, major histocompatibility complex; PD-1, programmed cell death protein 1; PD-L1, programmed cell death 1 ligand 1; TCR, T-cell receptor. Used with permission from Batlevi CL, Matsuki E, Brentjens RJ, Younes A. (2016) Novel immunotherapies in lymphoid malignancies. *Nat Rev Clin Oncol* 13, 25–40 [100]

Table 5.1 Monoclonal antibodies with regulatory approval or under investigation in B-NHL

Target antigen	Antibody	Type	Stage of investigation in B-NHL	Ongoing clinical trials in childhood B-NHL (sponsor)
CD19	SGN-CD19A	ADC	Phase I/II	NCT01786096: Phase I including BL and B-LBL (Seattle Genetics, Inc.)
	SAR3419	ADC	Phase II	None
CD20	Rituximab	Naked	Approved for B-NHL	NCT01859819: Phase II in aggressive B-NHL (NYMC)
				NCT01595048: Phase III in aggressive B-NHL (COG/Gustave Roussy)
				NCT00001337: Phase II in PMBL (NCI)
				NCT02419469: Phase II including BL (M.D. Anderson)
				NCT01700946: Phase II in r/r B-LBL (St. Jude)
				NCT01516567: Phase II in PMBL (NCI)
				NCT01760226: Phase II in PMBL (Baylor)
				NCT01046825: Phase II/III in aggressive B-NHL (St. Jude)
	Ofatumumab	Naked	Approved for CLL; Phase II/III in B-NHL	NCT02419469: Phase II including BL (M.D. Anderson)
				NCT02199184: Phase II including r/r Burkitt leukemia (M.D. Anderson)
	Obinutuzumab	Naked	Approved for CLL; Phase II/III in B-NHL	NCT02393157: Phase II in r/r B-NHL (NYMC)
	^{90}Y-Ibritumomab tiuxetan	RIC	Approved in r/r and as consolidation in FL	None

Table 5.1 (continued)

Target antigen	Antibody	Type	Stage of investigation in B-NHL	Ongoing clinical trials in childhood B-NHL (sponsor)
CD22	Epratuzumab	Naked	Phase II/III	None
	^{90}Y-Epratuzumab	RIC	Phase I/II	None
	Pinatuzumab vedotin	ADC	Phase II	None
CD30	Brentuximab vedotin	ADC	Phase I/II	None
CD79b	Polatuzumab vedotin	ADC	Phase I/II	None
CD3/CD19	Blinatumomab	Bispecific	Phase I/II	None
CTLA4	Ipilimumab	Naked	Phase I/II	NCT02304458: Phase I/II including r/r B-NHL (with nivolumab) (NCI)
PD-1	Pidilizumab	Naked	Phase II	None
	Nivolumab	Naked	Phase I/II	NCT02304458: Phase I/II including r/r B-NHL (with ipilimumab) (NCI)
	Pembrolizumab	Naked	Phase I/II	NCT02332668: Phase I/II including r/r B-NHL (Merck)

NHL non-Hodgkin lymphoma, *r/r* relapsed/refractory, *BL* Burkitt lymphoma, *B-LBL* B-lymphoblastic lymphoma, *ALCL* anaplastic large cell lymphoma, *HL* Hodgkin lymphoma, *ADC* antibody drug conjugate, *RIC* radioimmunoconjugate, *r/r* relapsed/refractory, *NCI* National Cancer Institute, *NYMC* New York Medical College, *COG* Children's Oncology Group

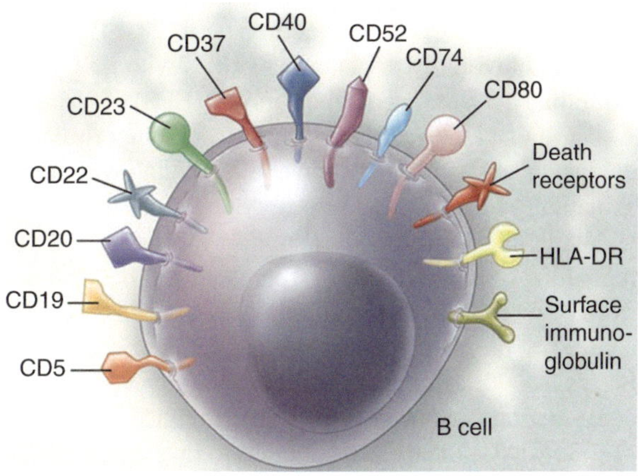

Fig. 5.2 Cell surface antigens on the B cell. The B cell has a large number of associated cell-surface antigens that can be exploited as targets for monoclonal-antibody therapy. The presence of CD5 on the surface of B cells varies according to histologic type. From Cheson BD, Leonard JP. (2008) Monoclonal antibody therapy for B-cell non-Hodgkin's lymphoma. *N Engl J Med* 359, 613–626 [144]

While all evidence points to a survival advantage with the addition of rituximab to chemotherapy in adult B-NHL, the question is still unsettled in paediatric B-NHL; though the data on rituximab use in pediatric B-NHL continues to grow. Rituximab was first investigated in paediatric B-NHL in the setting of relapsed/refractory disease in combination with ifosfamide, carboplatin and etoposide (R-ICE). In the Children's Oncology Group (COG) study, R-ICE led to an overall response rate (ORR) of 60% in 20 patients with relapsed/refractory diffuse large B-cell lymphoma (DLBCL), BL or mature B-cell acute lymphocytic leukaemia (B-ALL) [8]. Of note, 8 of the 12 responders were survivors 13–30 months from study entry with no survivors in the non-responders and a median survival of only 2.5 months, highlighting the significant chemoresistant state of relapsed tumours in childhood B-NHL and the need to develop novel approaches to treating relapsed/refractory disease.

In the up-front setting, rituximab has been formally studied in several trials. The first study of rituximab in *de novo* paediatric B-NHL was undertaken by the German Berlin-Frankfurt-Munster (BFM) group. In a window study of a single dose of rituximab with only a 5 day response assessment period, 45% of children with B-NHL responded to single agent rituximab [9]. While the study did not meet the pre-set target for response rate, the goal was ambitious considering the short assessment period, and overall the study demonstrated activity of rituximab in the setting of *de novo* paediatric B-NHL. The COG undertook a pilot study to investigate the addition of rituximab to FAB/LMB 96 backbone chemotherapy in FAB Group B and C patients. Based on evidence suggesting improved responses in adult patients that achieved higher peak plasma rituximab levels, the study utilized a dose-dense approach with the addition of two rituximab doses prior to each of two induction cycles and one rituximab dose prior to each of two consolidation cycles with Group C patients then receiving four additional maintenance cycles [10, 11]. There was no significant difference in toxicity noted with rituximab administration in combination with chemotherapy suggesting rituximab can be safely given to children receiving intensive B-NHL chemotherapy [12, 13]. Additionally, survival outcomes compared favorably to historical values with 45 Group B and 40 Group C patients exhibiting a 3-year event-free survival (EFS) of 95% and 90%, respectively [12, 13]. A pharmacokinetic analysis demonstrated that rituximab exhibited similar pharmacokinetics to those reported in adults, though with a trend toward higher peak levels and a higher rate of clearance in younger children [14].

While these three studies support the safety and potential efficacy of rituximab in treating paediatric B-NHL, there had still been no definitive evidence of the superiority of rituximab containing regimens for B-NHL in pediatrics. Considering the significant improvements in treating paediatric B-NHL with long term survival rates exceeding 90%, undertaking such a study would require a large collaboration to achieve adequate power to detect a difference. Thus, a large international cooperative group Phase III study was initiated to investigate the addition of rituximab to FAB/LMB-96 backbone chemotherapy in a randomised fashion in higher risk (high lactate dehydrogenase [LDH]) Group B and Group C patients (NCT01595048). Though the goal for accrual was not yet met, accrual was halted prematurely after an observed improvement in 1 year EFS in the rituximab arm suggesting a possible superiority of the rituximab containing regimen (Gross, personal communication). Though follow-up is ongoing, this finding suggests a likely benefit of rituximab at least in the high-risk setting. Incorporated within the same trial is a Phase II study of the dose adjusted EPOCH-R (rituximab, etoposide, prednisone, vincristine, cyclophosphamide and doxorubicin) regimen in children with primary mediastinal large B-cell lymphoma (PMBL) (NCT01516567). This regimen has shown significant promise in the treatment of this unique B-NHL subtype in studies performed in adults with 96% of 51 patients in complete remission (CR) after follow-up ranging from 10 months to 14 years in a recent report [15].

While the benefit of rituximab in improving outcomes in higher risk disease continues to be debated, another area of investigation includes the possibility of therapeutic de-intensification with the addition of rituximab. Multi-agent chemotherapy regimens utilised for paediatric B-NHL are associated with a high rate of acute toxicity, in particular mucositis and infectious complications/febrile neutropenia, and include anthracyclines, though generally at fairly low cumulative dose levels [16, 17]. While de-escalation of chemotherapy in a very curable disease remains a controversial issue, one potential application of rituximab would be to decrease cytotoxic chemotherapy associated with acute and/or late toxicities by the incorporation of rituximab into chemotherapy regimens for lower risk patients. The ongoing Reduced Burden of Oncologic Therapy (REBOOT) trial sponsored by the Childhood, Adolescent and Young Adult NHL Translational Research and Treatment (CAN TREAT) consortium is investigating a 60% reduction in the doxorubicin dose in Group B childhood, adolescent and young adult patients with the addition of rituximab to FAB/LMB-96 based chemotherapy while also investigating the addition of rituximab to standard Group C therapy with both groups also receiving less total intrathecal chemotherapy doses with the addition of intrathecal liposomal cytarabine (NCT01859819). While accrual is ongoing, in an initial report on 24 patients accrued (18 Group B and 6 Group C), the failure-free survival and overall survival (OS) are 100% with a median time from study entry of 52 weeks (6–152 weeks) [18].

Though incorporation of rituximab into chemotherapy regimens has led to a significant improvement in survival in adult B-NHL, resistance to repeat treatment in relapsed/refractory disease has been identified as a concern. In FL patients who initially responded to rituximab, less than half responded upon retreatment [19]. Additionally, the CORAL study, investigating outcomes in adults with relapsed/refractory DLBCL, reported significantly inferior EFS observed in patients previously treated with a rituximab containing regimen upon subsequent treatment with R-ICE or R-DHAP (rituximab, dexamethasone, cytarabine and cisplatin) [20]. This highlights the imperative need for novel targeted approaches to treatment of B-NHL, especially as rituximab usage increases in the upfront setting in childhood B-NHL. These novel approaches include next generation monoclonal antibodies targeting a variety of cell surface antigens currently either approved or under investigation in various B-NHL types. Many of these surface antigens are nearly ubiquitously expressed on the surface of childhood B-NHL tumour cells [21].

Several second and third generation monoclonal antibodies targeting CD20 continue to be developed. These include both naked and radio-immunoconjugate antibodies. Two naked antibodies, ofatumumab and obinutuzumab, already have regulatory approval for specific indications in chronic lymphocytic leukemia (CLL). Two radio-immunoconjugates, ^{131}I-tositumomab and ^{90}Y-ibritumomab tiuxetan (^{90}Y-IT), also have regulatory approval for consolidative therapy in indolent B-NHL, though production of ^{131}I-tositumomab was recently discontinued by the manufacturer due to its limited utilisation.

Ofatumumab is a fully human monoclonal antibody targeting a unique epitope incorporating the small and large extracellular loops of the CD20 antigen [22]. Possibly related to this more membrane proximal binding, ofatumumab has demonstrated enhanced complement dependent cytotoxicity (CDC) activity as compared to rituximab in pre-clinical testing [23–25]. It is currently approved by the FDA for use in fludarabine and alemtuzumab refractory CLL and in untreated CLL for patients not eligible for fludarabine-based therapy [26, 27]. It also recently gained an additional indication for extended therapy in relapsed/refractory CLL patients currently in complete or partial response following at least two prior treatment regimens. Despite promising pre-clinical findings and activity in CLL, clinical trials investigating the use of ofatumumab in B-NHL have led to underwhelming results, including similar response rates to rituximab when compared head to head in combination with DHAP chemotherapy in relapsed/refractory DLBCL, diminishing enthusiasm for ofatumumab in treatment of the more aggressive B-NHL types seen in children [28].

Obinutuzumab is a humanised type II anti-CD20 monoclonal antibody with a glycoengineered Fc portion enhancing its affinity for Fc receptors including in the setting of Fc receptor polymorphisms known to inhibit rituximab binding [29]. In pre-clinical investigations, obinutuzumab exhibited enhanced antibody dependent cellular cytotoxicity (ADCC) and direct induction of cell death compared to rituximab (and other type I antibodies like ofatumumab), with limited CDC activity while also prolonging survival compared to rituximab in mouse models of aggressive B-NHL including in rituximab-resistant models [29–31]. Clinically, similar to ofatumumab, obinutuzumab has demonstrated efficacy in the treatment of CLL and is currently approved for the treatment of previously untreated CLL in combination with chlorambucil [32]. When compared head to head to rituximab, obinutuzumab has exhibited promising activity in both indolent and aggressive adult B-NHL. In the randomised Phase II GAUSS trial, obinutuzumab therapy led to a higher ORR compared to rituximab (42% vs. 24%) in 149 relapsed/refractory indolent B-NHL patients, though there was no difference in progression-free survival (PFS) [33]. The Phase II GAUGIN study investigated obinutuzumab monotherapy in relapsed/refractory mantle cell lymphoma (MCL) or DLBCL. Obinutuzumab led to a 32% ORR in 19 patients in the higher of two dose levels tested [34]. This included responses in 4/12 (33%) patients deemed rituximab refractory. Pre-clinical studies using obinutuzumab have demonstrated it to be significantly better than rituximab in rituximab-sensitive and -resistant Burkitt lymphoma [35]. Based on these pre-clinical results, obinituzumab use in relapsed/refractory childhood B-NHL is being investigated in a trial sponsored by the CAN TREAT consortium combining obinutuzumab with ICE chemotherapy (NCT02393157).

While the use of anti-CD20 radioimmunoconjugates has been approved for use in adults with FL, limited data exists on their use in children. Currently, ^{90}Y-IT is indicated for consolidation in the front-line and may be effective as a part of myeloablative regimens for aggressive B-NHLs [36]. The main toxicity concerns include hematological toxicity which is generally associated with prior cytotoxic chemotherapy and the presence of bone marrow involvement with radiation nephritis being another possible concern. In children, ^{90}Y-IT was studied in a Phase I COG trial in relapsed/refractory B-NHL. While no dose-limiting toxicity or excessive radiation exposure was identified, there were also no responses noted in the five heavily pre-treated study patients [37].

5.2.2 *Alternative Cell Surface Targets of Monoclonal Antibody Therapy for B-NHL*

5.2.2.1 CD19

CD19 is expressed on nearly all B-cell malignancies and antibody drug conjugate (ADC) monoclonal antibodies have been developed that target CD19. Coltuximab ravtansine (SAR3419) is a humanised anti-CD19 conjugated with maytansinoid, a potent inhibitor of tubulin polymerisation [38]. In a Phase I study in 44 adults with relapsed/refractory B-NHL, SAR3419 led to an ORR of 30% [39]. In initial reports of findings in Phase II testing in adults with relapsed/refractory DLBCL, a single agent ORR of 44% was observed in 41 patients with acceptable toxicity; while, in combination with rituximab, only 31% of 52 patients achieved an objective response, though response rates were significantly higher in patients with relapsed vs. primary refractory disease (58% vs. 12%) in this high-risk population [40, 41]. A second immunoconjugate targeting CD19, denintuzumab mafodotin (SGN-CD19A), has also been tested in relapsed/refractory B-NHL. SGN-CD19A is conjugated with the microtubule stabilising agent monomethyauristatin F (MMAF). In two ongoing Phase I trials in relapsed/refractory B-NHL, 33% of 12 adult patients with BL/leukemia or B-lymphoblastic lymphoma (B-LBL) (NCT01786096) and 62 adult patients with DLBCL, MCL or FL (NCT01786135) responded, once again with higher response rates in relapsed patients [42, 43]. However, no responses have been observed in the nine paediatric patients with BL/leukemia reported to date [44]. High rates of superficial microcystic keratopathy were reported in both trials (56% and 84%, respectively), though generally managed with topical steroids with improvement/resolution. A Phase II study is underway investigating denintuzumab mafodotin in combination with R-ICE vs. R-ICE alone in adults with relapsed/refractory DLBCL (NCT02592876).

5.2.2.2 CD22

CD22 is another B-cell associated antigen frequently expressed on B-NHL cells. Two forms of the anti-CD22 antibody epratuzumab, one a naked antibody and the other a ^{90}Y radioconjugated form, have been investigated in B-NHL. Epratuzumab appears to have a unique mechanism of action from rituximab and may function synergistically with rituximab based on pre-clinical testing [45]. Single agent treatment with the unconjugated version of epratuzumab in Phase I/II trials led to ORRs of 43% in 14 FL though only 15% in 33 DLBCL patients [46, 47]. In combination with rituximab in FL or R-CHOP in DLBCL, combination therapy led to ORRs of 88% and 96%, respectively [48, 49]. When conjugated with ^{90}Y, epratuzumab therapy led to a promising ORR of 62% in 64 adults with relapsed/refractory B-NHL [50]. Though epratuzumab has been studied by the COG in relapsed/refractory childhood B-ALL, no data exists on its use in childhood B-NHL.

Pinatuzumab vedotin is an anti-CD22 ADC conjugated with the microtubule stabiliser monomethylauristatin E (MMAE). An initial Phase I trial of pinatuzumab vedotin alone or in combination with rituximab identified peripheral neuropathy as a significant toxicity with 12 of the 62 patients (19%) discontinuing treatment due to peripheral neuropathy, though this was reversible in many patients. Promising activity was observed with 41% of 29 DLBCL patients and 50% of 14 indolent B-NHL patients responding to single agent treatment though with no increased activity noted in combination with rituximab [51]. The Phase II ROMULUS study is investigating pinatuzumab vedotin in combination with rituximab in a randomized fashion with rituximab combined with another MMAE conjugated ADC targeting CD79B, polatuzumab vedotin, in relapsed/refractory B-NHL. The pinatuzumab vedotin-rituximab combination led to an ORR of 57% (24/42) in DLBCL and 62% (13/21) in FL [52]. Toxicities include diarrhea, neutropenia and peripheral neuropathy with 35 patients discontinuing treatment due to peripheral neuropathy.

Another conjugated anti-CD22 antibody inotuzumab ozogamicin has also exhibited promise in B-ALL, however, Phase 3 trials in B-NHL were halted prematurely due to either poor enrollment (NCT00562965) or lack of efficacy (NCT01232556) [53, 54].

5.2.2.3 CD79B

The B-cell receptor, composed of a heterodimer of CD79A and CD79B in combination with surface immunoglobulin, is nearly uniformly expressed on the surface of B-NHL cells. As previously mentioned, polatuzumab vedotin is an anti-CD79B antibody conjugated with MMAE. Following an initial Phase I dose finding study in B-NHL and CLL, with the most common toxicity being primarily hematological in nature, a phase II expansion cohort continued to enroll B-NHL patients for treatment with polatuzumab vedotin as a single agent or in combination with rituximab. In all patients treated at the recommended phase II dose, responses were observed in 14 of 25 (56%) DLBCL and 7 of 15 (47%) FL patients [55]. Seven of the nine

(78%) patients treated with the rituximab combination responded. In the ROMULUS study, in combination with rituximab in relapsed/refractory B-NHL, polatuzumab vedotin resulted in an ORR of 56% (22/39) in DLBCL and 70% (14/20) in FL patients [52].

5.2.2.4 CD30

While generally more consistently expressed on other lymphoma subtypes (e.g. T-cell, PMBL or Hodgkin lymphoma [HL]), CD30 is also frequently expressed on the surface of B-NHL cells. Brentuximab vedotin (Bv) is a CD30-targeted antibody conjugated to an auristatin E derivative (MMAE) through a linker that is stable in plasma, but labile in the presence of lysosomal enzymes (Fig. 5.3). One B-NHL subtype with higher rates of CD30 expression is PMBL. In a phase I trial of upfront therapy in PMBL with Bv in combination with rituximab, cyclophosphamide, doxorubicin and prednisone, the combination led to an ORR of 100% in nine PMBL and one grey zone lymphoma. PFS and OS were also 100% though at a short median follow-up of only 8 months at the time of the report [56]. Phase II studies are ongoing (NCT02423291, NCT01994850). While CD30 expression is generally lower on other B-NHL types, Bv has demonstrated activity in DLBCL including in the setting of minimal CD30 expression. In a phase 2 study in relapsed/refractory adult DLBCL, 44% of 49 DLBCL responded with no correlation between response and CD30 expression level, other than all responders having some degree of detectable

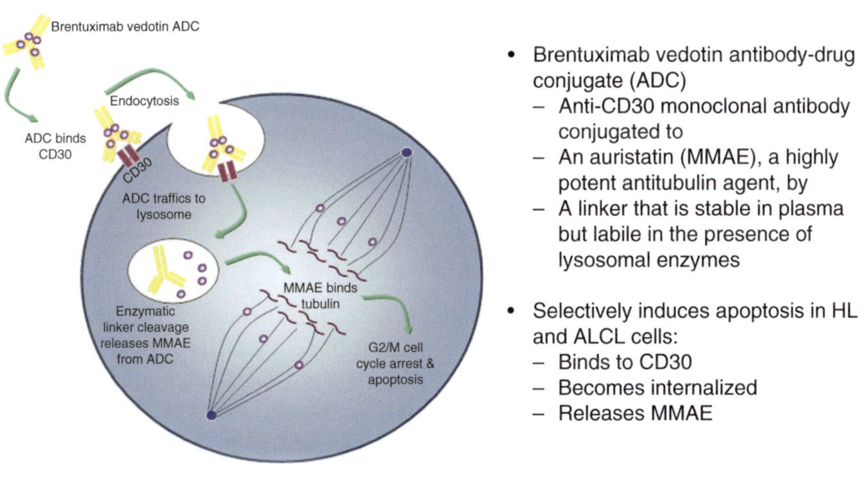

Fig. 5.3 Brentuximab vedotin mechanisms of action. Brentuximab vedotin (Bv) is an anti-CD30 ADC conjugated with the microtubule stabiliser monomethylauristatin E (MMAE). In a Phase I trial and ongoing Phase II studies of upfront therapy in PMBL and DLBCL, Bv has demonstrated activity with no correlation between response and CD30 expression levels. This may represent a low threshold of CD30 expression required for Bv activity or a bystander effect of free MMAE released following binding to CD30 positive cells in the tumour microenvironment

CD30 using a computer assisted scoring technique [57]. This may represent a low threshold of CD30 expression required for Bv activity or a bystander effect of free MMAE released following binding to CD30 positive cells in the tumour microenvironment. In DLBCL in the upfront setting, Bv has been evaluated in combination with R-CHOP in adults with high-risk DLBCL with a CR rate of 69% overall [58]. Patients with CD30 positivity by immunohistochemistry (IHC) appeared to have a higher CR and 12 month PFS rate (76% and 82%) compared to those that were CD30 negative (63% and 56%). Though, as evidenced by the previous study that utilised a computer assisted scoring system, detection of CD30 by standard IHC may not be reliable at low levels. Investigation of Bv in B-NHL is ongoing (NCT01805037, NCT01703949).

5.2.2.5 CD38

CD38 is a cell surface marker that is predominantly expressed on plasma cell neoplasms, such as multiple myeloma (MM). Though more limited, CD38 expression has also been reported in other hematological malignancies including ALL, AML and NHL. A recent report described CD38 expression in pediatric hematological malignancies [59]. Relative to normal plasma cells or MM cells, CD38 expression was lower in B-cell precursor ALL, AML and NHL, but above that of negative control and CLL cells with the highest expression noted in the mature B-cell NHL Burkitt lymphoma cases. Monoclonal antibodies targeting CD38 have demonstrated pre-clinial activity through induction of ADCC and CDC, including in mature B-NHL cell lines, *in vitro* and *in* vivo [60]. Recently, an anti-CD38 monoclonal antibody, daratumumab, was approved for use in MM [61]. Clinical investigation into the activity of the anti-CD38 monoclonal antibodies daratumumab and isatuximab is currently ongoing in other B-cell malignancies including B-NHL and ALL (NCT02413489, NCT02999633).

5.2.3 *Bispecific Monoclonal Antibodies*

A novel application of monoclonal antibody therapy is the use of multivalent antibodies targeting multiple cell surface proteins. Blinatumomab is a bispecific T-cell engaging (BiTE) antibody targeting both CD19 and CD3 inducing activation of CD3+ cytotoxic T-cells in the presence of CD19+ B-cells (Fig. 5.4). While blinatumomab has been extensively investigated in B-ALL, these studies generally excluded extramedullary disease so little data exists in B-LBL. In adult B-NHL, a phase I trial investigated blinatumomab in 38 relapsed/refractory B-NHL patients leading to an ORR of 29% with all seven patients in the highest dose group exhibiting a response [62]. Most of the responses were observed in indolent NHL types. In phase II testing in aggressive B-NHL, an ORR of 43% was observed in 21 relapsed/

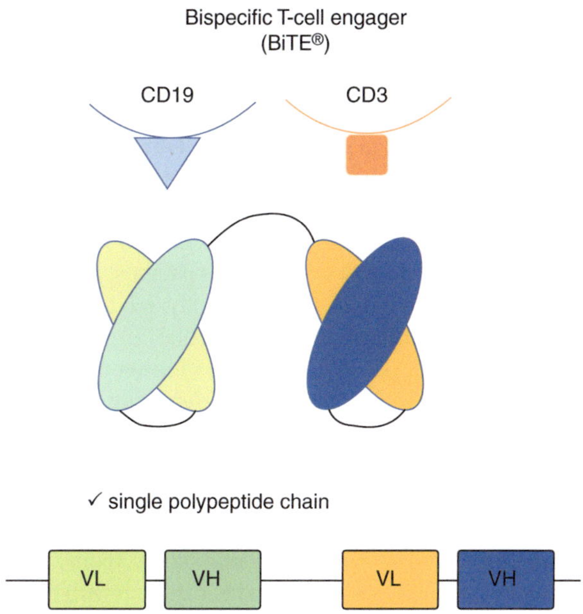

Fig. 5.4 Blinatumomab mechanisms of action. Blinatumomab is a novel application of a multivalent antibody that targets multiple cell surface proteins. It is a bispecific T-cell engaging (BiTE) antibody targeting both CD19 and CD3 inducing activation of CD3+ cytotoxic T-cells in the presence of CD19+ B-cells

refractory adult DLBCL patients [63]. Significant toxicities include neurotoxicity, the cause of which is not well understood, but which can be diminished by the co-administration of corticosteroids; and cytokine release syndrome (CRS), which can also be managed with supportive care and the use of the anti-IL6 monoclonal antibody tocilizumab [64, 65]. The role of such T-cell engaging antibody therapies with the emergence of cellular therapies, including chimeric antigen receptor T-cell therapies, continues to be investigated; though the "off the shelf" nature of the antibody based products is one clear benefit.

5.2.4 *Checkpoint Inhibitors*

One mechanism of tumour survival/proliferation is through the avoidance of host immune surveillance. One approach to enhancing immune surveillance is with antibodies targeting the checkpoint inhibitors cytotoxic T-lymphocyte-associated antigen-4 (CTLA-4), programmed cell death protein 1 (PD-1) and the PD-1 ligands PD-L1/PD-L2 expressed on the surface of CD4, CD8 and T_{reg} cells or, in the case of PD-L1/2, on the surface of tumour/tumour infiltrating cells [66]. These negative regulators of immune function inhibit anti-tumour T-cell function, thus their inhibition can lead to tumour regression. By enhancing immune function, though, antibodies targeting checkpoint inhibitors can also lead to immune related adverse events and exacerbation of autoimmune processes [67]. Several checkpoint inhibitor antibodies have recently gained approval for treatment of malignancies and continue to be investigated in relapsed/refractory B-NHL. Ipilimumab, an anti-CTLA-4 antibody, demonstrated tumour regression in relapsed/refractory FL or DLBCL and has been safely administered in combination with rituximab in early Phase I results [68, 69]. Of note, when utilised after stem-cell transplant (SCT), no significant increase in graft-versus-host disease was noted [70]. Pidilizumab, targeting PD-1, has demonstrated safety and activity in relapsed/refractory DLBCL after SCT, with responses noted in half of the 35 patients with measurable disease post-SCT; and in combination with rituximab in relapsed/refractory FL where the combination led to an ORR of 66% in 29 patients, including a CR rate of 52% [71, 72]. Nivolumab, another anti-PD-1 antibody, led to an ORR of 28% in a population of 29 heavily pre-treated B-NHL patients [73]. Pembrolizumab, another anti-PD-1 antibody, exhibited a 40% ORR (1 CR) in ten adults with heavily pre-treated PMBL [74]. Thus, a variety of antibodies targeting immune checkpoint pathways have demonstrated efficacy in B-NHL and continue to be investigated in numerous ongoing trials. In children, the COG is investigating nivolumab as a single agent and in combination with ipilimumab, a combination that has demonstrated efficacy in advanced melanoma, in children with relapsed/refractory solid tumours including lymphoma (NCT02304458). In an industry sponsored trial, pembrolizumab is also being investigated in children with PD-L1 positive tumours including lymphomas (NCT02332668).

5.3 Anaplastic Large Cell Lymphoma

ALCL is defined by large, pleomorphic, multinucleated cells or cells with eccentric horseshoe-shaped nuclei and abundant clear to basophilic cytoplasm with an area of eosinophilia near the nucleus. These hallmark cells commonly resemble Reed-Sternberg cells. The majority of ALCLs have been shown to be of the T-cell phenotype and are associated with a characteristic genetic alteration involving the ALK locus on chromosome 2 and expression of CD30 on the malignant cell. Accumulating evidence indicates that the immune system plays a major role in both the pathogenesis and final control of anaplastic lymphoma kinase (ALK)-positive ALCL [75–77].

In recent trials with very diverse first-line chemotherapy regimens in terms of the duration of treatment as well as the number and cumulative doses of drugs, there are reported similar EFS rates of about 65%–75% in children, adolescents and young adults [78–81]. No intervention has been able to improve on the approximate failure rate of 25%–30% that exists regardless of treatment strategy. There is currently no gold standard for the treatment of relapses. One of the unique features of ALCL compared to other pediatric NHL is its sensitivity to chemotherapy after recurrence leading to a survival rate of more than 85% in most series [79]. ALK inhibitors such as crizotinib are promising drugs [82, 83], but the role of crizotinib in the treatment of ALCL still has to be defined. The role of the immune system in the control of ALCL makes monoclonal antibody therapy particularly attractive.

5.3.1 Monoclonal Antibodies Targeting CD30

There have been two pivotal phase I studies of Bv involving patients with relapsed ALCL. Younes published the first phase I study using Bv given every 3 weeks to patient with refractory or relapsed CD30 positive lymphomas, including ALCL (NCT00430846) [84]. Of the 45 patients enrolled, 33 (73%) had previously received a SCT. Despite this high amount of pre-treatment, toxicity was tolerable and the vast majority of toxicities were Grade 1 or 2. In the second phase I dose escalation study, Fanale et al. gave Bv on Days 1, 8, and 15, of each 28-day cycle at doses ranging from 0.4 to 1.4 mg/kg [85]. Forty-four patients were enrolled including five with systemic ALCL, and one with peripheral T-cell lymphoma not-otherwise-specified. The maximum tolerated dose (MTD) was found to be 1.2 mg/ kg. Tumour regression occurred in 85% of patients and the overall objective response rate was 59% (n = 24), with 34% (n = 14) CRs. The median duration of response was not reached at a median follow-up of 45 weeks on study [85]. In these early phase I trials, 6/7 patients with ALCL had a CR and one had stable disease [84, 85].

A phase II multicenter trial using Bv 1.8 mg/kg every 3 weeks for patients over 12 years of age with relapsed or refractory ALCL has recently been completed (NCT00866047). Bv was administered over 30 min as an outpatient every 3 weeks. A total of 58 patients were enrolled with an ORR of 86% (53% CR, 33% partial response [PR]) and 97% of patients demonstrated tumour reduction. There was no difference between those patients who had ALK-positive versus ALK-negative ALCL. The responses have been durable, with the median duration of CR for patients off treatment not having been reached. Adverse events were manageable with a toxicity profile similar to the phase I studies [86]. This has led to the accelerated FDA approval of Bv in systemic ALCL after failure of multi-agent chemotherapy.

Combination chemotherapy with Bv and standard-dose CHOP chemotherapy or cyclophosphamide, doxorubicin and prednisone without vincristine (CHP) has been trialed (NCT01309789). Patients received sequential treatment with Bv 1.8 mg/kg (two cycles) followed by CHOP (six cycles) or Bv 1.8 mg/kg plus CHP (Bv+CHP) for six cycles. Responders then received single-agent Bv for eight to ten additional cycles (total of 16 cycles). The MTD of Bv in combination with CHP chemotherapy was 1.8 mg/kg administered every 3 weeks. All treated patients (100%) achieved an objective response, with 23 (88%) of 26 evaluable patients achieving a CR [87]. On the basis of these promising results, a randomised trial of Bv with CHP chemotherapy compared with CHOP chemotherapy in the first-line management of patients with CD30+ T-cell NHL is currently in progress (NCT01777152). The role of Bv and crizotinib added to front line treatment of ALCL is also currently being evaluated in a prospective trial by the COG in children and adolescents (NCT01979536).

5.4 Hodgkin Lymphoma

While cure rates for paediatric HL remain among the highest in paediatric oncology, this often comes with a significant cost in the form of delayed effects of therapy or secondary malignancy. Although the initial 5 year OS is excellent utilising combined modality chemotherapy and radiation, it is estimated that 1300–1500 patients with HL will continue to die each year [88]. In addition, Castellino et al. reporting for Children's Cancer Survivor Study Group, recently demonstrated excess secondary neoplasms and cardiovascular disease after more than 20 years, in childhood HL survivors with a 27% increase in additional mortality in 5 year HL survivors [89]. Various strategies have been developed to address the challenge of maintaining current OS rates for low and intermediate stage patients while further improving HL treatment outcomes in those with advanced stage disease, and minimising long-term morbidities for all. Personalised therapy will be needed based on risk factor assessment, response-based therapy adaptations and incorporation of new agents such as targeted monoclonal antibodies with improved toxicity profiles to upfront and relapsed/refractory therapy protocols.

5.4.1 Monoclonal Antibodies Targeting CD30

HL is typically characterised by rare Hodgkin Reed Sternberg (HRS) cells comprising about 5% of the tumour volume resting in a reactive infiltrate composed of lymphocytes, histiocytes, eosinophils, and plasma cells [1]. These surrounding benign, reactive, inflammatory cells contribute to HRS cell growth and survival through cytokine release. Novel therapeutics for HL are able to capitalise on this unique pathophysiology by modulating the microenvironment [1].

CD30 is a highly expressed cell surface antigen on HRS cells and can be targeted with the anti-CD30 ADC Bv. Bv selectively induces apoptosis in HL cells by binding to CD30, internalizing, and releasing MMAE. Younes et al. published a pivotal Phase II trial of a multicenter, open-label study of Bv in relapsed/refractory HL (NCT00848926) [90]. Single agent Bv was given every 21 days at a dose of 1.8 mg/ kg to patients who had undergone prior autologous SCT for a maximum of 16 cycles. There were a total of 102 patients treated and overall Bv was well-tolerated with minimal toxicity. The majority of patients (98%) showed objective responses to therapy with most of them having 50% or greater reduction in tumour size. The ORR was 75% with CR in 34% of patients [90]. They were able to show durable remissions with a follow-up time of 3 years the median OS and PFS were 40.5 months and 9.3 months, respectively. Those who achieved a CR had improved outcomes with 3-year OS and PFS rates of 73% (95% confidence interval [CI]: 57%, 88%) and 58% (95% CI: 41%, 76%), respectively. Of these patients, 47% remained progression-free after a median of 53.3 months (range, 29.0 to 56.2 months) of observation [91]. The major toxicity of Bv was peripheral neurotoxicity due to the anti-tubulin toxin once released from antibody linkage. The German Hodgkin Study Group published their experience with Bv used as single agent in 45 patients with refractory or relapsed CD30 HL. In 34 very heavily pretreated patients, they reported an objective response rate of 60%, with 22% CRs and a median duration of response of 8 months (NCT01026233) [92]. Moskowitz et al. also reported the results of the AETHERA trial, a randomised, double-blind, placebo-controlled, phase 3 trial utilising Bv as consolidation in patients with unfavourable-risk relapsed or primary refractory classic HL who had undergone autologous SCT (NCT01100502). Patients were assigned to treatment vs. placebo for up to 16 cycles every 3 weeks following transplant. Of the 329 patients, median PFS by independent review was 42.9 months (95% CI 30.4–42.9) for patients in the Bv group compared with 24.1 months (11.5–not estimable) for those in the placebo group [93]. Bv has also been investigated following allogeneic hematopoietic SCT (alloHSCT). Gopal et al. evaluated Bv in 25 HL patients with recurrent disease after alloHSCT (NCT00947856). Patients received a median of 9 (range, 5–19) prior regimens and a majority had refractory disease at the time of enrollment. Patients again received 1.2 or 1.8 mg/kg of Bv intravenously (IV) every 3 weeks. Overall and complete response rates were 50% and 38%, respectively, among 24 evaluable patients. Median time to response was 8.1 weeks, with a median PFS of 7.8 months [94]. Additional trials are ongoing assessing the use of Bv in the post-transplant setting (Table 5.2).

Table 5.2 Monoclonal antibodies under investigation in childhood, adolescent and young adult CD30+ lymphomas

Target antigen	Antibody	Type	Stage of investigation	Ongoing clinical trials in CD30+ lymphoma (sponsor)
CD30	Brentuximab	ADC	Phase I	NCT01900496: Pilot Study of Rituximab and Brentuximab Vedotin With Deferred BMT for Relapsed Classical Hodgkin Lymphoma (Sidney Kimmel Comprehensive Cancer Center)
			Phase I/II	NCT01805037: A Phase I-II Trial of Brentuximab Vedotin Plus Rituximab as Frontline Therapy for Patients With CD30+ and/or EBV+ Lymphomas (Northwestern University) NCT01492088: A Phase 1/2 Study of Brentuximab Vedotin in Paediatric Patients With Relapsed or Refractory Systemic Anaplastic Large-Cell Lymphoma or Hodgkin Lymphoma (Millenium Pharmaceuticals, Inc) NCT02098512: A Multicenter Pilot Study of Reduced Intensity Conditioning and Allogeneic Stem Cell Transplantation Followed by Targeted Immunotherapy in Children, Adolescents and Young Adults With Poor Risk CD30+ Hodgkin Lymphoma (New York Medical College)

(continued)

Table 5.2 (continued)

Target antigen	Antibody	Type	Stage of investigation	Ongoing clinical trials in CD30+ lymphoma (sponsor)
			Phase II	NCT02398240: A Pilot Study of Risk Adapted Therapy Utilizing Upfront Brentuximab With Combination Chemotherapy in the Treatment of Children, Adolescents and Young Adults With Newly Diagnosed Hodgkin Lymphoma (New York Medical College) NCT01920932: Adcetris Substituting Vincristine in the OEPA/COPDac Regimen [Treatment Group 3 (TG3) of Euro-Net C1] With Low Dose Tailored-Field Radiation Therapy for Unfavorable Risk Pediatric Hodgkin Lymphoma (St Judes Research Hospital) NCT01868451: A Pilot Study of Brentuximab Vedotin Combined With AVD Chemotherapy and Involved-Site Radiotherapy in Patients With Newly Diagnosed Early Stage, Unfavorable Risk Hodgkin Lymphoma (Memorial Sloan Kettering Cancer Center) NCT01979536: A Randomized Phase II Trial of Brentuximab Vedotin (SGN35, NSC# 749710), or Crizotinib (NSC#749005, Commercially Labeled) in Combination With Chemotherapy for Newly Diagnosed Patients With Anaplastic Large Cell Lymphoma (NCI) NCT01393717: A Phase II Study of Brentuximab Vedotin as Salvage Therapy for Hodgkin Lymphoma Prior to Autologous Hematopoietic Stem Cell Transplantation (City of Hope) NCT02169505: Safety and Efficacy of Brentuximab Vedotin Maintenance After Allogeneic Stem Cell Transplantation in High Risk CD30+ Lymphoma (Hodgkin Lymphoma and Anaplastic Large Cell Lymphoma) (MD Anderson)

Table 5.2 (continued)

Target antigen	Antibody	Type	Stage of investigation	Ongoing clinical trials in CD30+ lymphoma (sponsor)
			Phase III	NCT02166463: A Randomized Phase III Study of Brentuximab Vedotin (SGN-35) for Newly Diagnosed High-Risk Classical Hodgkin Lymphoma (cHL) in Children and Adolescents (NCI) NCT01777152: A Randomized, Double-blind, Placebo-controlled, Phase 3 Study of Brentuximab Vedotin and CHP (A+CHP) Versus CHOP in the Frontline Treatment of Patients With CD30-positive Mature T-cell Lymphomas (Seattle Genetics, Inc)
CD20	Rituximab	Naked	Phase I	NCT01900496: Pilot Study of Rituximab and Brentuximab Vedotin With Deferred BMT for Relapsed Classical Hodgkin Lymphoma (Sidney Kimmel Comprehensive Cancer Center)
			Phase I/II	NCT01805037: A Phase I-II Trial of Brentuximab Vedotin Plus Rituximab as Frontline Therapy for Patients With CD30+ and/or EBV+ Lymphomas (Northwestern University)
			Phase II	NCT02398240: A Pilot Study of Risk Adapted Therapy Utilizing Upfront Brentuximab and Rituximab with Combination Chemotherapy in the Treatment of Children, Adolescents and Young Adults With Newly Diagnosed Hodgkin Lymphoma (New York Medical College)
PD-1	Nivolumab	Naked	Phase I	NCT01592370: A Phase I Dose Escalation Study to Investigate the Safety, Pharmacokinetics, Immunoregulatory Activity, and Preliminary Antitumour Activity of Anti-Programmed-Death 1 (PD-1) Antibody (Nivolumab, BMS936558) and the Combination of Nivolumab and Ipilimumab or Nivolumab and Lirilumab in Subjects With Relapsed or Refractory Haematologic Malignancy (Bristol-Myers Squibb)

(continued)

Table 5.2 (continued)

Target antigen	Antibody	Type	Stage of investigation	Ongoing clinical trials in CD30+ lymphoma (sponsor)
			Phase I/II	NCT02572167: A Phase 1/2 Study Evaluating Brentuximab Vedotin in Combination With Nivolumab in Patients With Relapsed or Refractory Hodgkin Lymphoma After Failure of Frontline Therapy (Seattle Genetics, Inc) NCT02304458: A Phase 1/2 Study of Nivolumab (IND#124729) in Children, Adolescents, and Young Adults With Recurrent or Refractory Solid Tumors as a Single Agent and in Combination With Ipilimumab (NCI)
			Phase II	NCT02181738: Non-Comparative, Multi-Cohort, Single Arm, Open-Label, Phase 2 Study of Nivolumab in Classical Hodgkin Lymphoma Subjects (Bristol-Myers Squibb)
	Pembrolizumab	Naked	Phase I	NCT01953692: A Phase Ib Multi-Cohort Trial of MK-3475 (Pembrolizumab) in Subjects With Hematologic Malignancies (Merck Sharp & Dohme Corp)
			Phase II	NCT02453594: A Phase II Clinical Trial of MK-3475 (Pembrolizumab) in Subjects With Relapsed or Refractory (R/R) Classical Hodgkin Lymphoma (Merck Sharp & Dohme Corp) NCT02408042: A Phase Ib/II Study of Pembrolizumab With Chemotherapy in Patients With Advanced Lymphoma (Western Regional Medical Center) NCT02362997: A Phase 2 Study of Pembrolizumab (MK-3475) After Autologous Stem Cell Transplantation in Patients With Relapsed/Refractory Classical Hodgkin Lymphoma and Diffuse Large B Cell Lymphoma (Dana Farber Cancer Institute)

Ongoing trials are exploring this agent not only in the relapsed and refractory setting but in up-front therapy for advanced disease as a substitute for bleomycin in the ABVD regimen (ABvVD) [95, 96]. The first reported Phase I, open label, dose escalation study looked at newly diagnosed, CD30-positive patients with HL who with higher risk disease. Patients received doses of 0.6, 0.9, or 1.2 mg/kg Bv IV every 2 weeks with either ABVD or AVD (ABVD modified regimen without the inclusion of bleomycin) for up to six cycles (NCT01060904). Overall, 21 (95%) of 22 patients given Bv and ABVD achieved CR, as did 24 (96%) of 25 patients given Bv and AVD. While overall toxicities were minimal in both groups, they found an unacceptable rate of pulmonary toxicity in patients who received both brentuximab and bleomycin [95, 97]. Additional Phase III trials are in progress to determine whether the addition of Bv to up-front combination chemotherapy can enhance overall outcomes while minimising short- and long-term toxicities and potentially eliminating need for radiation therapy (Table 5.2).

5.4.2 Monoclonal Antibodies Targeting CD20

The Johns Hopkins group recently reported that within classical (cHL) cell lines, a small population of clonotypic B cells circulated in most patients with newly diagnosed cHL, including those with limited-stage disease, and had the same immunoglobulin gene rearrangements as lymph node-derived HRS cells [98]. These findings support the observed activity of rituximab in HL, even in those patients whose HRS cells lack CD20 expression [97]. Younes et al. first reported a phase 2 study in newly diagnosed advanced stage HL treated with rituximab 375 mg/m^2 weekly for 6 weeks and standard ABVD for 6 cycles (NCT00504504). With a median follow-up duration of 68 months (range, 26–110), the 5-year EFS and OS rates were 83% and 96%, respectively. The most frequent treatment-related grade 3 or 4 adverse events were neutropenia (23%), fatigue (9%), and nausea (8%) [97]. A second multicenter phase 2 study combining rituximab with ABVD in advanced stage patients looked at the behavior of circulating clonotypic B-cells in addition to clinical outcomes (NCT00369681). Rituximab-ABVD again was generally well-tolerated. While only 8% of the patients had confirmed CD20+ HRS cells, after 6 cycles 81% of patients were in CR. Only 8% of patients required radiation therapy for residual disease. The actuarial 3-year EFS and OS rates were 83% and 98%, respectively [99]. Of particular interest, it was found that persistence of detectable circulating clonotypic B-cells was associated with a greater relapse frequency ($P < .05$) [98]. Thus, both studies conclude that rituximab-ABVD and its effect on clonotypic B-cells warrant additional study in cHL.

5.4.3 Checkpoint Inhibitors and Hodgkin Lymphoma

HL may represent a unique target for PD-1 blockade therapy (Fig. 5.1). This disease is characterised by an extensive inflammatory immune cell infiltrate as well as genetic alterations in chromosome 9p24 that leads to PDL1 and PDL2 copy gain and associated overexpression of these PD-1 ligands. Its association with Epstein-Barr virus infection also presents an additional mechanism of upregulating PD-1 ligand expression [100]. Phase I studies of the checkpoint inhibitors nivolumab and pembrolizumab have both demonstrated exciting results in patients with HL. Nivolumab (NCT01592370) given at 1 mg/kg or 3 mg/kg in weeks 1 and 4, and then every 2 weeks thereafter until disease progression showed an ORR of 87% in 23 patients: 6 (26%) had a CR, 14 (61%) had a PR [101]. Additionally, three (13%) patients had stable disease. The PFS rate at 24 weeks was 86% [101]. The patients included in this study were heavily pre-treated with 78% having received Bv, and 78% had undergone autologous SCT. A second cohort combining Nivolumab with additional checkpoint inhibitors is ongoing (Table 5.2). Pembrolizumab has also demonstrated efficacy and safety in patients with relapsed/refractory HL. Preliminary results have been reported from the ongoing, multicenter, open-label, Phase 1b clinical trial of pembrolizumab (NCT01953692) in patients with prior exposure to Bv and/or autologous SCT. Pembrolizumab was given as a single-agent 10 mg/kg administered every 2 weeks until confirmed tumour progression, excessive toxicity, or completion of 2 years of therapy. Of the study patients, 67% were enrolled in the study after a relapse following autologous SCT and all patients had previously received Bv. Overall, three patients (20%) had a CR at 12 weeks. Five additional patients (33%) had PR as best overall response, for an ORR of 53%. Four patients (27%) experienced progressive disease, although all four experienced a decrease in their overall tumour burden [102]. Six patients obtained stable disease. Other immune-checkpoint-targeting antibodies in development include anti-PD-L1 and anti-4-1BB antibodies.

5.5 Humoral Immunotherapy for Paediatric Acute Leukaemias

The use of monoclonal antibodies (mAbs) is an attractive therapeutic strategy for acute leukemias. Leukaemia cells express multiple human differentiation antigens that are uncommonly found on other normal cells [103]. They thereby serve as ideal targets for the development of anti-cancer agents with a limited side-effect profile [104]. The development of mAbs conjugated with chemotherapy, radiotherapy, cytokines, or even toxins to enhance tumor cell kill has provided an added boost to the potential of humoral immunotherapy. Additionally, the novel development of bi-specific mAbs has successfully linked tumour cells with immune effector cells such as T or NK cells. Numerous targets for mAb therapy exist in acute leukemias

Table 5.3 Unconjugated and conjugated monoclonal antibodies (moAb) in paediatric acute leukaemias

Target antigen leukaemia	Unconjugated MoAb	Origin	Conjugated MoAb	Origin
CD19			SAR3419	Humanized
ALL			Blinatumomab (BiTE)	Mouse
	Rituximab	Chimeric		
	Ofatumumab	Human	90Y-Ibritumomab Tiuxetan	Mouse
CD20	Obinutuzumab	Humanized	1311-Tositumomab	Mouse
ALL	Veltuzumab	Humanized		
	AME-133	Humanized		
			Inotuzumab Ozogamicin	Humanized
			CAT-3888 (BL22)	Mouse
CD22	Epratuzumab	Humanized	Moxetumomab Pasudotox	Mouse
ALL			90Y-Epratuzumab Tetraxetan	Humanized
CD33			Gemtuzumab ozogamicin (NCT02221310, NCT02117297)	Humanized
AML			AMG 330 (BiTE)	Hamster
CD52	Alemtuzumab	Humanized		
ALL				
CD7			scFvCD7:sTRAIL	Murine
ALL				

Abbreviations: *CD* cluster of differentiation, *BiTE* Bi-specific T-cell Engagers, *ALL* acute lymphoblastic leukaemia, *AML* acute myelogenous leukaemia

(Table 5.3). For B-cell ALL, current strategies focus on targeting CD22, CD19, and CD20 (Fig. 5.2), while for acute myeloid leukemia (AML) focus on CD33. This section will expand more on the development of humoral immunotherapy targeting these specific antigens.

5.5.1 *Monoclonal Antibodies for Acute Lymphoblastic Leukaemia*

5.5.1.1 CD22

The presence of CD22 shifts from the cytoplasmic domain in developing B-cells to the cell surface in later stages of B-cell development [105]. The humanised moAb epratuzumab targets the extracellular domain of CD22 which is expressed in >95% of children with B-cell ALL. Its mechanisms of tumour cell kill include ADCC, phosphorylation of the CD22 antigen, and the inhibition of cell proliferation [106].

Paediatric data on epratuzumab were generated from COG trials in patients with relapsed B-cell ALL. The Phase I data demonstrated promising results. Epratuzumab was given alone twice weekly for four doses, and then weekly for an additional four doses in combination with standard re-induction chemotherapy. Of 15 patients, nine achieved CR, with seven having no evidence of minimal residual disease (MRD) [107]. Phase II data however, did not yield equally convincing results. It utilised epratuzumab twice weekly for eight total doses in combination with the same standard re-induction chemotherapy regimen. There was no distinct increase in the rate of achieving a second CR in comparison to historical controls. For those patients that achieved CR though, 42% were MRD negative, compared to only 25% achieved MRD-negative disease status in historical controls [108].

Building on of the epratuzumab experience, a conjugated anti-CD22 mAb was developed named inotuzumab ozogamicin. Another humanized mAb, it conjugates with calicheamicin, an anti-tumor antibiotic. Combined adult/paediatric data on incorporated three children amongst 49 patients; the ORR in the cohort was 57%; CR was achieved in 18% of patients [109].

Other recently developed conjugated anti-CD22 mAbs include CAT-3888 (BL22) and its second generation successor moxetumomab pasudotox (formerly known as CAT-8015 or HA22). They are both conjugated with a truncated form of the pseudomonas exotoxin A. Exhibiting a higher affinity for CD22, moxetumomab pasudotox, has produced promising preclinical and clinical results [110, 111]. Based upon these data, a multicenter clinical trial evaluating moxetumomab pasudotox in paediatric ALL prior to alloHSCT was set-up, but terminated prematurely due to unexpected toxicity.

Another agent in development conjugates epratuzumab with the radioisotope yttrium 90 (^{90}Y-epratuzumab tetraxetan). However, it has only been studied in clinical trials for adults with relapsed or refractory ALL and the experience with this agent in children is limited. Currently, there are no clinical trials utilising this radioisotope conjugated mAb in children, but potential use in the future may center on its incorporation in to pre-alloHSCT conditioning regimens.

5.5.1.2 CD19

Similar to CD22, CD19 is another antigen that is present on the majority of pre-B ALL cells, and another target for moAb immunotherapy with great potential. As discussed in the section on B-cell NHL, SAR3419 is a humanised moAb conjugated with maytansinoid, a tubulin polymerisation inhibitor. Other conjugated anti-CD19 moAbs have been developed but due to limitations from toxicity and availability, they have not been well incorporated into the clinical setting [112].

Initially evaluated in pre-clinical studies with B-cell NHL [113], data has been established with SAR3419 in CD19$^+$ ALL xenograft models as well [114]. Based upon favorable results, clinical trials were developed in adults with refractory/relapsed B cell NHL and demonstrated reduction in tumour size in 74% of patients, including seven out of fifteen patients who were refractory to rituximab [115]. A phase II trial evaluating SAR3419 in relapsed/refractory CD19$^+$ ALL (NCT01440179) is currently underway.

A lot of excitement has been generated by studies with the BiTE antibody blinatumomab. Blinatumomab has shown remarkable efficacy in adults with MRD-positive B-cell ALL. Sixteen of twenty-one patients with persistence or relapse of MRD achieved MRD-remission after treatment with a 4-week continuous infusion of blinatumomab. With a median follow-up of 405 days, the probability of relapse-free survival in this cohort was 78% [116]. Subsequently, long-term follow-up data from this study (median 33 months) was performed demonstrating a 61% relapse-free survival. Twelve patients are in a sustained CR: six of nine that went on to receive alloHSCT, in addition to six of eleven who did not receive alloHSCT. This included four out of six patients (with Philadelphia chromosome-negative disease) who received no further therapy after blinatumomab [117].

Based on these favorable outcomes in adults, blinatumomab is currently being studied in children with refractory ALL, with second or later bone marrow relapse, or with marrow relapse after alloHSCT. The MTD has been established at 15 μg/m^2/day given as a continuous IV infusion over 28 days, followed by a 14-day treatment-free interval. CRS has been an important dose-limiting toxicity in the paediatric trial; in adults central nervous system-related toxicity was also notable. To reduce the risk of CRS, a dose-escalating approach was utilised, giving 5 μg/m^2/day for the first 7 days, followed by an escalation to the MTD of 15 μg/m^2/day. None of the 11 patients treated on the dose escalation protocol experienced CRS and the ORR was 41%, with 32% of patients achieving CR [118]. Data from a phase II clinical trial investigating the efficacy, safety, and tolerability of blinatumomab in paediatric and adolescent patients with relapsed/refractory B-cell ALL has been presented (NCT01471782) [119]. Additionally, a case series of three paediatric ALL patients achieved CR with blinatumomab despite having relapsed post-alloHSCT [120]. The COG is currently enrolling a randomised phase III risk-stratified clinical trial investigating the use of blinatumomab in combination with re-induction chemotherapy either as a bridge to alloHSCT (in high and intermediate-risk patients) or as definitive therapy in in low-risk patients with relapsed B-cell ALL (NCT02101853).

5.5.1.3 CD20

Typically considered an antigen associated with mature B-cells (see section on mature B-NHL), CD20 is expressed in just under 50% of childhood B-cell precursor ALL patients. In a cohort of 353 patients with ALL, 169 demonstrated CD20 expression on >20% lymphoblasts. Outcomes were similar for patients with and without CD20 expression [121]. Although the use of anti-CD20 mAb therapy in pediatric malignancies has focused on mature B-NHL, multiple clinical trials have investigated their efficacy in ALL adults [122, 123]. There is a potential role for anti-CD20 immunotherapy in CD20$^+$ pediatric ALL in combination with other mAbs plus multi-agent chemotherapy.

While the novel type II anti-CD20 mAb obinutuzumab has established efficacy in clinical trials for CLL and B-NHL, more recently, it has been investigated in xenograft models for B-cell ALL where it successfully achieved significantly improved decrease in tumour luminescence as well as a statistically significant survival advantage compared with rituximab (at equal doses) and with lower doses of obinutuzumab [35]. These pre-clinical data in B-cell precursor ALL mouse models may serve as a foundation to further investigate anti-CD20 mAbs in the treatment of the subset of $CD20^+$ B-cell precursor ALL patients.

5.6 Other Monoclonal Antibodies

Although not commonly utilised in the setting of anti-leukemia therapy, alemtuzumab is a humanised mAb targeting CD52. Its major therapeutic role is to provide *in vivo* T-cell depletion in conditioning regimens prior to alloHSCT. However, because CD52 is expressed on the majority of both T and B-ALL cells, it does serve as a potential target for humoral immunotherapy. Its efficacy appeared equivocal in a small Phase II COG clinical trial evaluating alemtuzumab in 13 patients with relapsed ALL; only one patient achieved CR [124]. However, there remains a potential role for alemtuzumab to be incorporated into conditioning regimens for ALL patients undergoing alloHSCT. While cyclophosphamide and total body irradiation have been the mainstays in conditioning regimens for alloHSCT in paediatric ALL for many years, there is a role for targeted conditioning regimens to exert a dual benefit in eradicating ALL cells while simultaneously performing myeloablation and immune suppression in preparation for alloHSCT. Favorable outcomes have been established in both adult and paediatric ALL employing alemtuzumab, with the added benefit of lower rates of graft-versus-host-disease [125, 126].

As this section of this review illustrates, there has been great emphasis on developing mAb therapy for B-cell ALL, with much less progress on the frontiers of T-cell disease. One potential agent in development for T-cell ALL is an anti-CD7 mAb linked to the tumour necrosis factor-related apoptosis-inducing ligand (TRAIL). It demonstrated potent CD7-restricted apoptosis in a variety of malignant T-cell lines, including blood cell samples from patients with T-cell ALL [127]. However, it has yet to even be tested in animal models.

5.7 Monoclonal Antibodies for Acute Myeloid Leukaemia

Development of mAb immunotherapy in AML has focused on the antigen target CD33. Although several other targets have been pursued over the years, pre-clinical and clinical data have not fostered much hope for success in targeting antigens such as CD45, CD66, CD123, FLT3, KIR, VEGF, and CD52 [128]. Several clinical studies though, demonstrate clinical efficacy with the anti-CD33 conjugated mAb gemtuzumab ozogamicin, a recombinant humanised monoclonal antibody (IgG4). Coupled to the antibiotic calicheamicin, gemtuzumab has had a bittersweet history in clinical trials. The manufacturer voluntarily withdrew gemtuzumab in 2010 at the request of the FDA because of a combination of lack of efficacy combined with increased toxicity including serious hepatotoxicity including sinusoidal obstruction syndrome and a high rate of fatal hemorrhage (CNS and pulmonary) exhibited in a randomized phase III trial for adults with AML [129]. However, since then multiple clinical trials in both adult and pediatric AML have demonstrated the safety and efficacy of gemtuzumab and prompted the development of clinical trials focusing on its use in combination with chemotherapy as well as with alloHSCT [128].

CD33 is an optimal target as it is expressed in the leukemic cells in approximately 80–90% of children with AML [130]. Furthermore, increased CD33 expression has been associated with high-risk genetic mutations like FLT3/ITD [131]. The safety and efficacy of gemtuzumab has been demonstrated in pediatric clinical trials for relapsed/refractory disease both in the setting of single-agent use [132, 133] as well as in combination with multi-agent chemotherapy [134]. Additionally, phase III data from the COG demonstrated that the combination of gemtuzumab with up-front chemotherapy regimens in newly diagnosed children and adolescents with AML is safe and resulted in a reduced risk for relapse [135]. To further expand on the COG up-front study, the use of gemtuzumab reduced risk in patients with FLT3/ITD AML [136] and cancelled out the negative prognostic impact of high CD33 expression [137]. Finally, gemtuzumab has been combined with alloHSCT in children and adolescents with established safety and efficacy. For children with very poor-risk AML in refractory relapse, induction failure, and CR3, gemutuzumab was incorporated into the myeloablative conditioning regimen [138]. For children and adolescents with AML in CR1/CR2, gemtuzumab was combined as a post-transplant consolidation therapy in patients receiving a reduced-intensity conditioning regimen [139]. These studies are still currently ongoing in a Phase II setting (NCT02221310 and NCT02117297).

Ultimately, the options for mAb immunotherapy for AML are significantly less than in B-cell ALL, however gemtuzumab has been incorporated in novel ways to provide benefit to a significant subset of patients in a disease with relatively low curative rates in comparison to the majority of other childhood malignancies. Novel developments in BiTE immunotherapy that engage both CD33 and CD3 have offered some exciting pre-clinical data, with AMG 330 emerging as the agent with significant potential for development [140–143]. Breakthroughs in novel therapeutic strategies for AML are desperately needed, and it will be important to monitor how the BiTE moAb clinical trials unfold.

5.8 Conclusion

In summary, monoclonal antibodies or antibody conjugate therapy shows significant promise in the treatment of paediatric hematological malignancies. Future studies will determine the role to improve EFS, reduce acute and late morbidity and/or increase response after relapse in children with haematological malignancies.

Acknowledgements The authors would like to thank Erin Morris, RN, for her expert editorial assistance in the draft of this review.

References

1. Batlevi CL, Younes A. Novel therapy for Hodgkin lymphoma. Hematol Am Soc Hematol Educ Program. 2013, 2013:394–9.
2. Maloney DG, Grillo-Lopez AJ, White CA, Bodkin D, Schilder RJ, Neidhart JA, Janakiraman N, Foon KA, Liles TM, Dallaire BK, Wey K, Royston I, Davis T, Levy R. IDEC-C2B8 (Rituximab) anti-CD20 monoclonal antibody therapy in patients with relapsed low-grade non-Hodgkin's lymphoma. Blood. 1997;90:2188–95.
3. Czuczman MS, Grillo-Lopez AJ, White CA, Saleh M, Gordon L, LoBuglio AF, Jonas C, Klippenstein D, Dallaire B, Varns C. Treatment of patients with low-grade B-cell lymphoma with the combination of chimeric anti-CD20 monoclonal antibody and CHOP chemotherapy. J Clin Oncol. 1999;17:268–76.
4. Coiffier B, Lepage E, Briere J, Herbrecht R, Tilly H, Bouabdallah R, Morel P, Van Den Neste E, Salles G, Gaulard P, Reyes F, Lederlin P, Gisselbrecht C. CHOP chemotherapy plus rituximab compared with CHOP alone in elderly patients with diffuse large-B-cell lymphoma. N Engl J Med. 2002;346:235–42.
5. Pfreundschuh M, Trumper L, Osterborg A, Pettengell R, Trneny M, Imrie K, Ma D, Gill D, Walewski J, Zinzani PL, Stahel R, Kvaloy S, Shpilberg O, Jaeger U, Hansen M, Lehtinen T, Lopez-Guillermo A, Corrado C, Scheliga A, Milpied N, Mendila M, Rashford M, Kuhnt E, Loeffler M. CHOP-like chemotherapy plus rituximab versus CHOP-like chemotherapy alone in young patients with good-prognosis diffuse large-B-cell lymphoma: a randomised controlled trial by the MabThera International Trial (MInT) Group. Lancet Oncol. 2006;7:379–91.
6. Rizzieri DA, Johnson JL, Byrd JC, Lozanski G, Blum KA, Powell BL, Shea TC, Nattam S, Hoke E, Cheson BD, Larson RA, the Alliance for Clinical Trials In O. Improved efficacy using rituximab and brief duration, high intensity chemotherapy with filgrastim support for Burkitt or aggressive lymphomas: cancer and Leukemia Group B study 10 002. Br J Haematol. 2014;165:102–11.
7. Hoelzer D, Walewski J, Döhner H, Viardot A, Hiddemann W, Spiekermann K, Serve H, Dührsen U, Hüttmann A, Thiel E, Dengler J, Kneba M, Schaich M, Schmidt-Wolf IGH, Beck J, Hertenstein B, Reichle A, Domanska-Czyz K, Fietkau R, Horst H-A, Rieder H, Schwartz S, Burmeister T, Gökbuget N. Improved outcome of adult Burkitt lymphoma/leukemia with rituximab and chemotherapy: report of a large prospective multicenter trial. Blood. 2014;124:3870–9.
8. Griffin TC, Weitzman S, Weinstein H, Chang M, Cairo M, Hutchison R, Shiramizu B, Wiley J, Woods D, Barnich M, Gross TG, Children's Oncology G. A study of rituximab and ifosfamide, carboplatin, and etoposide chemotherapy in children with recurrent/refractory B-cell (CD20+) non-Hodgkin lymphoma and mature B-cell acute lymphoblastic leukemia: a report from the Children's Oncology Group. Pediatr Blood Cancer. 2009;52:177–81.
9. Meinhardt A, Burkhardt B, Zimmermann M, Borkhardt A, Kontny U, Klingebiel T, Berthold F, Janka-Schaub G, Klein C, Kabickova E, Klapper W, Attarbaschi A, Schrappe M, Reiter A, Berlin-Frankfurt-Munster g. Phase II window study on rituximab in newly diagnosed pediatric mature B-cell non-Hodgkin's lymphoma and Burkitt leukemia. J Clin Oncol. 2010;28:3115–21.
10. Jäger U, Fridrik M, Zeitlinger M, Heintel D, Hopfinger G, Burgstaller S, Mannhalter C, Oberaigner W, Porpaczy E, Skrabs C, Einberger C, Drach J, Raderer M, Gaiger A, Putman M, Greil R. Rituximab serum concentrations during immuno-chemotherapy of follicular lymphoma correlate with patient gender, bone marrow infiltration and clinical response. Haematologica. 2012;97:1431–8.
11. Berinstein NL, Grillo-Lopez AJ, White CA, Bence-Bruckler I, Maloney D, Czuczman M, Green D, Rosenberg J, McLaughlin P, Shen D. Association of serum Rituximab (IDEC-C2B8) concentration and anti-tumor response in the treatment of recurrent low-grade or follicular non-Hodgkin's lymphoma. Ann Oncol. 1998;9:995–1001.

12. Goldman S, Smith L, Anderson JR, Perkins S, Harrison L, Geyer MB, Gross TG, Weinstein H, Bergeron S, Shiramizu B, Sanger W, Barth M, Zhi J, Cairo MS. Rituximab and FAB/LMB 96 chemotherapy in children with Stage III/IV B-cell non-Hodgkin lymphoma: a Children's Oncology Group report. Leukemia. 2013;27:1174–7.
13. Goldman S, Smith L, Galardy P, Perkins SL, Frazer JK, Sanger W, Anderson JR, Gross TG, Weinstein H, Harrison L, Shiramizu B, Barth M, Cairo MS. Rituximab with chemotherapy in children and adolescents with central nervous system and/or bone marrow-positive Burkitt lymphoma/leukaemia: a Children's Oncology Group Report. Br J Haematol. 2014;167(3):394–401.
14. Barth MJ, Goldman S, Smith L, Perkins S, Shiramizu B, Gross TG, Harrison L, Sanger W, Geyer MB, Giulino-Roth L, Cairo MS. Rituximab pharmacokinetics in children and adolescents with de novo intermediate and advanced mature B-cell lymphoma/leukaemia: a Children's Oncology Group report. Br J Haematol. 2013;162:678–83.
15. Dunleavy K, Pittaluga S, Maeda LS, Advani R, Chen CC, Hessler J, Steinberg SM, Grant C, Wright G, Varma G, Staudt LM, Jaffe ES, Wilson WH. Dose-Adjusted EPOCH-Rituximab Therapy in Primary Mediastinal B-Cell Lymphoma. N Engl J Med. 2013;368:1408–16.
16. Patte C, Auperin A, Gerrard M, Michon J, Pinkerton R, Sposto R, Weston C, Raphael M, Perkins SL, McCarthy K, Cairo MS, Committee FLIS. Results of the randomized international FAB/LMB96 trial for intermediate risk B-cell non-Hodgkin lymphoma in children and adolescents: it is possible to reduce treatment for the early responding patients. Blood. 2007;109:2773–80.
17. Cairo MS, Gerrard M, Sposto R, Auperin A, Pinkerton CR, Michon J, Weston C, Perkins SL, Raphael M, McCarthy K, Patte C. Results of a randomized international study of high-risk central nervous system B non-Hodgkin lymphoma and B acute lymphoblastic leukemia in children and adolescents. Blood. 2007;109:2736–43.
18. Goldman S, Barth MJ, Oesterheld JE, Heym K, Harrison L, Nickerson B, El-Mallawany N, Hochberg J, Cairo MS Preliminary results of a reduced burden of therapy trial by incorporation of rituximab and intrathecal liposomal cytarabine in children, adolescents and young adults with intermediate (FAB Group B) and high risk (FAB Group C) mature B-cell lymphoma/leukemia. In: 2016 ASCO Annual Meeting, Chicago, IL, June 3–7, 2016 2016 (abstract).
19. Davis TA, Grillo-Lopez AJ, White CA, McLaughlin P, Czuczman MS, Link BK, Maloney DG, Weaver RL, Rosenberg J, Levy R. Rituximab anti-CD20 monoclonal antibody therapy in non-Hodgkin's lymphoma: safety and efficacy of re-treatment. J Clin Oncol. 2000;18:3135–43.
20. Gisselbrecht C, Glass B, Mounier N, Singh Gill D, Linch DC, Trneny M, Bosly A, Ketterer N, Shpilberg O, Hagberg H, Ma D, Briere J, Moskowitz CH, Schmitz N. Salvage regimens with autologous transplantation for relapsed large B-cell lymphoma in the rituximab era. J Clin Oncol. 2010;28:4184–90.
21. Perkins SL, Lones MA, Davenport V, Cairo MS. B-Cell non-Hodgkin's lymphoma in children and adolescents: surface antigen expression and clinical implications for future targeted bioimmune therapy: a children's cancer group report. Clin Adv Hematol Oncol. 2003;1:314–7.
22. Teeling JL, French RR, Cragg MS, van den Brakel J, Pluyter M, Huang H, Chan C, Parren PW, Hack CE, Dechant M, Valerius T, van de Winkel JG, Glennie MJ. Characterization of new human CD20 monoclonal antibodies with potent cytolytic activity against non-Hodgkin lymphomas. Blood. 2004;104:1793–800.
23. Barth MJ, Hernandez-Ilizaliturri FJ, Mavis C, Tsai PC, Gibbs JF, Deeb G, Czuczman MS. Ofatumumab demonstrates activity against rituximab-sensitive and -resistant cell lines, lymphoma xenografts and primary tumour cells from patients with B-cell lymphoma. Br J Haematol. 2012;156:490–8.
24. Beum PV, Lindorfer MA, Beurskens F, Stukenberg PT, Lokhorst HM, Pawluczkowycz AW, Parren PW, van de Winkel JG, Taylor RP. Complement activation on B lymphocytes opsonized with rituximab or ofatumumab produces substantial changes in membrane structure preceding cell lysis. J Immunol. 2008;181:822–32.

25. Pawluczkowycz A, Beurskens F, Beum P, Lindorfer M, van de Winkel J, Parren P, Taylor R. Binding of submaximal C1q promotes complement-dependent cytotoxicity (CDC) of B cells opsonized with anti-CD20 mAbs ofatumumab (OFA) or rituximab (RTX): considerably higher levels of CDC are induced by OFA than by RTX. J Immunol. 2009;183:749–58.
26. Jain N, O'Brien S. Initial treatment of CLL: integrating biology and functional status. Blood. 2015;126:463–70.
27. Lemery SJ, Zhang J, Rothmann MD, Yang J, Earp J, Zhao H, McDougal A, Pilaro A, Chiang R, Gootenberg JE, Keegan P, Pazdur R. U.S. Food and Drug Administration approval: ofatumumab for the treatment of patients with chronic lymphocytic leukemia refractory to fludarabine and alemtuzumab. Clin Cancer Res. 2010;16:4331–8.
28. van Imhoff GW, McMillan A, Matasar MJ, Radford J, Ardeshna KM, Kuliczkowski K, Kim W, Hong X, Soenderskov Goerloev J, Davies A, Caballero Barrigón MD, Ogura M, Fennessy M, Liao Q, van der Holt B, Lisby S, Lin TS, Hagenbeek A. Ofatumumab versus rituximab salvage chemoimmunotherapy in relapsed or refractory diffuse large b-cell lymphoma: the orcharrd study. J Clin Oncol. 2017;35(5):544–51.
29. Mossner E, Brunker P, Moser S, Puntener U, Schmidt C, Herter S, Grau R, Gerdes C, Nopora A, van Puijenbroek E, Ferrara C, Sondermann P, Jager C, Strein P, Fertig G, Friess T, Schull C, Bauer S, Dal Porto J, Del Nagro C, Dabbagh K, Dyer MJ, Poppema S, Klein C, Umana P. Increasing the efficacy of CD20 antibody therapy through the engineering of a new type II anti-CD20 antibody with enhanced direct and immune effector cell-mediated B-cell cytotoxicity. Blood. 2010;115:4393–402.
30. Alduaij W, Ivanov A, Honeychurch J, Cheadle EJ, Potluri S, Lim SH, Shimada K, Chan CH, Tutt A, Beers SA, Glennie MJ, Cragg MS, Illidge TM. Novel type II anti-CD20 monoclonal antibody (GA101) evokes homotypic adhesion and actin-dependent, lysosome-mediated cell death in B-cell malignancies. Blood. 2011;117:4519–29.
31. Awasthi A, Ayello J, van de Ven C, Elmacken M, Reggio C, Barth MJ, Cairo MS. Comparative study of obinutuzumab (GA101) vs. rituximab against CD20+ rituximab-sensitive and -resistant burkitt (BL) and acute lymphoblastic leukemia (B-ALL): potential targeted therapy in patients with high risk BL and pre-B-ALL. Blood. 2014;124:2251.
32. Lee HZ, Miller BW, Kwitkowski VE, Ricci S, DelValle P, Saber H, Grillo J, Bullock J, Florian J, Mehrotra N, Ko CW, Nie L, Shapiro M, Tolnay M, Kane RC, Kaminskas E, Justice R, Farrell AT, Pazdur R. U.S. Food and drug administration approval: obinutuzumab in combination with chlorambucil for the treatment of previously untreated chronic lymphocytic leukemia. Clin Cancer Res. 2014;20:3902–7.
33. Sehn LH, Goy A, Offner FC, Martinelli G, Caballero MD, Gadeberg O, Baetz T, Zelenetz AD, Gaidano G, Fayad LE, Buckstein R, Friedberg JW, Crump M, Jaksic B, Zinzani PL, Padmanabhan Iyer S, Sahin D, Chai A, Fingerle-Rowson G, Press OW. Randomized phase II trial comparing obinutuzumab (GA101) with rituximab in patients with relapsed CD20+ indolent B-cell non-Hodgkin lymphoma: final analysis of the GAUSS study. J Clin Oncol. 2015;33(30):3467–74.
34. Morschhauser FA, Cartron G, Thieblemont C, Solal-Celigny P, Haioun C, Bouabdallah R, Feugier P, Bouabdallah K, Asikanius E, Lei G, Wenger M, Wassner-Fritsch E, Salles GA. Obinutuzumab (GA101) monotherapy in relapsed/refractory diffuse large b-cell lymphoma or mantle-cell lymphoma: results from the phase II GAUGUIN study. J Clin Oncol. 2013;31:2912–9.
35. Awasthi A, Ayello J, Van de Ven C, Elmacken M, Sabulski A, Barth MJ, Czuczman MS, Islam H, Klein C, Cairo MS. Obinutuzumab (GA101) compared to rituximab significantly enhances cell death and antibody-dependent cytotoxicity and improves overall survival against CD20(+) rituximab-sensitive/−resistant Burkitt lymphoma (BL) and precursor B-acute lymphoblastic leukaemia (pre-B-ALL): potential targeted therapy in patients with poor risk CD20(+) BL and pre-B-ALL. Br J Haematol. 2015;171:763–75.
36. Witzig TE, Gordon LI, Cabanillas F, Czuczman MS, Emmanouilides C, Joyce R, Pohlman BL, Bartlett NL, Wiseman GA, Padre N, Grillo-Lopez AJ, Multani P, White CA. Randomized controlled trial of yttrium-90-labeled ibritumomab tiuxetan radioimmunotherapy versus rituximab immunotherapy for patients with relapsed or refractory low-grade, follicular, or transformed B-cell non-Hodgkin's lymphoma. J Clin Oncol. 2002;20:2453–63.

37. Cooney-Qualter E, Krailo M, Angiolillo A, Fawwaz RA, Wiseman G, Harrison L, Kohl V, Adamson PC, Ayello J, vande Ven C, Perkins SL, Cairo MS. A phase I study of 90yttrium-ibritumomab-tiuxetan in children and adolescents with relapsed/refractory CD20-positive non-Hodgkin's lymphoma: a Children's Oncology Group study. Clin Cancer Res. 2007;13:5652s–60s.
38. Blanc V, Bousseau A, Caron A, Carrez C, Lutz RJ, Lambert JM. SAR3419: an anti-CD19-maytansinoid immunoconjugate for the treatment of B-cell malignancies. Clin Cancer Res. 2011;17:6448–58.
39. Ribrag V, Dupuis J, Tilly H, Morschhauser F, Laine F, Houot R, Haioun C, Copie C, Varga A, Lambert J, Hatteville L, Ziti-Ljajic S, Caron A, Payrard S, Coiffier B. A dose-escalation study of SAR3419, an anti-CD19 antibody maytansinoid conjugate, administered by intravenous infusion once weekly in patients with relapsed/refractory B-cell non-Hodgkin lymphoma. Clin Cancer Res. 2014;20:213–20.
40. Trneny M, Verhoef G, Dyer MJ, Patti DBY, Canales M, López A, Awan F, Montgomery P, Janikova A, Barbui AM, Sulek K, Terol MJ, Radford JA, Siraudin L, Hatteville L, Schwab S, Oprea C, Gianni AM. Starlyte phase II study of coltuximab ravtansine (CoR, SAR3419) single agent: clinical activity and safety in patients (pts) with relapsed/refractory (R/R) diffuse large B-cell lymphoma (DLBCL; NCT01472887). Journal of Clinical Oncology, 2014 ASCO Annual Meeting Abstracts. 2014;32:8506.
41. Thieblemont C, de Guibert S, Dupuis J, Ribrag V, Bouabdallah R, Morschhauser F, Cartron G, Le Gouill S, Casasnovas O, Holte H, Hatteville L, Zilocchi C, Oprea C, Tilly H. Phase II study of anti-CD19 antibody drug conjugate (SAR3419) in combination with rituximab: clinical activity and safety in patients with relapsed/refractory diffuse large B-cell lymphoma (NCT01470456). Blood. 2013;122:4395.
42. Moskowitz CH, Fanale MA, Shah BD, Advani RH, Chen R, Kim S, Kostic A, Liu T, Peng J, Forero-Torres A. A phase 1 study of denintuzumab mafodotin (SGN-CD19A) in relapsed/refactory B-lineage non-Hodgkin lymphoma. Blood. 2015;126:182.
43. Fathi AT, Borate U, DeAngelo DJ, O'Brien MM, Trippett T, Shah BD, Hale GA, Foran JM, Silverman LB, Tibes R, Cramer S, Pauly M, Kim S, Kostic A, Huang X, Pan Y, Chen R. A phase 1 study of denintuzumab mafodotin (SGN-CD19A) in adults with relapsed or refractory B-lineage acute leukemia (B-ALL) and highly aggressive lymphoma. Blood. 2015;126:1328.
44. Fathi AT, Chen R, Trippett TM, O'Brien MM, DeAngelo DJ, Shah BD, Cooper TM, Foran JM, Hale GA, Pressey J, Silverman LB, Tibes R, Kim S, Albertson TM, Sandalic L, Zhao B, Borate U. Interim Analysis of a Phase 1 Study of the Antibody-Drug Conjugate SGN-CD19A in Relapsed or Refractory B-Lineage Acute Leukemia and Highly Aggressive Lymphoma. Blood. 2014;124:963.
45. Coleman M, Goldenberg DM, Siegel AB, Ketas JC, Ashe M, Fiore JM, Leonard JP. Epratuzumab: targeting B-cell malignancies through CD22. Clin Cancer Res. 2003;9:3991S–4S.
46. Leonard JP, Coleman M, Ketas JC, Chadburn A, Ely S, Furman RR, Wegener WA, Hansen HJ, Ziccardi H, Eschenberg M, Gayko U, Cesano A, Goldenberg DM. Phase I/II trial of epratuzumab (humanized anti-CD22 antibody) in indolent non-Hodgkin's lymphoma. J Clin Oncol. 2003;21:3051–9.
47. Leonard JP, Coleman M, Ketas JC, Chadburn A, Furman R, Schuster MW, Feldman EJ, Ashe M, Schuster SJ, Wegener WA, Hansen HJ, Ziccardi H, Eschenberg M, Gayko U, Fields SZ, Cesano A, Goldenberg DM. Epratuzumab, a humanized anti-CD22 antibody, in aggressive non-Hodgkin's lymphoma: phase I/II clinical trial results. Clin Cancer Res. 2004;10:5327–34.
48. Micallef IN, Maurer MJ, Wiseman GA, Nikcevich DA, Kurtin PJ, Cannon MW, Perez DG, Soori GS, Link BK, Habermann TM, Witzig TE. Epratuzumab with rituximab, cyclophosphamide, doxorubicin, vincristine, and prednisone chemotherapy in patients with previously untreated diffuse large B-cell lymphoma. Blood. 2011;118:4053–61.
49. Grant BW, Jung SH, Johnson JL, Kostakoglu L, Hsi E, Byrd JC, Jones J, Leonard JP, Martin SE, Cheson BD. A phase 2 trial of extended induction epratuzumab and rituximab for previously untreated follicular lymphoma: CALGB 50701. Cancer. 2013;119:3797–804.

50. Morschhauser F, Kraeber-Bodere F, Wegener WA, Harousseau JL, Petillon MO, Huglo D, Trumper LH, Meller J, Pfreundschuh M, Kirsch CM, Naumann R, Kropp J, Horne H, Teoh N, Le Gouill S, Bodet-Milin C, Chatal JF, Goldenberg DM. High rates of durable responses with anti-CD22 fractionated radioimmunotherapy: results of a multicenter, phase I/II study in non-Hodgkin's lymphoma. J Clin Oncol. 2010;28:3709–16.
51. Chen AI, Lebovic D, Brunvand MW, Goy A, Chang JE, Hochberg E, Yalamanchili S, Kahn R, Lu D, Chai A, Chu Y-W, Cheson BD. Final results of a phase I study of the anti-CD22 antibody-drug conjugate (ADC) DCDT2980S with or without rituximab (RTX) in patients (Pts) with relapsed or refractory (R/R) B-cell non-Hodgkin's lymphoma (NHL). Blood. 2013;122:4399.
52. Morschhauser F, Flinn I, Advani RH, Diefenbach CS, Kolibaba K, Press OW, Sehn LH, Chen AI, Salles G, Tilly H, Cheson BD, Assouline S, Dreyling M, Hagenbeek A, Zinzani PL, Yalamanchili S, Lu D, Jones C, Jones S, Chu Y-W, Sharman JP. Updated results of a phase II randomized study (ROMULUS) of polatuzumab vedotin or pinatuzumab vedotin plus rituximab in patients with relapsed/refractory non-Hodgkin lymphoma. Blood. 2014;124:4457.
53. Rytting M, Triche L, Thomas D, O'Brien S, Kantarjian H. Initial experience with CMC-544 (inotuzumab ozogamicin) in pediatric patients with relapsed B-cell acute lymphoblastic leukemia. Pediatr Blood Cancer. 2014;61:369–72.
54. Wagner-Johnston ND, Goy A, Rodriguez MA, Ehmann WC, Hamlin PA, Radford J, Thieblemont C, Suh C, Sweetenham J, Huang Y, Sullivan ST, Vandendries ER, Gisselbrecht C. A phase 2 study of inotuzumab ozogamicin and rituximab, followed by autologous stem cell transplant in patients with relapsed/refractory diffuse large B-cell lymphoma. Leuk Lymphoma. 2015;56(10):2863–9.
55. Palanca-Wessels MC, Czuczman M, Salles G, Assouline S, Sehn LH, Flinn I, Patel MR, Sangha R, Hagenbeek A, Advani R, Tilly H, Casasnovas O, Press OW, Yalamanchili S, Kahn R, Dere RC, Lu D, Jones S, Jones C, Chu YW, Morschhauser F. Safety and activity of the anti-CD79B antibody-drug conjugate polatuzumab vedotin in relapsed or refractory B-cell non-Hodgkin lymphoma and chronic lymphocytic leukaemia: a phase 1 study. Lancet Oncol. 2015;16:704–15.
56. Svoboda J, Strelec LE, Nasta SD, Landsburg DJ, Mato AR, Pro B, Barta SK, Shah NN, Nagle SJ, Chong EA, Napier E, Garrett S, Schuster SJ. Brentuximab vedotin in combination with multi-agent chemotherapy is well tolerated and shows promising activity as frontline treatment for primary mediastinal B-cell lymphoma. Blood. 2015;126:2694.
57. Jacobsen ED, Sharman JP, Oki Y, Advani RH, Winter JN, Bello CM, Spitzer G, Palanca-Wessels MC, Kennedy DA, Levine P, Yang J, Bartlett NL. Brentuximab vedotin demonstrates objective responses in a phase 2 study of relapsed/refractory DLBCL with variable CD30 expression. Blood. 2015;125:1394–402.
58. Yasenchak CA, Halwani A, Advani R, Ansell S, Budde LE, Burke JM, Farber CM, Holkova B, Fayad LE, Kolibaba KS, Knapp M, Li M, Manley TJ, Patel-Donnelly D, Seetharam M, Yimer HA, Bartlett NL. Brentuximab vedotin with RCHOP as frontline therapy in patients with high-intermediate/high-risk diffuse large B cell lymphoma (DLBCL): results from an Ongoing Phase 2 Study. Blood. 2015;126:814.
59. Bras AE, Beishuizen A, Langerak AW, Jongen-Lavrencic M, te Marvelde JG, van den Heuvel-Eibrink MM, Zwaan CM, van Dongen JJM, van der Velden VHJ. CD38 expression in paediatric leukaemia and lymphoma: implications for antibody targeted therapy. Br J Haematol. 2016; doi:10.1111/bjh.14310.
60. de Weers M, Tai Y-T, van der Veer MS, Bakker JM, Vink T, Jacobs DCH, Oomen LA, Peipp M, Valerius T, Slootstra JW, Mutis T, Bleeker WK, Anderson KC, Lokhorst HM, van de Winkel JGJ, Parren PWHI. Daratumumab, a novel therapeutic human CD38 monoclonal antibody, induces killing of multiple myeloma and other hematological tumors. J Immunol. 2011;186:1840–8.
61. Lee HC, Weber DM. Advances and practical use of monoclonal antibodies in multiple myeloma therapy. ASH Education Program Book. 2016, 2016:512–20.
62. Bargou R, Leo E, Zugmaier G, Klinger M, Goebeler M, Knop S, Noppeney R, Viardot A, Hess G, Schuler M, Einsele H, Brandl C, Wolf A, Kirchinger P, Klappers P, Schmidt M,

Riethmuller G, Reinhardt C, Baeuerle PA, Kufer P. Tumor regression in cancer patients by very low doses of a T cell-engaging antibody. Science. 2008;321:974–7.

63. Viardot A, Goebeler M-E, Hess G, Neumann S, Pfreundschuh M, Adrian N, Zettl F, Libicher M, Sayehli C, Stieglmaier J, Zhang A, Nagorsen D, Bargou RC. Phase 2 study of bispecific T-cell engager (BiTE®) antibody blinatumomab in relapsed/refractory diffuse large B cell lymphoma. Blood. 2016;127(11):1410–6.
64. Teachey DT, Rheingold SR, Maude SL, Zugmaier G, Barrett DM, Seif AE, Nichols KE, Suppa EK, Kalos M, Berg RA, Fitzgerald JC, Aplenc R, Gore L, Grupp SA. Cytokine release syndrome after blinatumomab treatment related to abnormal macrophage activation and ameliorated with cytokine-directed therapy. Blood. 2013;121:5154–7.
65. Oak E, Bartlett NL. Blinatumomab for the treatment of B-cell lymphoma. Expert Opin Investig Drugs. 2015;24:715–24.
66. Eyre TA, Collins GP. Immune checkpoint inhibition in lymphoid disease. Br J Haematol. 2015;170:291–304.
67. Page DB, Postow MA, Callahan MK, Allison JP, Wolchok JD. Immune modulation in cancer with antibodies. Annu Rev Med. 2014;65:185–202.
68. Ansell SM, Hurvitz SA, Koenig PA, LaPlant BR, Kabat BF, Fernando D, Habermann TM, Inwards DJ, Verma M, Yamada R, Erlichman C, Lowy I, Timmerman JM. Phase I study of ipilimumab, an anti-CTLA-4 monoclonal antibody, in patients with relapsed and refractory B-cell non-Hodgkin lymphoma. Clin Cancer Res. 2009;15:6446–53.
69. Galligan BM, Tsao-Wei D, Groshen S, Kirschabum M, O'Donnell R, Kaesberg PR, Siddiqui T, Popplewell L, Sikander A, Myo H, Chen R, DiPersio JF, Palmisiano ND, Claxton DF, Newman EM, Tuscano J. Efficacy and safety of combined rituximab and ipilimumab to treat patients with relapsed/refractory CD20+ B-cell lymphoma. Blood. 2015;126:3977.
70. Bashey A, Medina B, Corringham S, Pasek M, Carrier E, Vrooman L, Lowy I, Solomon SR, Morris LE, Holland HK, Mason JR, Alyea EP, Soiffer RJ, Ball ED. CTLA4 blockade with ipilimumab to treat relapse of malignancy after allogeneic hematopoietic cell transplantation. Blood. 2009;113:1581–8.
71. Westin JR, Chu F, Zhang M, Fayad LE, Kwak LW, Fowler N, Romaguera J, Hagemeister F, Fanale M, Samaniego F, Feng L, Baladandayuthapani V, Wang Z, Ma W, Gao Y, Wallace M, Vence LM, Radvanyi L, Muzzafar T, Rotem-Yehudar R, Davis RE, Neelapu SS. Safety and activity of PD1 blockade by pidilizumab in combination with rituximab in patients with relapsed follicular lymphoma: a single group, open-label, phase 2 trial. Lancet Oncol. 2014;15:69–77.
72. Armand P, Nagler A, Weller EA, Devine SM, Avigan DE, Chen YB, Kaminski MS, Holland HK, Winter JN, Mason JR, Fay JW, Rizzieri DA, Hosing CM, Ball ED, Uberti JP, Lazarus HM, Mapara MY, Gregory SA, Timmerman JM, Andorsky D, Or R, Waller EK, Rotem-Yehudar R, Gordon LI. Disabling immune tolerance by programmed death-1 blockade with pidilizumab after autologous hematopoietic stem-cell transplantation for diffuse large B-cell lymphoma: results of an international phase II trial. J Clin Oncol. 2013;31:4199–206.
73. Lesokhin AM, Ansell SM, Armand P, Scott EC, Halwani A, Gutierrez M, Millenson MM, Cohen AD, Schuster SJ, Lebovic D, Dhodapkar MV, Avigan D, Chapuy B, Ligon AH, Rodig SJ, Cattry D, Zhu L, Grosso JF, Kim SY, Shipp MA, Borrello I, Timmerman J. Preliminary results of a phase I study of nivolumab (BMS-936558) in patients with relapsed or refractory lymphoid malignancies. Blood. 2014;124:291.
74. Zinzani PL, Ribrag V, Moskowitz CH, Michot J-M, Kuruvilla J, Balakumaran A, Snyder E, Marinello P, Shipp MA, Armand P. Phase 1b study of PD-1 blockade with pembrolizumab in patients with relapsed/refractory primary mediastinal large B-cell lymphoma (PMBCL). Blood. 2015;126:3986.
75. Stein H, Foss HD, Durkop H, Marafioti T, Delsol G, Pulford K, Pileri S, Falini B. CD30(+) anaplastic large cell lymphoma: a review of its histopathologic, genetic, and clinical features. Blood. 2000;96:3681–95.
76. Chiarle R, Voena C, Ambrogio C, Piva R, Inghirami G. The anaplastic lymphoma kinase in the pathogenesis of cancer. Nat Rev Cancer. 2008;8:11–23.

77. Lamant L, McCarthy K, d'Amore E, Klapper W, Nakagawa A, Fraga M, Maldyk J, Simonitsch-Klupp I, Oschlies I, Delsol G, Mauguen A, Brugieres L, Le Deley MC. Prognostic impact of morphologic and phenotypic features of childhood ALK-positive anaplastic large-cell lymphoma: results of the ALCL99 study. J Clin Oncol. 2011;29:4669–76.
78. Alexander S, Kraveka JM, Weitzman S, Lowe E, Smith L, Lynch JC, Chang M, Kinney MC, Perkins SL, Laver J, Gross TG, Weinstein H. Advanced stage anaplastic large cell lymphoma in children and adolescents: results of ANHL0131, a randomized phase III trial of APO versus a modified regimen with vinblastine: a report from the children's oncology group. Pediatr Blood Cancer. 2014;61:2236–42.
79. Brugieres L, Quartier P, Le Deley MC, Pacquement H, Perel Y, Bergeron C, Schmitt C, Landmann J, Patte C, Terrier-Lacombe MJ, Delsol G, Hartmann O. Relapses of childhood anaplastic large-cell lymphoma: treatment results in a series of 41 children—a report from the French society of pediatric oncology. Ann Oncol. 2000;11:53–8.
80. Le Deley MC, Rosolen A, Williams DM, Horibe K, Wrobel G, Attarbaschi A, Zsiros J, Uyttebroeck A, Marky IM, Lamant L, Woessmann W, Pillon M, Hobson R, Mauguen A, Reiter A, Brugieres L. Vinblastine in children and adolescents with high-risk anaplastic large-cell lymphoma: results of the randomized ALCL99-vinblastine trial. J Clin Oncol. 2010;28:3987–93.
81. Lowe EJ, Sposto R, Perkins SL, Gross TG, Finlay J, Zwick D, Abromowitch M. Intensive chemotherapy for systemic anaplastic large cell lymphoma in children and adolescents: final results of Children's Cancer Group Study 5941. Pediatr Blood Cancer. 2009;52:335–9.
82. Gambacorti Passerini C, Farina F, Stasia A, Redaelli S, Ceccon M, Mologni L, Messa C, Guerra L, Giudici G, Sala E, Mussolin L, Deeren D, King MH, Steurer M, Ordemann R, Cohen AM, Grube M, Bernard L, Chiriano G, Antolini L, Piazza R. Crizotinib in advanced, chemoresistant anaplastic lymphoma kinase-positive lymphoma patients. J Natl Cancer Inst. 2014;106:djt378.
83. Mosse YP, Lim MS, Voss SD, Wilner K, Ruffner K, Laliberte J, Rolland D, Balis FM, Maris JM, Weigel BJ, Ingle AM, Ahern C, Adamson PC, Blaney SM. Safety and activity of crizotinib for paediatric patients with refractory solid tumours or anaplastic large-cell lymphoma: a Children's Oncology Group phase 1 consortium study. Lancet Oncol. 2013;14:472–80.
84. Younes A, Bartlett NL, Leonard JP, Kennedy DA, Lynch CM, Sievers EL, Forero-Torres A. Brentuximab vedotin (SGN-35) for relapsed CD30-positive lymphomas. N Engl J Med. 2010;363:1812–21.
85. Fanale MA, Forero-Torres A, Rosenblatt JD, Advani RH, Franklin AR, Kennedy DA, Han TH, Sievers EL, Bartlett NL. A phase I weekly dosing study of brentuximab vedotin in patients with relapsed/refractory CD30-positive hematologic malignancies. Clin Cancer Res. 2012;18:248–55.
86. Pro B, Advani R, Brice P, Bartlett NL, Rosenblatt JD, Illidge T, Matous J, Ramchandren R, Fanale M, Connors JM, Yang Y, Sievers EL, Kennedy DA, Shustov A. Brentuximab vedotin (SGN-35) in patients with relapsed or refractory systemic anaplastic large-cell lymphoma: results of a phase II study. J Clin Oncol. 2012;30:2190–6.
87. Fanale MA, Horwitz SM, Forero-Torres A, Bartlett NL, Advani RH, Pro B, Chen RW, Davies A, Illidge T, Huebner D, Kennedy DA, Shustov AR. Brentuximab vedotin in the front-line treatment of patients with CD30+ peripheral T-cell lymphomas: results of a phase I study. J Clin Oncol. 2014;32:3137–43.
88. Johnston LJ, Horning SJ. Autologous hematopoietic cell transplantation in Hodgkin's disease. Biol Blood Marrow Transplant. 2000;6:289–300.
89. Castellino SM, Geiger AM, Mertens AC, Leisenring WM, Tooze JA, Goodman P, Stovall M, Robison LL, Hudson MM. Morbidity and mortality in long-term survivors of Hodgkin lymphoma: a report from the Childhood Cancer Survivor Study. Blood. 2011;117:1806–16.
90. Younes A, Gopal AK, Smith SE, Ansell SM, Rosenblatt JD, Savage KJ, Ramchandren R, Bartlett NL, Cheson BD, de Vos S, Forero-Torres A, Moskowitz CH, Connors JM, Engert A, Larsen EK, Kennedy DA, Sievers EL, Chen R. Results of a pivotal phase II study of brentuximab vedotin for patients with relapsed or refractory Hodgkin's lymphoma. J Clin Oncol. 2012;30:2183–9.

91. Gopal AK, Chen R, Smith SE, Ansell SM, Rosenblatt JD, Savage KJ, Connors JM, Engert A, Larsen EK, Chi X, Sievers EL, Younes A. Durable remissions in a pivotal phase 2 study of brentuximab vedotin in relapsed or refractory Hodgkin lymphoma. Blood. 2015;125:1236–43.
92. Rothe A, Sasse S, Goergen H, Eichenauer DA, Lohri A, Jager U, Bangard C, Boll B, von Bergwelt Baildon M, Theurich S, Borchmann P, Engert A. Brentuximab vedotin for relapsed or refractory CD30+ hematologic malignancies: the German Hodgkin Study Group experience. Blood. 2012;120:1470–2.
93. Moskowitz CH, Nademanee A, Masszi T, Agura E, Holowiecki J, Abidi MH, Chen AI, Stiff P, Gianni AM, Carella A, Osmanov D, Bachanova V, Sweetenham J, Sureda A, Huebner D, Sievers EL, Chi A, Larsen EK, Hunder NN, Walewski J. Brentuximab vedotin as consolidation therapy after autologous stem-cell transplantation in patients with Hodgkin's lymphoma at risk of relapse or progression (AETHERA): a randomised, double-blind, placebo-controlled, phase 3 trial. Lancet. 2015;385:1853–62.
94. Gopal AK, Ramchandren R, O'Connor OA, Berryman RB, Advani RH, Chen R, Smith SE, Cooper M, Rothe A, Matous JV, Grove LE, Zain J. Safety and efficacy of brentuximab vedotin for Hodgkin lymphoma recurring after allogeneic stem cell transplantation. Blood. 2012;120:560–8.
95. Younes A, Connors JM, Park SI, Fanale M, O'Meara MM, Hunder NN, Huebner D, Ansell SM. Brentuximab vedotin combined with ABVD or AVD for patients with newly diagnosed Hodgkin's lymphoma: a phase 1, open-label, dose-escalation study. Lancet Oncol. 2013;14:1348–56.
96. Ansell SM, Connors JM, Park SI, O'Meara MM, Younes A. Frontline therapy with brentuximab vedotin combined with ABVD or AVD in patients with newly diagnosed advanced stage Hodgkin lymphoma. ASH Ann Meet Abstr. 2012;120:798.
97. Younes A, Oki Y, McLaughlin P, Copeland AR, Goy A, Pro B, Feng L, Yuan Y, Chuang HH, Macapinlac HA, Hagemeister F, Romaguera J, Samaniego F, Fanale MA, Dabaja BS, Rodriguez MA, Dang N, Kwak LW, Neelapu SS, Fayad LE. Phase 2 study of rituximab plus ABVD in patients with newly diagnosed classical Hodgkin lymphoma. Blood. 2012;119:4123–8.
98. Jones RJ, Gocke CD, Kasamon YL, Miller CB, Perkins B, Barber JP, Vala MS, Gerber JM, Gellert LL, Siedner M, Lemas MV, Brennan S, Ambinder RF, Matsui W. Circulating clonotypic B cells in classic Hodgkin lymphoma. Blood. 2009;113:5920–6.
99. Kasamon YL, Jacene HA, Gocke CD, Swinnen LJ, Gladstone DE, Perkins B, Link BK, Popplewell LL, Habermann TM, Herman JM, Matsui WH, Jones RJ, Ambinder RF. Phase 2 study of rituximab-ABVD in classical Hodgkin lymphoma. Blood. 2012;119:4129–32.
100. Batlevi CL, Matsuki E, Brentjens RJ, Younes A. Novel immunotherapies in lymphoid malignancies. Nat Rev Clin Oncol. 2016;13:25–40.
101. Ansell SM, Lesokhin AM, Borrello I, Halwani A, Scott EC, Gutierrez M, Schuster SJ, Millenson MM, Cattry D, Freeman GJ, Rodig SJ, Chapuy B, Ligon AH, Zhu L, Grosso JF, Kim SY, Timmerman JM, Shipp MA, Armand P. PD-1 blockade with nivolumab in relapsed or refractory Hodgkin's lymphoma. N Engl J Med. 2015;372:311–9.
102. Moskowitz CH, Ribrag V, Michot JM, Martinelli G, Zinzani PL, Gutierrez M, De Maeyer G, Jacob A, Giallella K, Anderson J, Derosier M, Wang J, Yang Z, Rubin E, Rose S, Shipp M, Armand P. PD-1 blockade with the monoclonal antibody pembrolizumab (MK-3475) in patients with classical Hodgkin lymphoma after brentuximab vedotin failure: preliminary results from a phase 1b study (KEYNOTE-013). Blood. 2014;124:290.
103. Shah NN, Dave H, Wayne AS. Immunotherapy for pediatric leukemia. Front Oncol. 2013;3:166.
104. Barth M, Raetz E, Cairo MS. The future role of monoclonal antibody therapy in childhood acute leukaemias. Br J Haematol. 2012;159:3–17.
105. Gudowius S, Recker K, Laws HJ, Dirksen U, Troger A, Wieczorek U, Furlan S, Gobel U, Hanenberg H. Identification of candidate target antigens for antibody-based immunotherapy in childhood B-cell precursor ALL. Klin Padiatr. 2006;218:327–33.
106. Carnahan J, Stein R, Qu Z, Hess K, Cesano A, Hansen HJ, Goldenberg DM. Epratuzumab, a CD22-targeting recombinant humanized antibody with a different mode of action from rituximab. Mol Immunol. 2007;44:1331–41.

107. Raetz EA, Cairo MS, Borowitz MJ, Blaney SM, Krailo MD, Leil TA, Reid JM, Goldenberg DM, Wegener WA, Carroll WL, Adamson PC, Children's Oncology Group Pilot S. Chemoimmunotherapy reinduction with epratuzumab in children with acute lymphoblastic leukemia in marrow relapse: a Children's Oncology Group Pilot Study. J Clin Oncol. 2008;26:3756–62.
108. Raetz EA, Cairo MS, Borowitz MJ, Lu X, Devidas M, Reid JM, Goldenberg DM, Wegener WA, Zeng H, Whitlock JA, Adamson PC, Hunger SP, Carroll WL. Re-induction chemoimmunotherapy with epratuzumab in relapsed acute lymphoblastic leukemia (ALL): phase II results from Children's Oncology Group (COG) study ADVL04P2. Pediatr Blood Cancer. 2015;62:1171–5.
109. Kantarjian H, Thomas D, Jorgensen J, Jabbour E, Kebriaei P, Rytting M, York S, Ravandi F, Kwari M, Faderl S, Rios MB, Cortes J, Fayad L, Tarnai R, Wang SA, Champlin R, Advani A, O'Brien S. Inotuzumab ozogamicin, an anti-CD22-calecheamicin conjugate, for refractory and relapsed acute lymphocytic leukaemia: a phase 2 study. Lancet Oncol. 2012;13:403–11.
110. Mussai F, Campana D, Bhojwani D, Stetler-Stevenson M, Steinberg SM, Wayne AS, Pastan I. Cytotoxicity of the anti-CD22 immunotoxin HA22 (CAT-8015) against paediatric acute lymphoblastic leukaemia. Br J Haematol. 2010;150:352–8.
111. Wayne AS, Bhojwani D, Silverman LB, Richards K, Stetler-Stevenson M, Shah NN, Jeha S, Pui CH, Buzoianu M, FitzGerald DJ, Kreitman RJ, Ibrahim R, Pastan I. A novel anti-CD22 immunotoxin, moxetumomab pasudotox: phase I study in pediatric acute lymphoblastic leukemia (ALL). Blood (ASH Annual Meeting Abstracts). 2011;118:248.
112. Smith MA. Update on developmental therapeutics for acute lymphoblastic leukemia. Curr Hematol Malig Rep. 2009;4:175–82.
113. Al-Katib AM, Aboukameel A, Mohammad R, Bissery MC, Zuany-Amorim C. Superior antitumor activity of SAR3419 to rituximab in xenograft models for non-Hodgkin's lymphoma. Clin Cancer Res. 2009;15:4038–45.
114. Carol H, Szymanska B, Evans K, Boehm I, Houghton PJ, Smith MA, Lock RB. The anti-CD19 antibody-drug conjugate SAR3419 prevents hematolymphoid relapse postinduction therapy in preclinical models of pediatric acute lymphoblastic leukemia. Clin Cancer Res. 2013;19:1795–805.
115. Younes A, Kim S, Romaguera J, Copeland A, Farial Sde C, Kwak LW, Fayad L, Hagemeister F, Fanale M, Neelapu S, Lambert JM, Morariu-Zamfir R, Payrard S, Gordon LI. Phase I multidose-escalation study of the anti-CD19 maytansinoid immunoconjugate SAR3419 administered by intravenous infusion every 3 weeks to patients with relapsed/refractory B-cell lymphoma. J Clin Oncol. 2012;30:2776–82.
116. Topp MS, Kufer P, Gokbuget N, Goebeler M, Klinger M, Neumann S, Horst HA, Raff T, Viardot A, Schmid M, Stelljes M, Schaich M, Degenhard E, Kohne-Volland R, Bruggemann M, Ottmann O, Pfeifer H, Burmeister T, Nagorsen D, Schmidt M, Lutterbuese R, Reinhardt C, Baeuerle PA, Kneba M, Einsele H, Riethmuller G, Hoelzer D, Zugmaier G, Bargou RC. Targeted therapy with the T-cell-engaging antibody blinatumomab of chemotherapy-refractory minimal residual disease in B-lineage acute lymphoblastic leukemia patients results in high response rate and prolonged leukemia-free survival. J Clin Oncol. 2011;29:2493–8.
117. Topp MS, Gokbuget N, Zugmaier G, Degenhard E, Goebeler ME, Klinger M, Neumann SA, Horst HA, Raff T, Viardot A, Stelljes M, Schaich M, Kohne-Volland R, Bruggemann M, Ottmann OG, Burmeister T, Baeuerle PA, Nagorsen D, Schmidt M, Einsele H, Riethmuller G, Kneba M, Hoelzer D, Kufer P, Bargou RC. Long-term follow-up of hematologic relapse-free survival in a phase 2 study of blinatumomab in patients with MRD in B-lineage ALL. Blood. 2012;120:5185–7.
118. von Stackelberg A, Zugmaier G, Handgretinger R, Locatelli F, Rizzari C, Trippett TM, Borkhardt A, Rheingold SR, Bader BD, Cooper TM, DuBois SG, O'Brien MM, Zwaan CM, Holland C, Mergen N, Fischer A, Zhu M, Hijazi Y, Whitlock JA, Gore L. A phase 1/2 study of blinatumomab in pediatric patients with relapsed/refractory B-cell precursor acute lymphoblastic leukemia. Blood (ASH Annual Meeting Abstracts). 2013;122:70.

119. Gore L, Zugmaier G, Handgretinger R, Locatelli F, Trippett TM, Rheingold SR, Bader P, Borkhardt A, Cooper TM, O'Brien MM, Zwaan CM, Fischer A, Whitlock J, Von Stackelberg A. Cytological and molecular remissions with blinatumomab treatment in second or later bone marrow relapse in pediatric acute lymphoblastic leukemia (ALL). J Clin Oncol. 2013;31:10007.
120. Handgretinger R, Zugmaier G, Henze G, Kreyenberg H, Lang P, von Stackelberg A. Complete remission after blinatumomab-induced donor T-cell activation in three pediatric patients with post-transplant relapsed acute lymphoblastic leukemia. Leukemia. 2011;25:181–4.
121. Jeha S, Behm F, Pei D, Sandlund JT, Ribeiro RC, Razzouk BI, Rubnitz JE, Hijiya N, Howard SC, Cheng C, Pui CH. Prognostic significance of CD20 expression in childhood B-cell precursor acute lymphoblastic leukemia. Blood. 2006;108:3302–4.
122. Jandula BM, Nomdedeu J, Marin P, Vivancos P. Rituximab can be useful as treatment for minimal residual disease in bcr-abl-positive acute lymphoblastic leukemia. Bone Marrow Transplant. 2001;27:225–7.
123. Thomas DA, O'Brien S, Faderl S, Garcia-Manero G, Ferrajoli A, Wierda W, Ravandi F, Verstovsek S, Jorgensen JL, Bueso-Ramos C, Andreeff M, Pierce S, Garris R, Keating MJ, Cortes J, Kantarjian HM. Chemoimmunotherapy with a modified hyper-CVAD and rituximab regimen improves outcome in de novo Philadelphia chromosome-negative precursor B-lineage acute lymphoblastic leukemia. J Clin Oncol. 2010;28:3880–9.
124. Angiolillo AL, AL Y, Reaman G, Ingle AM, Secola R, Adamson PC. A phase II study of Campath-1H in children with relapsed or refractory acute lymphoblastic leukemia: a Children's Oncology Group report. Pediatr Blood Cancer. 2009;53:978–83.
125. Patel B, Kirkland KE, Szydlo R, Pearce RM, Clark RE, Craddock C, Liakopoulou E, Fielding AK, Mackinnon S, Olavarria E, Potter MN, Russell NH, Shaw BE, Cook G, Goldstone AH, Marks DI. Favorable outcomes with alemtuzumab-conditioned unrelated donor stem cell transplantation in adults with high-risk Philadelphia chromosome-negative acute lymphoblastic leukemia in first complete remission. Haematologica. 2009;94:1399–406.
126. Veys P, Wynn RF, Ahn KW, Samarasinghe S, He W, Bonney D, Craddock J, Cornish J, Davies SM, Dvorak CC, Duerst RE, Gross TG, Kapoor N, Kitko C, Krance RA, Leung W, Lewis VA, Steward C, Wagner JE, Carpenter PA, Eapen M. Impact of immune modulation with in vivo T-cell depletion and myleoablative total body irradiation conditioning on outcomes after unrelated donor transplantation for childhood acute lymphoblastic leukemia. Blood. 2012;119:6155–61.
127. Bremer E, Samplonius DF, Peipp M, van Genne L, Kroesen BJ, Fey GH, Gramatzki M, de Leij LF, Helfrich W. Target cell-restricted apoptosis induction of acute leukemic T cells by a recombinant tumor necrosis factor-related apoptosis-inducing ligand fusion protein with specificity for human CD7. Cancer Res. 2005;65:3380–8.
128. Gasiorowski RE, Clark GJ, Bradstock K, Hart DN. Antibody therapy for acute myeloid leukaemia. Br J Haematol. 2014;164:481–95.
129. Petersdorf SH, Kopecky KJ, Slovak M, Willman C, Nevill T, Brandwein J, Larson RA, Erba HP, Stiff PJ, Stuart RK, Walter RB, Tallman MS, Stenke L, Appelbaum FR. A phase 3 study of gemtuzumab ozogamicin during induction and postconsolidation therapy in younger patients with acute myeloid leukemia. Blood. 2013;121:4854–60.
130. Creutzig U, Harbott J, Sperling C, Ritter J, Zimmermann M, Loffler H, Riehm H, Schellong G, Ludwig WD. Clinical significance of surface antigen expression in children with acute myeloid leukemia: results of study AML-BFM-87. Blood. 1995;86:3097–108.
131. Pollard JA, Alonzo TA, Loken M, Gerbing RB, Ho PA, Bernstein ID, Raimondi SC, Hirsch B, Franklin J, Walter RB, Gamis A, Meshinchi S. Correlation of CD33 expression level with disease characteristics and response to gemtuzumab ozogamicin containing chemotherapy in childhood AML. Blood. 2012;119:3705–11.
132. Arceci RJ, Sande J, Lange B, Shannon K, Franklin J, Hutchinson R, Vik TA, Flowers D, Aplenc R, Berger MS, Sherman ML, Smith FO, Bernstein I, Sievers EL. Safety and efficacy

of gemtuzumab ozogamicin in pediatric patients with advanced CD33+ acute myeloid leukemia. Blood. 2005;106:1183–8.
133. Zwaan CM, Reinhardt D, Zimmerman M, Hasle H, Stary J, Stark B, Dworzak M, Creutzig U, Kaspers GJ, International BFMSGoPAML. Salvage treatment for children with refractory first or second relapse of acute myeloid leukaemia with gemtuzumab ozogamicin: results of a phase II study. Br J Haematol. 2010;148:768–76.
134. Aplenc R, Alonzo TA, Gerbing RB, Lange BJ, Hurwitz CA, Wells RJ, Bernstein I, Buckley P, Krimmel K, Smith FO, Sievers EL, Arceci RJ, Children's Oncology G. Safety and efficacy of gemtuzumab ozogamicin in combination with chemotherapy for pediatric acute myeloid leukemia: a report from the Children's Oncology Group. J Clin Oncol. 2008;26:2390–3295.
135. Gamis AS, Alonzo TA, Meshinchi S, Sung L, Gerbing RB, Raimondi SC, Hirsch BA, Kahwash SB, Heerema-McKenney A, Winter L, Glick K, Davies SM, Byron P, Smith FO, Aplenc R. Gemtuzumab ozogamicin in children and adolescents with de novo acute myeloid leukemia improves event-free survival by reducing relapse risk: results from the randomized phase III Children's Oncology Group trial AAML0531. J Clin Oncol. 2014;32:3021–32.
136. Tarlock K, Alonzo TA, Gerbing R, Raimondi SC, Hirsch BA, Sung L, Pollard JA, Aplenc R, Loken MR, Gamis A, Meshinchi S. Gemtuzumab ozogamicin reduces relapse risk in FLT3/ITD acute myeloid leukemia: a report from the Children's Oncology Group. Clin Cancer Res. 2015;22(8):1951–7.
137. Pollard J, Alonzo TA, Gerbing RB, Raimondi SC, Hirsch B, Aplenc R, Gamis AS, Loken MR, Meshinchi S. Negative prognostic impact of high CD33 expression is negated with the use of gemtuzumab ozogamicin: a report from the Children's Oncology Group. Blood (ASH Annual Meeting Abstracts). 2013;122:491.
138. Satwani P, Bhatia M, Garvin JH Jr, George D, Dela Cruz F, Le Gall J, Jin Z, Schwartz J, Duffy D, van de Ven C, Foley S, Hawks R, Morris E, Baxter-Lowe LA, Cairo MS. A Phase I study of gemtuzumab ozogamicin (GO) in combination with busulfan and cyclophosphamide (Bu/Cy) and allogeneic stem cell transplantation in children with poor-risk CD33+ AML: a new targeted immunochemotherapy myeloablative conditioning (MAC) regimen. Biol Blood Marrow Transplant. 2012;18:324–9.
139. Zahler S, Bhatia M, Ricci A, Roy S, Morris E, Harrison L, van de Ven C, Fabricatore S, Wolownik K, Cooney-Qualter E, Baxter-Lowe LA, Luisi P, Militano O, Kletzel M, Cairo MS. A phase I study of reduced-intensity conditioning and allogeneic stem cell transplantation followed by dose escalation of targeted consolidation immunotherapy with gemtuzumab ozogamicin in children and adolescents with CD33 acute myeloid leukemia. Biol Blood Marrow Transplant. 2016;22(4):698–704.
140. Friedrich M, Henn A, Raum T, Bajtus M, Matthes K, Hendrich L, Wahl J, Hoffmann P, Kischel R, Kvesic M, Slootstra JW, Baeuerle PA, Kufer P, Rattel B. Preclinical characterization of AMG 330, a CD3/CD33-bispecific T-cell-engaging antibody with potential for treatment of acute myelogenous leukemia. Mol Cancer Ther. 2014;13:1549–57.
141. Harrington KH, Gudgeon CJ, Laszlo GS, Newhall KJ, Sinclair AM, Frankel SR, Kischel R, Chen G, Walter RB. The broad anti-AML activity of the CD33/CD3 BiTE antibody construct, AMG 330, is impacted by disease stage and risk. PLoS One. 2015;10:e0135945.
142. Krupka C, Kufer P, Kischel R, Zugmaier G, Bogeholz J, Kohnke T, Lichtenegger FS, Schneider S, Metzeler KH, Fiegl M, Spiekermann K, Baeuerle PA, Hiddemann W, Riethmuller G, Subklewe M. CD33 target validation and sustained depletion of AML blasts in long-term cultures by the bispecific T-cell-engaging antibody AMG 330. Blood. 2014;123:356–65.
143. Laszlo GS, Gudgeon CJ, Harrington KH, Dell'Aringa J, Newhall KJ, Means GD, Sinclair AM, Kischel R, Frankel SR, Walter RB. Cellular determinants for preclinical activity of a novel CD33/CD3 bispecific T-cell engager (BiTE) antibody, AMG 330, against human AML. Blood. 2014;123:554–61.
144. Cheson BD, Leonard JP. Monoclonal antibody therapy for B-cell non-Hodgkin's lymphoma. N Engl J Med. 2008;359:613–26.

Chapter 6
Monoclonal Antibodies Directly Targeting Antigens on Solid Tumours

Holger N. Lode

Abstract Monoclonal antibodies (Mabs) are a highly versatile class of anti-cancer agents that emerged after a long journey of development from discovery in 1975 to clinical applicability and finally to approved drugs for cancer immunotherapy in the late 1990s. The number of approved Mabs in adult oncology is dramatically increasing over the years. Although approval rates in paediatric indications stay far behind, the clinical utility of Mabs in paediatric oncology is clearly acknowledged and will be discussed in the following chapters with focus on neuroblastoma.

Keywords Monoclonal antibodies • Ganglioside GD2 • Neuroblastoma • Anti-GD2 antibodies • Fc receptor

6.1 Introduction

Monoclonal antibodies specifically targeting tumour-associated antigens on solid tumours have shown promising results in the treatment of cancer [1]. Important mechanisms of action mediated by such antibodies are the activation of complement-dependent- (CDC) and antibody-dependent cellular cytotoxicity (ADCC). CDC is induced through binding of a serine protease complex C1 to the Fc domains of two or more Ab binding to antigens expressed on tumour cells. This classical complement pathway results in an activation cascade resulting in the membrane attack complex disrupting the target cell. ADCC is a result of Fc-gamma receptor (FcγR) mediated interaction with effector immune cells such as natural killer (NK) cells, macrophages and granulocytes [1]. The binding of FcγR to Fc domain induces both release of granzymes and perforin from effector cells leading to a target cell lysis and Fc-dependent tumour cell phagocytosis. One important mechanism that engages the immune is antibody-dependent cellular phagocytosis (ADCP) of the malignant cells by macrophages. The uptake of tumor cells by

H.N. Lode, M.D.
Pediatric Hematology and Oncology, University Medicine Greifswald, Greifswald, Germany
e-mail: lode@uni-greifswald.de

J.C. Gray, A. Marabelle (eds.), *Immunotherapy for Pediatric Malignancies*,
https://doi.org/10.1007/978-3-319-43486-5_6

ADCP culminates in the establishment of vacuoles that are referred to as phagosomes. During maturation, late endosomes and lysosomes fuse with the phagosome to form phagolysosomes. The pH is lowered into the range of 4.5, and the phagosome becomes highly oxidative with generation of reactive oxygen species (ROS) that mediate killing of phagocytosed cancer cells [2]. In addition to the array of immune effector functions engaged by monoclonal antibodies, there are a variety of direct effects that include the induction of apoptosis or inhibition of cell growth by blocking the binding of a ligand to its growth factor receptor [1]. The latter mechanism plays, for example, an important role in anti-EGFR mAb therapy, which is effective in patients with wild-type RAS, but because of various mutations in EGFR signalling routes intracellular signalling sustains even in the absence of ligand binding.

In paediatric oncology, the most advanced concept to target antigens on solid tumours are monoclonal antibodies directed against disialoganglioside GD2 which have emerged as an important treatment option for neuroblastoma, a malignancy characterized by high expression of GD2 on tumour cells [3, 4].

6.2 GD2 Directed Monoclonal Antibody Immunotherapy in Neuroblastoma

In the development of novel immunotherapies for malignant disease, one goal is to find tumor targets that are not widely shared by normal cells. One such target is the carbohydrate disialoganglioside antigen GD2. Several high risk tumors frequently express GD2, making it an attractive target for relatively tumor-specific therapies such as antibody therapy. Disialoganglioside GD2 is ranked in the top 20% (12/75) of tumor-associated antigens in a priority list published by the National Cancer Institute [5]. Expression of GD2 in normal tissues is mostly restricted to neurons that are protected from the effects of intravenous monoclonal antibodies by the blood-brain barrier. However, GD2 is also expressed to a limited extent on normal nerve fibers.

Neuroblastoma is the most common GD2 expressing tumor in childhood and due to its nature remains one of the major challenges in pediatric oncology. Most patients with neuroblastoma are young (median age at diagnosis between 17 and 22 months) and commonly present already with metastatic disease.

The GD2 molecule is also expressed on several other high risk tumors, importantly on approximately 50% of melanomas, as well as on approximately 50% of tumor samples from osteosarcoma and soft tissue sarcomas [6, 7]. In all cases, the tumor-selective expression of this molecule makes GD2 an attractive target for tumor-specific immunotherapy. Therapies using various anti- GD2 -antibodies have been assessed in phase I, phase II and phase III trials, and their safety profile has been established.

6.3 Development of Anti-GD2 Antibodies for the Treatment of Pediatric Malignancies

There are two major streams of clinical developments originating from two research groups engaged in the development of anti-GD2 antibodies. The first report of a monocolonal anti-GD2 antibody describes murine monoclonal antibody 126 (IgM) [8], which was produced against cultured human neuroblastoma cells (LAN-1) and it was found to be specifically directed to disialoganglioside (GD2) antigen. This antibody was and still is broadly used for diagnostic purposes all over the world. As this antibody is an IgM isotype, the development as a cancer therapeutic was not further pursued. One year later further murine monoclonal antibodies were produced against human neuroblastoma cells with specificity against GD2, and one of them was designated 3F8 (IgG3) [9] and 14.18 (IgG3) [10, 11], respectively. High-risk NB patients have been successfully treated with antibodies from both these lines of development. This chapter focusses on the 14.18 antibody family.

The first version of monoclonal antibody 14.18 directed against disialoganglioside GD2 of was a murine IgG3 isotype [11]. As murine IgG3 isotypes are difficult to handle, and generally have poor ADCC effector function, a murine IgG2a class switch variant of 14.18, called 14.G2a, was prepared [12].

The murine antibody 14.G2a was tested in phase I clinical trials and anti-tumor responses were demonstrated. In view of the fact that murine antibodies are generally limited by the development of Human Anti-Mouse Antibody (HAMA) responses in patients, a human/murine chimeric mAb ch14.18 [13] was generated using the murine variable genes of 14.18 and the human constant IgG1 and κ genes, known to effectively mediate antibody dependent cellular cytotoxicity (ADCC) and to maintain complement dependent cytotoxicity (CDC). The antibody was produced in SP2/0 non secreting murine hybridoma cells (ch14.18/SP2/0) and subjected to preclinical evaluation. It has been shown that ch14.18/SP2/0 antibody induces killing of neuroectodermal tumor cells in vitro mediated by ADCC and CDC [14].

After a series of reports concerning effects on survival, the first results of a randomized clinical trial of the chimeric GD2 antibody ch14.18 in combination with Interleukin-2 (IL2) and Granulocyte Macrophage Colony-stimulating Factor (GM-CSF) were recently published and indicated a 2-year EFS of 66% compared to 46% in favor of the immunotherapy arm [15]. This trial led to the approval of ch14.18/SP2/0 (dinutuximab) by FDA for the treatment of children with neuroblastoma. The results regarding the ch14.18 regimen suggest that the toxicity profile (including pain, allergic reactions, and vascular leakage syndrome) is substantial, but manageable and that this treatment may be used for high-risk patients in future [16].

However, it clearly has to be stated that the immunotherapy regimen was associated with important treatment-related clinical toxic effects [15]. Pain of high intensity (grade 3 and 4, where pain grade 3 refers to pain or severe pain or the use of analgesics severely interfering with the activities of daily living, and grade 4 pain refers to disabling pain) that is observed during the immunotherapy with any standard ch14.18 antibody (as well with other anti-GD2 antibodies) is the most debilitating negative side effect of the therapy. In order to maintain the well-being of the treated pediatric patients aggressive and preventive administration of high-dose opioids (morphine) is required as a bolus and by continuous infusion during the antibody treatment cycles in order to maintain effective opioid plasma concentrations.

This pain is associated with anti-GD2 antibody binding to GD2 on nerve cells. The pain occurs in the abdominal region and in lower extremities, requiring the use of morphine for pain relief in all patients. Although the mechanism of pain induction is not entirely clear, immunohistochemical studies of bowel tissue with anti-GD2 antibody revealed staining of fine nerve fibers, suggesting the expression of GD2 on nerve fibers. Pain is likely to result from the binding of anti-GD2 antibody to those nerve fibers with subsequent inflammation [17]. In animal models, which approximate the pain associated with anti-GD2 Ab in humans in terms of timing and quality, anti-GD2-specific biding to Aδ and C pain fibers results in decreased mechanical stimulus thresholds [18]. Therefore, clinical use of anti-GD2 Ab therapy requires heavy co-administration of analgesic drugs including intravenous morphine in order to make this treatment tolerable.

Several modifications of the GD2 antibody ch14.18 (produced in NS0, SP2/0 and CHO cells) have been and are currently used in various nonclinical and clinical studies. Following the change to the state of the art expression host for monoclonal antibodies, namely Chinese Hamster Ovary cells (CHO), anti-GD2 antibody ch14.18/CHO was characterized in vitro as well as in preclinical animal models [19]. A comparison with other preparations of ch14.18 antibody from NS0 and SP2/0 cells revealed similar binding and effector functions, apart from the ADCC activity at low antibody concentrations of ch14.18/CHO which was superior. The affinity of the binding of ch14.18/CHO to the disialoganglioside antigen GD2 was not different compared to ch14.18/SP2/0 and ch14.18/NS0. It mediates both complement dependent cytotoxicity (CDC) and antibody dependent cellular cytotoxicity (ADCC) against GD2 positive neuroectodermal tumor cell lines in vitro.

Ch14.18/CHO was tested in a syngeneic neuroblastoma model. Dose dependent and antigen specific suppression of neuroblastoma metastases was demonstrated in mice treated with ch14.18/CHO. There was no difference in efficacy comparing to mice treated with ch14.18/SP2/0. Furthermore, there was no evidence of toxicity in mice treated with ch14.18/CHO as indicated by a stable body weight after treatment with ch14.18/CHO [19].

The structure of the ch14.18/CHO human/mouse chimeric anti-ganglioside GD2 antibody ch14.18 corresponds to the principle of a chimeric monoclonal antibody with approx. 30% mouse and 70% human sequences (lower left). Constant regions are derived from human IgG1. The 30% mouse sequences were used from murine IgG2a monoclonal antibody 14.G2a (Fig. 6.1, upper left). Humanized versions of 14.18 (Fig. 6.1, upper right) also are in early stages of development. A fully human version does not exist.

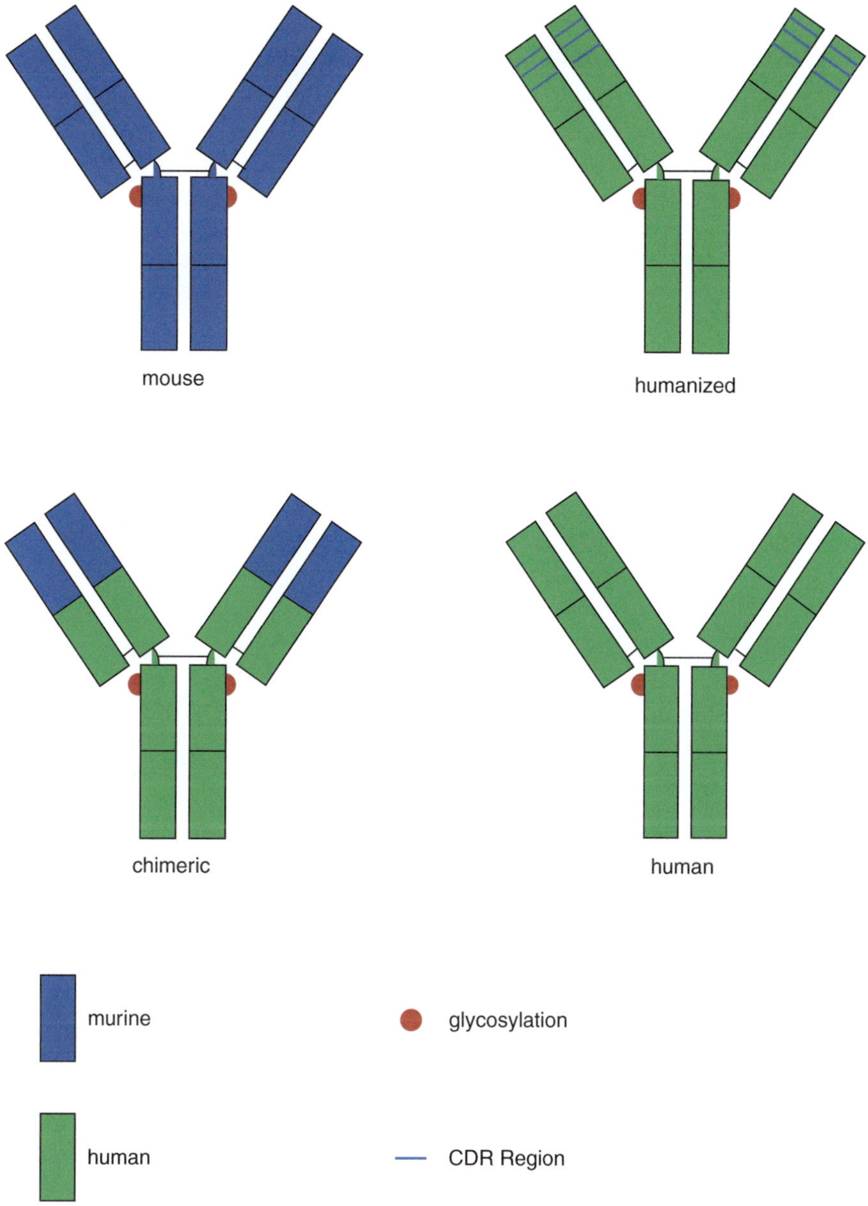

Fig. 6.1 Schematic structure of Mab-variants of the 14.18 family. The structure of the ch14.18/CHO human/mouse chimeric anti-ganglioside GD2 antibody ch14.18 corresponds to the principle of a chimeric monoclonal antibody with approx. 30% mouse and 70% human sequences (*lower left*). Constant regions are derived from human IgG1. The 30% mouse sequences were used from murine IgG2a monoclonal antibody 14.G2a (*upper left*). Humanized versions of 14.18 (*upper right*) also are in early stages of development. A fully human version does not exist. Glycosylation is an important asset to anti-ganglioside GD2 antibodies that impacts on pharmacokinetics, effector function and allergic side effects. The glycosylation pattern varies depending on the production system used for monoclonal antibodies

6.4 Results from Early Clinical Trials with Anti-GD2 Antibodies of the 14.18 Family

Clinical trials provide evidence that variants of the monoclonal antibody 14.18 directed against disialoganglioside GD2 are useful in passive immunotherapy of cancer. Therapeutic responses in patients with GD2-positive tumors have been obtained in clinical studies done with the murine IgG2 class switch variant of 14.18, called 14.G2a, and the human/murine chimeric mAb ch14.18 that was produced in SP2/0 non secreting murine hybridoma cells (ch14.18/SP2/0) as well as in Chinese Hamster Ovary (CHO) cells (ch14.18/CHO).

In several of these studies mAb therapy was given in combination with cytokines such as IL2 and GM-CSF as these cytokines demonstrated to augment natural killer cell-mediated and granulocyte mediated antibody-dependent cellular cytotoxicity (ADCC) in vitro and in vivo [20–23].

In the following an overview on the clinical data obtained with the various variants of the monoclonal antibody 14.18 will be provided.

6.4.1 *Murine Monoclonal Antibody 14.G2a*

Five phase I trials were conducted with the murine mAb 14.G2a (Table 6.1). In one of these studies 14.G2a was administered in combination with cytokines (IL2 and GM-CSF).

Already in these early phase clinical trials response rates were observed in patients who had no other treatment options. This was interpreted by investigators as a clear signal of clinical activity of this treatment concept.

However, there were no randomised controlled clinical trials performed with the murine 14.G2a antibody, to ultimately proof whether the observed response rates would translate into an improved outcome in patients treated with the antibody.

6.4.2 *Chimeric Monoclonal Antibody ch14.18/SP2/0*

The high rate of human anti-mouse immune responses in clinical trials with 14G2a and the progress in antibody engineering triggered the generation of a human/mouse chimeric antibody [13]. Ch14.18 was engineered using the murine variable genes of 14.18 and the human constant IgG1 and kappa genes, known to effectively mediate antibody dependent cellular cytotoxicity (ADCC) and to maintain complement dependent cytotoxicity (CDC). The antibody was produced in SP2/0 non secreting murine hybridoma cells (ch14.18/SP2/0) and subjected to preclinical evaluation. It has been shown that ch14.18/SP2/0 antibody induces killing of neuroectodermal tumour cells in vitro mediated by ADCC and CDC.

Several clinical trials have been performed with ch14.18/SP2/0 used as a single agent (Table 6.2) or in combination with cytokines (Table 6.3).

Table 6.1 Clinical trials with murine 14.G2a antibody

Reference/ protocol no	Phase	Indication	Design	Dosage regimen(s)	Duration	Population (male/female)	Results
[45]	I	Metastatic melanoma	Single centre, open-label, uncontrolled, dose-escalation	1–40 mg/day 14.G2a as 1-h i.v. infusion on days 1, 3, 5, and 8, up to a total dose of 10, 60, 80, 100 or 120 mg/course	1 course	12 adults (m/f)	1 PR, 1 MR, 1 SD
[17]	I	Stage 4 neuroblastoma	Single centre, open-label, uncontrolled	20–60 mg/m^2/day 14.G2a as 5-h i.v. infusion on 5–10 consecutive days, up to total doses of 100–400 mg/m^2/course	1 course	9 patients, 2–12 y (m/f)	2 CR, 2 PR; PK: $t\alpha½ = 0.7–2.0$ h $t\beta½ = 30.1–53.3$ h
[46]	I	Neuroecto-dermal tumors (melanoma, neuroblastoma, osteosarcoma)	Single centre, open-label, uncontrolled, dose-escalation	10, 20 or 40 mg/m^2/day 14.G2a as 24-h i.v. infusion over 5 consecutive days, up to a total dose of 50, 100 or 200 mg/m^2/course	1 course	18 patients (11 melanoma, 5neuroblastoma, 2 osteosarcoma), 4–72 y (m/f)	2 PR (neuroblastoma), 3 MR (2 melanoma, 1 osteosarcoma), 4 SD; MTD: 20 mg/m^2/day
[47]	I	Neuroblastoma, osteosarcoma	Single centre, open-label, uncontrolled, dose-escalation	5–100 mg/m^2/day 14.G2a as 5-h i.v. infusion on 5 consecutive days, up to a total dose of 25, 50, 100, 250 or 500 mg/m^2/course	1–2 courses	15 patients, 3–15 y (m/f)	PK: $t\alpha½ = 2.8 \pm 2.8$ h $t\beta½ = 18.3 \pm 11.8$ h
[48] CCG-0901	I/Ib	Refractory neuroblastoma, osteosarcoma	Multi-centre, open-label, uncontrolled, dose-escalation	Regimen A: 2, 10, 15, 20, 30, 40, or60 mg/m^2/day 14.G2a as 2-h i.v. infusion on days 8–12 + i.v. IL2 on days 1–4, 8–11, 15–18; total dose 14.G2a: 10–300 mg/m^2/course Regimen B: 15 mg/m^2/day 14.G2a as 2-h infusion on days 1–5 + regimen A (15 mg/m^2/day 14.G2a) in weeks 5–10; total dose 14.G2a: 75 mg/m^2/course Regimen C: regimen A (15 mg/m^2/day 14.G2a) + s.c. GM-CSF (days 1–19); total dose 14.G2a: 75 mg/m^2/course	1–3 courses	33 patients, 1–16 y (m/f)	1 CR (osteosarcoma), 1 PR (neuroblastoma), 7 SD decrease in the number of neuroblastoma cells in bone marrow in 3 patients; MTD: 15 mg/m^2/day

CR complete response, *MR* mixed response, *MTD* maximum tolerated dose, *PD* progressive disease, *PK* pharmacokinetics, *PR* partial response, *SD* stable disease

Table 6.2 Clinical trials with mAb ch14.18/SP2/0

Reference/ protocol no	Phase	Indication	Design, type of control	Dosage regimen(s)	Duration	Population (male/ female)	Results
[24]	I	Metastatic melanoma	Single centre, open-label, uncontrolled	5–45 mg/course (single dose) ch14.18/SP2/0 or 50 mg/day on 2 consecutive days, as 4-h i.v. infusion	1 course	13 adults	PK: tα½ = 24 ± 1 h, tβ½ = 181 ± 73 h
[25]	I	Stage 4 neuroblastoma	Single centre, open-label, uncontrolled, dose-escalation	30, 40 or 50 $mg/m^2/day$ ch14.18/SP2/0 as 8-h i.v. infusion over 55 consecutive days	1–4 courses	9 patients, 2–10 y (m/f)	2 CR, 2 PR, 1 minor response, 1 SD; MTD: 50 $mg/m^2/day$
[26]	I	Refractory neuroblastoma, osteosarcoma	Single-centre, open-label, uncontrolled, dose-escalation	Neuroblastoma: 10–100 $mg/m^2/day$ ch14.18/SP2/0 as 1- to 5-h i.v. infusion on 1 to 4 (consecutive) days; total doses: 10, 20, 50, 100 or 200 $mg/m^2/course$ Osteosarcoma: 50 $mg/m^2/day$ ch14.18/SP2/0 as 5-h i.v. infusion over 4 consecutive days	1–5 courses	10 patients with neuroblastoma, 2–11 y; 1 patient with osteosarcoma, 22 y (m/f)	1 PR, 4 MR, 1 SD PK: tα½ = 3.4 ± 3.1 h, tβ½ = 66.6 ± 27.4 h
[27] [28] NB90, NB97	II	Stage 4 neuroblastoma	Multi-centre, open-label, controlled, retrospective	20 $mg/m^2/day$ ch14.18/SP2/0 as 8- to 12-h i.v. infusion on 5 consecutive days in 2 month cycles	6 courses	334 patients (166 ch14.18/SP2/0; 99 MT; 69 no treatment), 1–20 y (m/f)	9-y-EFS ch14.18/SP2/0: 41±3% MT: 31±5% (p = 0.147) No treatment: 32±6% (p = 0.038) 9-y-OS ch14.18/SP2/0: 46±4% MT: 34±5% (p = 0.023) No treatment: 35±6% (p = 0.015)

CR complete response, *EFS* event free survival, *MR* mixed response, *MT* maintenance chemotherapy, *MTD* maximum tolerated dose, *OS* overall survival, *PR* partial response, *SD* stable disease

Table 6.3 Clinical trials with mAb ch14.18/SP2/0 in combination with cytokines

Reference/ Protocol no	Phase	Indication	Design	Dosage Regimen(s)	Duration	Population	Results
[30]	I	Metastatic melanoma	Single centre, open-label, uncontrolled, dose-escalation	15, 30, 45 or 60 mg/m^2 (single dose) ch14.18/SP2/0 as 4-h i.v. infusion + GM-CSF daily for a total of 14 days starting 1 day after ch14.18/SP2/0 treatment	1–2 courses	16 adults (m/f)	PK: $t½ = 123 \pm 29$ h MTD: 45 mg/m^2/day No response
[31]	1b	Refractory melanoma	Single centre,open-label, uncontrolled, dose-escalation	2, 5, 7.5 or 10 mg/m^2/day ch14.18/SP2/0 as daily 4-h i.v. infusion for 5 consecutive days before, during or following i.v. IL2	1–3 courses	24 patients, 29–75 y (m/f)	1 CR, 1 PR, 8 SD MTD: 7.5 mg/m^2/day
[23]	I	Neuroblastoma	Multi-centre, open-label, uncontrolled, dose-escalation	20, 30, 40 or 50 mg/m^2/day ch14.18/SP2/0 as 5- to 10-h i.v. infusion on 4 consecutive days + GMCSF	6 courses	19 patients, 2–15 y (m/f)	MTD: 40 mg/m^2/day × 4 days
[32] A0935A	I	Stage 4 neuroblastoma	Multi-centre, open-label, uncontrolled, dose-escalation	20, 25 or 40 mg/m^2/day ch14.18/SP2/0 as 5–20-h i.v. infusion on 4 consecutive days in 3 or 4 week cycles + GM-CSF (cycles 1, 3 and 5) + i.v. IL2 (cycles 2 and 4) + 13-cis-RA	3–6 courses	23 patients, 1–14 y (m/f)	MTD: 25 mg/m^2/day × 4 days
[49]	II	Recurrent/ refractory neuroblastoma	Open-label, uncontrolled	50 mg/m^2/day ch14.18/SP2/0 as 5-h i.v. infusion on 4 consecutive days + GM-CSF	-	32 patients	1 CR, 3 PRs, 1 MR
[15] ANBL0032 NCT00026312	III	Neuroblastoma	Multi-centre, open-label, randomized, controlled	13-cis-RA (standard therapy) ± 25 mg/m^2/day ch14.18/SP2/0 i.v. infusion on 4 consecutive days in 4-week cycles and in combination with alternating GM-CSF (cylces 1, 3 and 5) and i.v. IL2 (cycles 2 and 4)	6 courses 13-cis-RA ± 5 courses ch14.18 IT	226 patients (113 patients Standard, 113 patients ch14.18 IT), < 31 y (m/f)	2-y-EFS ch14.18 IT: 66±5% Standard: 46±5% ($p = 0.01$) 2-y-OS ch14.18 IT: 86±4% Standard: 75±5% ($p = 0.02$)

13-cis-RA 13-cis-retinoic acid, *CR* complete response, *EFS* event free survival, *MR* mixed response, *MTD* maximum tolerated dose, *OS* overall survival, *PR* partial response, *SD* stable disease, *IT* immunotherapy

6.4.3 *Treatment with Antibody ch14.18/SP2/0 Used as Single Agent*

The first single agent clinical trial with ch14.18/SP2/0 was conducted in 13 adult patients with antigen GD2 positive malignant melanoma [24] (Table 6.2). The antibody was given as a single dose of 5–100 mg. Infusion-related abdominal/pelvic pain syndrome was observed and treated with intravenous morphine for control. First pharmacokinetic data were reported (Table 6.2). Eight of thirteen patients developed a human anti chimeric antibody response directed at the variable region of ch14.18/SP2/0. Clinical antitumor responses were not observed but the antibody was detectable on tumor cells analyzed by fluorescent activated cell sorter.

With this reported first in man experience, ch14.18/SP2/0 was also assessed in paediatric indications, namely neuroblastoma and osteosarcoma [25, 26]. In the first trial, nine patients with stage 4 neuroblastoma were treated with 19 courses of human/mouse chimeric monoclonal antiganglioside GD2 antibody ch14.18 and a maximum tolerated dose (MTD) per injection of 50 mg/m^2/day was reported. None of the patients developed any evidence of human anti-mouse antibody (HAMA) response.

In the second trial, ten patients with refractory neuroblastoma and one patient with osteosarcoma were treated, and the toxicities were found to be dose-dependent and rarely noted at dosages of 20 mg/m^2 and less.

In contrast to melanoma patients, the use of ch14.18/SP2/0 induced responses in neuroblastoma patients in both trials and the conclusions were that clinical activity was observed and that further trials of ch14.18/SP2/0 were warranted in patients with neuroblastoma.

Subsequent to these early phase clinical trials, ch14.18/SP2/0 was assessed by the German cooperative group within the NB97 study. The antibody was given to patients with stage 4 neuroblastoma, older than 1 year who underwent consolidation treatment by high dose chemotherapy followed by autologous stem cell transplantation and who had completed initial treatment without event. Ch14.18/SP2/0 was scheduled in a dose of 20 mg/m^2 during 5 days in six cycles every 2 months (100 mg/m^2/cycle). The study was not randomized, but patients who did not receive ch14.18 for several reasons served as non-randomised controls. Of 334 assessable patients, 166 received ch14.18, 99 received 12-months of low-dose maintenance chemotherapy instead, and 69 patients received no additional treatment.

This retrospective analysis was initially reported in 2004 [27], and then re-analysed in 2011 [28].

In the first report in 2004 [27], univariate analysis revealed similar 3-year event-free survival (EFS) of 46.5% ± 4.1%, 44.4% ± 4.9%, 37.1% ± 5.9% for patients treated with antibody ch14.18, maintenance chemotherapy (MT), and no additional therapy, respectively (log-rank test, P = .314). For overall survival (OS), ch14.18 treatment (3-year OS, 68.5% ± 3.9%) was superior to MT (3-year OS, 56.6% ± 5.0%) or no additional therapy (3-year OS, 46.8% ± 6.2%; log-rank test, P = .018). As multivariate analysis failed to demonstrate an advantage of antibody treatment for EFS and OS it was concluded that ch14.18/SP2/0 had no clear impact on the outcome of patients.

However, in 2011 [28] the median observation time reached 11.11 years and results as well as the interpretation of the results changed. The 9-year event-free survival rates were 41 ± 4%, 31 ± 5%, and 32 ± 6% for ch14.18/SP2/0, NB90 MT, and no consolidation, respectively ($p = 0.098$). In contrast to the report in 2004, ch14.18/SP2/0 treatment improved the long-term outcome compared to no additional therapy ($p = 0.038$) and the overall survival was better in the ch14.18/SP2/0 treated group (9-y-OS 46 ± 4%) compared to NB90 MT (34 ± 5%, $p = 0.026$) and to no consolidation (35 ± 6%, $p = 0.019$). The conclusion from this follow-up analysis was that immunotherapy ch14.18/SP2/0 used as a single agent, without cytokine, may prevent late relapse.

In summary, although ch14.18/SP2/0 was never tested as a single immunotherapeutic agent against no ch14.18/SP2/0 treatment in a randomized trial, clinical activity observed in the Phase I studies [25, 26] and the efficacy reported in the Phase II retrospective analysis [27, 28] suggests single agent activity of this agent in neuroblastoma patients.

6.4.4 Combination of ch14.18/SP2/0 with Cytokines

The rationale for using ch14.18/SP2/0 in combination with cytokines was driven by preclinical and clinical research demonstrating an increased ADCC response when anti-GD2 antibodies were combined with interleukin-2 (IL-2) [21, 29] or GM-CSF [22]. Based on these findings several Phase I clinical trials were initiated first in adult patients with metastatic melanoma [30, 31] followed by studies in paediatric patients with neuroblastoma [23, 32] (Table 6.3).

In melanoma patients ($n = 24$), ch14.18/SP2/0 (dose level, 2–10 mg/m^2/day for 5 days) was combined with a continuous infusion of IL-2 (1.5×10^6 units/m^2/day) given 4 days/week for 3 weeks [31]. The ch14.18/SP2/0 antibody was scheduled to be given for 5 days, before, during, or following initial systemic IL-2 treatment. The ch14.18/SP2/0 MTD was 7.5 mg/m^2/day, and 15 patients were treated at that dose. Serum samples obtained following ch14.18/SP2/0 infusions induced in vitro antibody-dependent cellular cytotoxicity. Antitumor activity was seen (Table 6.3) and it was concluded that IL-2 and ch14.18/SP2/0 treatment induces immune activation in all, and antitumor activity in some, melanoma patients.

Anti-GD2 antibody ch14.18/SP2/0 was also tested in combination with GM-CSF in patients with metastatic malignant melanoma ($n = 16$) [30]. Patients receive escalating doses of ch14.18 (15–60 mg/m^2) administered intravenously for 4 h on day 1. Twenty-four hours later, subcutaneous injections of recombinant human GM-CSF (rhGM-CSF) were administered daily for a total of 14 days. Dose-limiting toxicity was observed at 60 mg/m^2 of antibody. Significant enhancement of in vitro and in vivo monocyte and neutrophil tumoricidal activity and antibody-dependent cellular cytotoxicity along with significant elevations in C-reactive protein and neopterin were observed. Despite these immunological and biological changes, no antitumor activity was seen. In short, the combination of ch14.18 and rhGM-CSF resulted in toxicity similar to that observed with ch14.18 alone without apparent improvement in tumor response.

In paediatric neuroblastoma patients (n = 19) who had recently completed hematopoietic stem-cell transplantation the MTD of ch14.18/SP2/0 in combination with GM-CSF was determined [23]. Patients received GM-CSF 250 μg/m²/day starting at least 3 days before and continued for 3 days after the completion of antibody treatment. Ch14.18/SP2/0 was applied in 5 h infusions daily for 4 consecutive days at dose levels of 20, 30, 40, and 50 mg/m²/d. Patients were allowed to receive up to six 4-day courses. A total of 79 courses were administered. Three dose-limiting toxicities were observed among six patients at 50 mg/m²/d. A HACA response was observed in 28% of patients. In conclusion, the treatment was manageable at the MTD of 40 mg/m²/day for 4 days when given in this schedule with GM-CSF.

Based on these clinical Phase I trials, it was concluded that ch14.18/SP2/0 can be administered in combination with IL2 or GMCSF with an acceptable and manageable toxicity profile, and that the approach to combine the antibody with cytokines warrants further evaluation in a prospective clinical trial.

At the time of planning such a prospective trial in the year 2000, a new cooperative group system for clinical research formed in North America. By the mid-1990s there were four cooperative groups focused on childhood cancer research. Two groups, the Children's Cancer Study Group (CCG) and the Paediatric Oncology Group (POG) studied a diverse array of childhood cancers including neuroblastoma, while two other groups, the Intergroup rhabdomyosarcoma Study Group (IRSG) and the National Wilms Tumour Study Group (NWTS) were cancer-specific. In 2000, these four paediatric groups voluntarily merged to create the Children's Oncology Group (COG).

At that time COG planned the ANBL0032 study aiming at a prospective randomized assessment of immunotherapy with ch14.18/SP2/0 in combination with cytokines (IL2; GM-CSF) in children with high risk neuroblastoma. In the process of study planning, COG could not make a clear decision as to which cytokine to prioritise for testing. Scientifically, there was no clear advantage of either cytokine over the other in preclinical testing or early phase clinical trials. As there were clinical research groups working with both combination approaches that were now unified under the roof of the COG, the group agreed to compromise by using ch14.18/SP2/0 with GMCSF and IL2 in alternating cycles.

This approach was first assessed in a Phase I trial [32] using 20, 25 or 40 mg/m²/day ch14.18/SP2/0 as 5–20-h i.v. infusion on 4 consecutive days in combination with s.c. GM-CSF (cycles 1, 3 and 5) or i.v. IL2 (cycles 2 and 4) and oral 13-cis-RA. The MTD of ch14.18/SP2/0 was determined to be 25 mg/m²/day for 4 days given concurrently with 4.5 × 10⁶ IU/m²/day of IL-2 for 4 days. IL-2 was also given at a dose of 3 × 10⁶ IU/m²/day for 4 days starting 1 week before ch14.18/SP2/0.

The schedule and dose from that Phase I study was then selected by COG to determine whether adding ch14.18, GM-CSF, and interleukin-2 to standard isotretinoin therapy after intensive multimodal therapy would improve outcomes in high-risk neuroblastoma [15]. Patients with high-risk neuroblastoma who had a response to induction therapy and stem-cell transplantation were randomly assigned, to receive standard therapy (six cycles of isotretinoin) or immunotherapy (six cycles of isotretinoin and five concomitant cycles of ch14.18 in combination with alternating GM-CSF and interleukin-2).

A total of 226 eligible patients were randomly assigned to a treatment group. The median duration of follow-up was 2.1 years. Immunotherapy was superior to standard therapy with regard to rates of event-free survival (66 ± 5% vs. 46 ± 5% at 2 years, P = 0.01) and overall survival (86 ± 4% vs. 75 ± 5% at 2 years, P = 0.02). In conclusion, immunotherapy with ch14.18, GM-CSF, and interleukin-2 was associated with a significantly improved outcome as compared with standard therapy in patients with high-risk neuroblastoma. The most recent analysis of this data (March 2014), showed a persistent OS benefit at 5 years (74.2 vs. 57%, p = 0.03), but by 3 years, the difference in EFS (62.8 vs. 50.9%) had lost significance (European Medicines Agency Assessment report 2015).

As this combination approach with three immunologically active substances it remains somewhat unclear which are essential for the observed effect. However, the study lead to the approval of this combined treatment by the Food and Drug Administration and the European Medicines Agency.

6.4.5 Development of the Monoclonal Antibody Ch14.18/CHO

In Europe, ch14.18/SP2/0 was not available for clinical trials in 2000. The production for clinical trials in the United States was established at The Frederick National Laboratory for Cancer Research (FNLCR), and it was not possible to either gain access to study drug for European investigators nor was it possible to transfer the production process to a European contract manufacturer.

Therefore, the International Society of Pediatric Oncology European Neuroblastoma Group (SIOPEN) commissioned a Good Manufacturing Practice (GMP) production of ch14.18 Ab in the most commonly used mammalian cell line for industrial production of recombinant protein therapeutics, Chinese hamster ovary (CHO) cells [19]. Such a major change in the antibody production process requires preclinical and clinical reevaluation, including its pharmacokinetics (PK) and pharmacodynamics (PD). For that reason, a Phase 1 bridging study was initiated to assess safety, PK and activity profiles of the recloned Ab ch14.18/CHO [33]. Analysis of 16 patients revealed that the toxicity profile, clinical activity and PK of ch14.18/CHO given as 8 h short term infusion (STI) on 5 consecutive days (5 × 20 mg/m^2) were comparable to ch14.18 produced in SP2/0 cells, allowing for approval of the use in Phase II and Phase III randomized clinical trials (Table 6.4).

The **Phase I** Study (EudraCT 2005-001267-63) (Table 6.4) was an investigator-initiated, phase I, multi-center, open-label, dose escalation study, designed to evaluate safety, immunologic activation, immunogenicity and antitumor responses, and to characterize the PK profile of ch14.18/CHO. According to the inclusion criteria

Table 6.4 Clinical trials with ch14.18/CHO short term infusion

EudraCT no. Sponsor no. Sponsor	Phase	Indication	Design	Dosage regimen(s)	Duration	Population	Status/results
2005–001267-63 SIOPENRNET001 St. Anna Kinderkrebs-forschung	I	Relapsed or refractory neuroblastoma	Multi-center, open-label, uncontrolled, dose-escalation	10, 20 or 30 mg/m²/day ch14.18/CHO administered as 8-h i.v. infusion on 5 consecutive days in 4–6-week cycles Total dose ch14.18/CHO per cycle: 50, 100 or 150 mg/m²	3 cycles	16 patients > 1y and ≤ 21y (m/f)	Completed; Confirmed responses in mIBG: 1 VGPR, 1 PR in 7 evaluable patients
2009–015936-14 University Hospital Tübingen	II	Relapsed or refractory neuroblastoma	Multi-center, open-label, uncontrolled	20 mg/m²/day ch14.18/CHO administered as 8-h i.v. infusion on 5 consecutive days in 4 week cycles + s.c. IL2 (cycles 4 to 6 only) Total dose ch14.18/CHO per cycle: 100 mg/m²	6 cycles	35 patients ≤ 21y (m/f)	Ongoing (14 patients enrolled as of April 17th, 2012)
2006–001489-17 SIOPENRNET003 HR-NBL-1/SIOPEN St. Anna Kinderkrebs-forschung	III	High-risk neuroblastoma	Multi-center, open-label, randomized, controlled	Study Protocol Amendment 2: 13-cis-RA ± 20 mg/m²/day ch14.18/CHO administered as 8-h i.v. infusion on 5 consecutive days in 4 week cycles Total dose ch14.18/CHO per cycle: 100 mg/m²	5 cycles	36 patients < 21y (m/f)	Completed; follow-up for EFS ongoing Confirmed responses in mIBG: 5 CR, 1 PR, 1 MR in 11 evaluable patients
2006–001489-17 SIOPENRNET003 HR-NBL-1/SIOPEN St. Anna Kinderkrebs-forschung				Study Protocol Amendment 4: 13-cis-RA + 20 mg/m²/day ch14.18/CHO administered as 8-h i.v. infusion on 5 consecutive days in 4 week cycles ± s.c. IL2 Total dose ch14.18/CHO per cycle: 100 mg/m²	5 cycles	400 patients < 21y (m/f)	Ongoing (293 patients enrolled as of September 14th, 2012)

13-cis-RA 13-cis-retinoic acid, *CR* complete response, *EFS* event-free survival, *mIBG* metaiodobenzylguanidine, *MRI* Magnetic Resonance Imaging, *PR* partial response, *SD* stable disease male and female patients 1–21 years of age with relapsed or refractory high-risk neuroblastoma were enrolled. Patients without progression of disease were allowed to receive up to 3 cycles of ch14.18/CHO [33].

Three dose levels were evaluated: 10, 20 and 30 mg/m²/day ch14.18/CHO, corresponding to total doses of 50, 100 and 150 mg/m²/cycle. 10 mg/m²/day ch14.18/CHO was considered to be the safe starting dose as this was 50% below the dose of a ch14.18 antibody produced in SP2/0 cells (ch14.18/SP2/0) that has already been investigated in a large cohort of patients [27] (Table 6.2).

The studied compound ch14.18/CHO was administered as an 8-h i.v. infusion for 5 consecutive days in 4–6 week cycles. The study was conducted in Austria, Germany and Italy. In the study, 16 patients with a median age of 7.6 years (range 3.8–17.3 years) were enrolled. Fourteen patients had stage 4, one stage 2b and one stage 3 disease at first diagnosis.

In total 41 cycles (10 × 3 cycles, 5 × 2 cycles, 1 × 1 cycle) were administered within the study period. Supportive care provided to patients followed written standards. In particular, the expected visceral pain was controlled by the preventive application of i.v. morphine via continuous infusion. In cases where a patient still experienced pain, the ch14.18/CHO infusion was interrupted for a 30 min period and a non-opioid analgesic was given as an adjunct. The standardized treatment regimen in cases of anaphylactic reactions included anti-histamines.

Compared to the first treatment cycle, fever and pain were less severe in subsequent cycles.

The safe dose was confirmed at 20 mg/m²/day. The dose level 30 mg/m²/day had a higher rate of fever, CRP elevations and acute allergic reactions. The high prevalence of hematologic abnormalities including leukopenia, thrombocytopenia, anemia, neutropenia and infection has not been reported in other trials. These findings were not associated with ch14.18/CHO treatment. They were related to the advanced stage neuroblastoma also including bone marrow metastases. There were no treatment related deaths, and all toxicities were reversible and similar to those reported for ch14.18/SP2/0 [15, 27].

Thirty-two cycles administered to 14 neuroblastoma patients could be evaluated for pharmacokinetic analyses. Furthermore, sera from 14 patients were screened for the development of Human Anti-Chimeric Antibodies (HACA) against ch14.18/CHO and antibodies directed specifically to the antigen binding variable regions of ch14.18/CHO (anti-idiotypic antibodies) by ELISA.

The analysis of ch14.18/CHO pharmacokinetics revealed a ß t½ of 76.9 h ± 52.5 h for ch14.18/CHO, which is comparable to t½ of ch14.18/SP2/0, that was reported to be 66.6 h ± 27.4 h [34] (Table 6.2).

The mean peak plasma concentration in patients treated with 20 mg/m² ch14.18/CHO (n = 8) was 16.5 μg/mL ± 5.9 μg/mL, ranging from 7.4 μg/mL to 26.6 μg/mL, compared to 19.3 μg/mL ± 6.0 μg/mL, ranging from 12.3 μg/mL to 23.7 μg/mL, in patients receiving ch14.18/SP2/0 at the 20 mg/m² dose level.

A comparison of half-lives between cycles indicated that there was a tendency towards accelerated half-lives in subsequent cycles. Therefore, in order to compare pharmacokinetics of ch14.18/CHO and ch14.18/SP2/0, only the first treatment cycles were taken into account. In three out of fourteen patients (21%) human anti-chimeric antibody responses were detected. HACA positive patients developed increasing titers over time, in subsequent cycles. The development of HACA was associated with decreased half-life and AUC in two of these three patients.

In contrast, HACA negative patients did not show a significant decrease of half-life or AUC over 3 cycles. All three patients who developed HACA were tested positive also for anti-idiotypic antibodies.

In six out of sixteen patients (38%) anti tumor responses were noted by the treating physicians. A central mIBG review confirmed responses in two out of seven patients (29%) with evaluable scans, one very good partial response (VGPR) (dose level 20 mg/m^2) and one partial response (PR) (dose level 30 mg/m^2).

With a median follow-up of 39 months, 11 out of 16 patients (69%) died from disease progression. There were no deaths reported while on protocol therapy or within 1 month following completion of protocol therapy.

The **Phase II** Study (EudraCT 2009-015936-14) is an investigator-initiated, multi-center, multinational, open-label trial. It is designed to evaluate safety, immunologic activation, pharmacokinetics and anti-tumor responses of ch14.18/CHO in combination with s.c. IL2 in patients with relapsed or refractory neuroblastoma after haploidentical stem cell transplantation.

Patients enrolled in this study receive 6 cycles of 20 mg/m^2/day ch14.18/CHO administered as an 8 h i.v. infusion for 5 consecutive days in 28-day cycles. This corresponds to a total dose of 100 mg/m^2/cycle ch14.18/CHO. IL2 is given in cycles 4–6.

Thirty-five evaluable male and female patients up to 21 years of age will be recruited. They are enrolled in two stages with the possibility of stopping the study early for lack of efficacy.

Treatment success is defined as a patient receiving the full protocol treatment, still alive 180 days after end of treatment without progression and without unacceptable toxicity and acute graft versus host disease (GvHD) ≥ Grade III or extensive chronic GvHD. The study is ongoing.

The **Phase III** study (EudraCT 2006-001489-17) is an investigator-initiated, multi-center, open-label, randomized, controlled trial. The design of the study was a fully powered Phase III clinical trial to compare ch14.18/CHO therapy with the standard treatment (13-cis RA).

This phase was activated in March 2006 (study protocol amendment 2), and the first patient was treated with ch14.18/CHO in the second quarter of 2009. Only 36 patients had been enrolled in Austria, Greece, Israel, Italy and Slovakia from March 2006 to July 2009. Eighteen patients were randomized to receive ch14.18/CHO and 13-cis-RA; the other eighteen patients received 13-cis-RA alone. After this short recruitment period of a few months, the immunotherapy scheme had to be revised, after data from clinical trial ANBL0032 conducted by the Children's Oncology Group (COG) became available. In view of the significant improvement in EFS and OS reported in this study, it was considered unacceptable to continue the European trial with the original randomisation, as it was considered that all patients should receive antibody.

In the COG study it was not possible to deduce which of the three agents used in the immunotherapy arm (ch14.18/SP2/0, IL2, GM-CSF) contributed to which extent to the observed efficacy. However, it was clear that the additional cyctokines (particularly IL-2) contributed to toxicity. It was therefore decided that all patients in the European trial should receive ch14.18/CHO antibody immunotherapy, and that the benefit of additional IL-2 should be tested in a randomised way. As intravenous IL2, as it was administered in the COG-study immunotherapy arm, is toxic and GM-CSF is not commercially available in Europe, it was decided to build on previous SIOPEN experience with s.c. IL2 [35], and patients were randomized to receive ch14.18/CHO with and without s.c.IL2 administration. All patients were treated with 13cis-RA.

The initial part of the study aimed to test immunotherapy with ch14.18/CHO, following myeloablative therapy (MAT), in addition to differentiation therapy with 13-cis-RA with respect to improve 3-year event-free survival (EFS) in male and female patients < 21 years of age with high-risk neuroblastoma compared to differentiation therapy with 13-cis-RA alone.

The revised study design was initiated in July 2009 (study protocol amendment 4) with the main objective to test the hypothesis that the addition of s.c. IL2 to immunotherapy with ch14.18/CHO in addition to differentiation therapy with 13-cis-RA following myeloablative therapy (MAT) and autologous stem cell rescue (SCR), improves EFS in patients with high-risk neuroblastoma.

Ireland, Israel, Italy, Norway, Spain, Switzerland and the UK already have been randomized to receive the revised immunotherapy scheme consisting of 13-cis-RA and ch14.18/CHO with or without s.c. IL2.

6.5 Long Term Infusion (LTI) of ch14.18/CHO

One major obstacle associated with anti-GD2 Ab therapies is the induction of neuropathic pain [15], which is an on-target side effect not observed with other human/mouse chimeric mAbs. In animal models, which approximate the pain associated with anti-GD2 Ab in humans in terms of timing and quality, GD2-specific binding to Aδ—and C pain fibres results in decreased mechanical stimulus thresholds. SIOPEN initiated a novel treatment schedule aiming at a reduction of toxicity. Instead of STI over 5 days (5 × 20 mg/m^2/d, 8 h infusion), neuroblastoma patient were treated by long term infusion with ch14.18/CHO (LTI Study, Table 6.5).

The LTI study (EudraCT 2009-018077-31) started as a phase I/II dose-finding study with a confirmatory phase, based on the continuous infusion scheme. It is an investigator-initiated, multi-centre, open-label, dose-escalation trial, designed to find a tolerable treatment schedule that reduces the pain-toxicity profile of ch14.18/CHO whilst maintaining immunomodulatory efficacy.

In the dose finding Phase, patients with relapsed/refractory neuroblastoma were planned to be treated with 7, 10 or 15 mg/m^2/day ch14.18/CHO administered by

Table 6.5 Clinical trials with ch14.18/CHO long term infusion

EudraCT no. Sponsor no. Sponsor	Phase	Indication	Design	Dosage regimen(s)	Duration	Population	Status/results
2009–018077-31 LTI Study St. Anna Kinderkrebs-forschung Vienna	I/II	Relapsed or refractory neuroblastoma	Multi-center, open-label, uncontrolled	7, 10 or 15 mg/m²/day ch14.18/CHO administered by continuous infusion over 10 to 21 days in five 35 to 50-day cycles (=100, 150 or 210 mg/m²/cycle). Treatment combined with 2 × 5 days s.c. IL2 (6 × 10⁶ IU/m²) (=60 mg/m²/cycle. 13-cis-RA (160 mg/m²/day; 14 days)	5 cycles	24 patients dose finding 20 patients confirmation 44 patients ≤ 21y (m/f)	Safe and effective dose: 10 mg/m²/day administered by continuous infusion over 10 days in 5 week intervals
	II expansion cohort			10 mg/m²/day ch14.18/CHO administered by continuous infusion over 10 days in five 35 day cycles (=100 mg/m²/cycle). Treatment combined with 2 × 5 days s.c. IL2 (6 × 10⁶ IU/m²) (=60 mg/m²/cycle. 13-cis-RA (160 mg/m²/day; 14 days)		80 patients	Recruitment completed
	II randomized cohort		Multi-center, open-label, controlled	Dosage as expansion cohort. ch14.18 ± IL2		160 patients	ongoing
2014–000588-42 Single agent study University Medicine Greifswald	II	Relapsed or refractory neuroblastoma	Multi-center, open-label, uncontrolled	10 mg/m²/day ch14.18/CHO; continuous infusion; 10 days; 35 day cycles (=100 mg/m²/cycle)	5 cycles	40 patients	ongoing
2006–00[illegible]489-17 SIOPENRNET003 HR-NBL-1/SIOPEN St. Anna Kinderkrebs-forschung Vienna	III	High-risk neuroblastoma	Multi-center, open-label, randomized, controlled	Study Protocol Amendment 6: 13-cis-RA + 20 mg/m²/day ch14.18/CHO administered as 10 day continuous i.v. infusion in 5 week cycles ± s.c. IL2 Total dose ch14.18/CHO/cycle: 100 mg/m²	5 cycles	400 patients < 21y (m/f)	ongoing

continuous infusion over 10–21 days in five 35 to 50-day cycles (= 100, 150 or 210 mg/m^2/cycle). Treatment combined with 2 × 5 days s.c. IL2 (6 × 10^6 IU/m^2) (= 60 mg/m^2/cycle. 13-cis-RA (160 mg/m^2/day; 14 days).

The study was activated in December 2011 and is ongoing in Austria, Germany, France, Israel, Italy, Poland, Belgium, Spain, Australia, Hong Kong and UK.

Secondary study objectives are to evaluate pain intensity and pain relief by appropriate medication with a validated self-report tool, to determine immunologic activation, immunogenicity and ch14.18/CHO pharmacokinetics, and to assess anti-tumour responses.

Furthermore, the chosen ch14.18/CHO infusion schedule is examined in an expansion cohort of 20 and further 80 patients to confirm the results from the dose schedule finding.

The LTI study was then transferred into a controlled trial in order to determine the role of IL2 in the long term continuous infusion setting of ch14.18/CHO and the trial is still ongoing.

A single agent Phase II study was initiated based on the scientific advice of competent authorities to confirm the results of the LTI study, but using ch14.18/CHO based on the continuous infusion scheme without IL2 and without 13-cis RA. The study is an open-label, multi-center trial, designed to evaluate the efficacy of ch14.18/CHO continuous infusion in patients with refractory or relapsed neuroblastoma. The primary endpoint is the overall response rate.

Secondary study objectives are to evaluate the pharmacodynamic activity (NK-cell activation, ADCC, CDC, sIL2-receptor, whole blood test) pharmacokinetics, immunogenicity (HAMA, HACA), and safety and tolerability specifically taking into account pain intensity and pain relief by appropriate medication.

Based on the favourable toxicity profile observed with LTI of ch14.18/CHO in ongoing Phase II studies, the Phase III study (EudraCT 2006-001489-17) was amended to test the LTI concept in frontline neuroblastoma patients randomizing LTI of ch14.18/CHO with and without IL2. This study is also ongoing.

6.6 Future Directions

Monoclonal antibodies with enhanced effector functions are of particular interest as future options to further increase the effect. In this respect, recombinant antibody-cytokine fusion proteins, i.e. immunocytokines (ICs) [36], and trifunctional antibodies (trAbs) [37] combining tumour specificity with a T-cell activating functionality are of particular interest. Both classes of antibody constructs are capable of linking innate with adaptive immunity. Immunocytokines achieve sufficient concentrations of cytokines in the tumour microenvironment to enhance the stimulation of a cellular immune response against tumours. This contrasts with passive immunotherapy by antibodies directed against tumour-associated antigens, which utilizes the natural effector mechanisms of antibodies to destroy tumour cells without additional stimulation. More important, immunocytokines provide a tool for active tumour immunotherapy by increasing the cytokine concentration in the tumour microenvironment and thereby potentiating immunogenicity of syngeneic tumours followed in some cases by T cell activation and a subsequent memory immune response. Immunocytokines are neither limited by a patient-specific modus operandi nor by the antigenic heterogeneity of tumour cells, because only a limited number of antigen sites are required as their docking sites. Once placed into the tumour microenvironment, immunocytokines are capable of activating and expanding a variety of immune effectors, including T lymphocytes, natural killer cells, macrophages, and granulocytes, and thereby eradicate tumour cells and their metastases. This effect can amplify insufficient T cell immune responses previously induced by a cancer vaccine and lead to effective tumour eradication followed by a long-lasting protective memory [38]. Trifunctional antibodies (trAbs) are promising novel anticancer biologics with a particular mode of action capable of linking innate with adaptive immunity [37]. Based on their unique structure, trifunctional IgG-like heterodimeric antibodies, consisting of nonhuman mouse and rat immunoglobulin halves are able to redirect T lymphocytes, as well as accessory cells, to the tumour site. This recruitment of immune cells is accompanied by cellular activation events elicited by anti-CD3, as well as Fcγ-receptor engagement of trAbs supported by a proinflammatory Th1-biased cytokine milieu. All necessary immunological factors required for long-term vaccination-like effects are stimulated along trAb-mediated therapeutic interventions. Thus, the concerted interplay of antibody-dependent cellular cytotoxicity plus the polyclonal T-cell cytotoxicity and Fcγ-receptor-driven induction of long-lasting immune responses after the initial tumour cell elimination represent the major hallmarks of trAb-mediated treatment of malignant diseases. For both classes of antibody constructs there are candidate molecules at different stages of clinical development. The IC hu14.18-IL2 was clinically evaluated in Phase I [39] and Phase II [40] clinical trials revealing an interesting toxicity profile and objective clinical responses in patients with disease evaluable only by MIBG and/or bone marrow histology. The trAb Ektomun [41] combining the specificity for GD2/GD_3 with a T-cell activating moiety has shown early signals of clinical activity in neuroblastoma patients.

Further options to explore the use of monoclonal antibodies targeting tumour-associated antigen GD2 relate to novel routes of administration, the use in combination with other established cancer therapeutics as well as expansion to other indications. In particular the challenge with CNS relapse in neuroblastoma and the limited penetration of the blood brain barrier by immunoglobulins has stimulated investigators to use intrathecal anti-GD2 antibodies for compartmental intrathecal radio-immunotherapy [42]. Also the application of anti-GD2 antibody in combination with chemotherapeutic agents as well as with other immune modulatory strategies including immune checkpoint blockade are important future developments with great potential to improve response rates and outcome of patients with this challenging disease. Finally, GD2 expression was described in other paediatric tumour entities, in particular sarcomas [43], including desmoblastic small round cell tumours [44] and in osteosarcoma [6]. With availability of anti-GD2 antibodies for clinical use, the development of this approach in paediatric sarcoma has the potential to advance treatment options also for these GD2 positive malignancies.

6.7 Summary

Targeting tumour-associated antigen GD2 is the most advanced treatment concept for solid tumours in paediatrics using monoclonal antibodies. Results are promising and have led to the approval of one anti-GD2 antibody (ch14.18/SP2/0, dinutuximab) for the treatment of neuroblastoma so far. Further developments address an improved toxicity profile and enhanced variants of the antibody to increase immune activation against tumour targets and thereby provide an opportunity to further improve outcome for children with GD2 positive paediatric cancers.

References

1. Shuptrine CW, Surana R, Weiner LM. Monoclonal antibodies for the treatment of cancer. Semin Cancer Biol. 2012;22:3–13.
2. Gul N, van EM. Antibody-dependent phagocytosis of tumor cells by macrophages: a potent effector mechanism of monoclonal antibody therapy of cancer. Cancer Res. 2015;75:5008–13.
3. Modak S, Cheung NK. Disialoganglioside directed immunotherapy of neuroblastoma. Cancer Investig. 2007;25:67–77.
4. Yang RK, Sondel PM. Anti-GD2 strategy in the treatment of neuroblastoma. Drugs Future. 2010;35:665.
5. Cheever MA, Allison JP, Ferris AS, Finn OJ, Hastings BM, Hecht TT, et al. The prioritization of cancer antigens: a national cancer institute pilot project for the acceleration of translational research. Clin Cancer Res. 2009;15:5323–37.
6. Heiner JP, Miraldi F, Kallick S, Makley J, Neely J, Smith-Mensah WH, et al. Localization of GD2-specific monoclonal antibody 3F8 in human osteosarcoma. Cancer Res. 1987;47:5377–81.
7. Chang HR, Cordon-Cardo C, Houghton AN, Cheung NK, Brennan MF. Expression of disialogangliosides GD2 and GD3 on human soft tissue sarcomas. Cancer. 1992;70:633–8.
8. Schulz G, Cheresh DA, Varki NM, Yu A, Staffileno LK, Reisfeld RA. Detection of ganglioside GD2 in tumor tissues and sera of neuroblastoma patients. Cancer Res. 1984;44:5914–20.
9. Cheung NK, Saarinen UM, Neely JE, Landmeier B, Donovan D, Coccia PF. Monoclonal antibodies to a glycolipid antigen on human neuroblastoma cells. Cancer Res. 1985;45:2642–9.
10. Cheresh DA, Rosenberg J, Mujoo K, Hirschowitz L, Reisfeld RA. Biosynthesis and expression of the disialoganglioside GD2, a relevant target antigen on small cell lung carcinoma for monoclonal antibody-mediated cytolysis. Cancer Res. 1986;46:5112–8.
11. Honsik CJ, Jung G, Reisfeld RA. Lymphokine-activated killer cells targeted by monoclonal antibodies to the disialogangliosides GD2 and GD3 specifically lyse human tumor cells of neuroectodermal origin. Proc Natl Acad Sci U S A. 1986;83:7893–7.
12. Mujoo K, Kipps TJ, Yang HM, Cheresh DA, Wargalla U, Sander DJ, et al. Functional properties and effect on growth suppression of human neuroblastoma tumors by isotype switch variants of monoclonal antiganglioside GD2 antibody 14.18. Cancer Res. 1989;49:2857–61.
13. Gillies SD, Lo KM, Wesolowski J. High-level expression of chimeric antibodies using adapted cDNA variable region cassettes. J Immunol Methods. 1989;125:191–202.

14. Mueller BM, Romerdahl CA, Gillies SD, Reisfeld RA. Enhancement of antibody-dependent cytotoxicity with a chimeric anti-GD2 antibody. J Immunol. 1990;144:1382–6.
15. AL Y, Gilman AL, Ozkaynak MF, London WB, Kreissman SG, Chen HX, et al. Anti-GD2 antibody with GM-CSF, interleukin-2, and isotretinoin for neuroblastoma. N Engl J Med. 2010;363:1324–34.
16. Ora I, Eggert A. Progress in treatment and risk stratification of neuroblastoma: impact on future clinical and basic research. Semin Cancer Biol. 2011;21:217–28.
17. Handgretinger R, Baader P, Dopfer R, Klingebiel T, Reuland P. Treuner, et al. A phase I study of neuroblastoma with the anti-ganglioside GD2 antibody 14.G2a. Cancer Immunol Immunother. 1992;35:199–204.
18. Xiao WH, AL Y, Sorkin LS. Electrophysiological characteristics of primary afferent fibers after systemic administration of anti-GD2 ganglioside antibody. Pain. 1997;69:145–51.
19. Zeng Y, Fest S, Kunert R, Katinger H, Pistoia V, Michon J, et al. Anti-neuroblastoma effect of ch14.18 antibody produced in CHO cells is mediated by NK-cells in mice. Mol Immunol. 2005;42:1311–9.
20. Lotze MT, Grimm EA, Mazumder A, Strausser JL, Rosenberg SA. Lysis of fresh and cultured autologous tumor by human lymphocytes cultured in T-cell growth factor. Cancer Res. 1981;41:4420–5.
21. Hank JA, Robinson RR, Surfus J, Mueller BM, Reisfeld RA, Cheung NK, et al. Augmentation of antibody dependent cell mediated cytotoxicity following in vivo therapy with recombinant interleukin 2. Cancer Res. 1990;50:5234–9.
22. Barker E, Reisfeld RA. A mechanism for neutrophil-mediated lysis of human neuroblastoma cells. Cancer Res. 1993;53:362–7.
23. Ozkaynak MF, Sondel PM, Krailo MD, Gan J, Javorsky B, Reisfeld RA, et al. Phase I study of chimeric human/murine anti-ganglioside G(D2) monoclonal antibody (ch14.18) with granulocyte-macrophage colony-stimulating factor in children with neuroblastoma immediately after hematopoietic stem-cell transplantation: a Children's Cancer Group Study. J Clin Oncol. 2000;18:4077–85.
24. Saleh MN, Khazaeli MB, Wheeler RH, Allen L, Tilden AB, Grizzle W, et al. Phase I trial of the chimeric anti-GD2 monoclonal antibody ch14.18 in patients with malignant melanoma. Hum Antibodies Hybridomas. 1992;3:19–24.
25. Handgretinger R, Anderson K, Lang P, Dopfer R, Klingebiel T, Schrappe M, et al. A phase I study of human/mouse chimeric antiganglioside GD2 antibody ch14.18 in patients with neuroblastoma. Eur J Cancer. 1995;31A:261–7.
26. AL Y, Uttenreuther-Fischer MM, Huang CS, Tsui CC, Gillies SD, Reisfeld RA, et al. Phase I trial of a human-mouse chimeric anti-disialoganglioside monoclonal antibody ch14.18 in patients with refractory neuroblastoma and osteosarcoma. J Clin Oncol. 1998;16:2169–80.
27. Simon T, Hero B, Faldum A, Handgretinger R, Schrappe M, Niethammer D, et al. Consolidation treatment with chimeric anti-GD2-antibody ch14.18 in children older than 1 year with metastatic neuroblastoma. J Clin Oncol. 2004;22:3549–57.
28. Simon T, Hero B, Faldum A, Handgretinger R, Schrappe M, Klingebiel T, et al. Long term outcome of high-risk neuroblastoma patients after immunotherapy with antibody ch14.18 or oral metronomic chemotherapy. BMC Cancer. 2011;11:21.
29. Hank JA, Surfus J, Gan J, Chew TL, Hong R, Tans K, et al. Treatment of neuroblastoma patients with antiganglioside GD2 antibody plus interleukin-2 induces antibody-dependent cellular cytotoxicity against neuroblastoma detected in vitro. J Immunother. 1994;15:29–37.
30. Murray JL, Kleinerman ES, Jia SF, Rosenblum MG, Eton O, Buzaid A, et al. Phase Ia/Ib trial of anti-GD2 chimeric monoclonal antibody 14.18 (ch14.18) and recombinant human granulocyte-macrophage colony-stimulating factor (rhGM-CSF) in metastatic melanoma. J Immunother Emphasis Tumor Immunol. 1996;19:206–17.
31. Albertini MR, Hank JA, Schiller JH, Khorsand M, Borchert AA, Gan J, et al. Phase IB trial of chimeric antidisialoganglioside antibody plus interleukin 2 for melanoma patients. Clin Cancer Res. 1997;3:1277–88.

32. Gilman AL, Ozkaynak MF, Matthay KK, Krailo M, AL Y, Gan J, et al. Phase I study of ch14.18 with granulocyte-macrophage colony-stimulating factor and interleukin-2 in children with neuroblastoma after autologous bone marrow transplantation or stem-cell rescue: a report from the Children's Oncology Group. J Clin Oncol. 2009;27:85–91.
33. Ladenstein R, Weixler S, Baykan B, Bleeke M, Kunert R, Katinger D, et al. Ch14.18 antibody produced in CHO cells in relapsed or refractory Stage 4 neuroblastoma patients: a SIOPEN Phase 1 study. MAbs. 2013;5:801–9.
34. Uttenreuther-Fischer MM, Huang CS, Yu AL. Pharmacokinetics of human-mouse chimeric anti-GD2 mAb ch14.18 in a phase I trial in neuroblastoma patients. Cancer Immunol Immunother. 1995;41:331–8.
35. Ladenstein R, Potschger U, Siabalis D, Garaventa A, Bergeron C, Lewis IJ, et al. Dose finding study for the use of subcutaneous recombinant interleukin-2 to augment natural killer cell numbers in an outpatient setting for stage 4 neuroblastoma after megatherapy and autologous stem-cell reinfusion. J Clin Oncol. 2011;29:441–8.
36. Sondel PM, Gillies SD. Current and potential uses of immunocytokines as cancer immunotherapy. Antibodies (Basel). 2012;1:149–71.
37. Hess J, Ruf P, Lindhofer H. Cancer therapy with trifunctional antibodies: linking innate and adaptive immunity. Future Oncol. 2012;8:73–85.
38. Lode HN, Reisfeld RA. Targeted cytokines for cancer immunotherapy [In Process Citation]. Immunol Res. 2000;21:279–88.
39. Osenga KL, Hank JA, Albertini MR, Gan J, Sternberg AG, Eickhoff J, et al. A phase I clinical trial of the hu14.18-IL2 (EMD 273063) as a treatment for children with refractory or recurrent neuroblastoma and melanoma: a study of the Children's Oncology Group. Clin Cancer Res. 2006;12:1750–9.
40. Shusterman S, London WB, Gillies SD, Hank JA, Voss SD, Seeger RC, et al. Antitumor activity of hu14.18-IL2 in patients with relapsed/refractory neuroblastoma: a Children's Oncology Group (COG) phase II study. J Clin Oncol. 2010;28:4969–75.
41. Chelius D, Ruf P, Gruber P, Ploscher M, Liedtke R, Gansberger E, et al. Structural and functional characterization of the trifunctional antibody catumaxomab. MAbs. 2010;2:309–19.
42. Kramer K, Kushner BH, Modak S, Pandit-Taskar N, Smith-Jones P, Zanzonico P, et al. Compartmental intrathecal radioimmunotherapy: results for treatment for metastatic CNS neuroblastoma. J Neuro-Oncol. 2010;97:409–18.
43. Dobrenkov K, Ostrovnaya I, Gu J, Cheung IY, Cheung NK. Oncotargets GD2 and GD3 are highly expressed in sarcomas of children, adolescents, and young adults. Pediatr Blood Cancer. 2016;63:1780–5.
44. Modak S, Gerald W, Cheung NK. Disialoganglioside GD2 and a novel tumor antigen: potential targets for immunotherapy of desmoplastic small round cell tumor. Med Pediatr Oncol. 2002;39:547–51.
45. Saleh MN, Khazaeli MB, Wheeler RH, Dropcho E, Liu T, Urist M, et al. Phase I trial of the murine monoclonal anti-GD2 antibody 14G2a in metastatic melanoma. Cancer Res. 1992;52:4342–7.
46. Murray JL, Cunningham JE, Brewer H, Mujoo K, Zukiwski AA, et al. Phase I trial of murine monoclonal antibody 14G2a administered by prolonged intravenous infusion in patients with neuroectodermal tumors. J Clin Oncol. 1994;12:184–93.
47. Uttenreuther-Fischer MM, Huang CS, Reisfeld RA, Yu AL. Pharmacokinetics of anti-ganglioside GD2 mAb 14G2a in a phase I trial in pediatric cancer patients. Cancer Immunol Immunother. 1995;41:29–36.
48. Frost JD, Hank JA, Reaman GH, Frierdich SRN, Seeger RC, Gan J, et al. Phase I/IB trial of murine monoclonal anti-GD2 antibody 14.G2a plus Il-2 in children with refractory neuroblastoma: a report of the children's cancer group. Cancer. 1997;80:317–33.
49. Yu AL, Batova A, Alvarado C, Rao VJ, Castleberry RP. Usefulness of a chimeric anti-GD2 (ch14.18) and GM-CSF for refractory neuroblastoma: a POG phase II study (Meeting abstract). ASCO Proceedings 1997.

Chapter 7
Monoclonal Antibodies Targeting the Immune System

Véronique Minard-Colin

Abstract Scientific advances during the past decades have demonstrated the critical role of host immune system in the elimination of cancer. Better knowledge of immune cancer evasion has enabled the development of new cancer immunotherapy targeted to inhibitory immune checkpoints: PD-1, PD-L1 and CTLA4. Dramatic results were obtained in advanced melanoma (34% survival at 5 years with anti-PD-1) and non-small cell lung cancer, and proof of efficacy has been demonstrated with PD-1/PD-L1 antibodies in more than 20 cancer types in adults. By contrast, there are still limited clinical trials focusing on immunotherapies targeting the host immune system in pediatric oncology although some outstanding results have been reported in specific tumor histology/genetic predisposition syndrome. The first phase 1 in children and adolescents with recurrent/refractory solid tumors has been recently published with anti-CTL4A (ipilimumab). Toxicity profile was similar to adults and 6 (18%) of patients experienced stable disease. Translational research will allow understanding and analyzing mechanisms of action of immune checkpoints regulators and define biomarkers predictive of response. These drugs are already challenging our practice like for evaluation of tumor response or for management of immune related toxicities. Many other immune checkpoints have been identified and could potentially be targeted in pediatric cancers. Future studies will help to identify predictive factors but also to coordinate these new immunotherapies with our classic treatment strategies.

Keywords Cancer • Children • Adolescents • Immune system • Immune checkpoint inhibitors • CTLA4 • PD-1 • PD-L1

V. Minard-Colin, M.D., Ph.D.
Département de Cancérologie de l'enfant et de l'adolescent, Institut Gustave Roussy, 114 rue Édouard-Vaillant, 94805 Villejuif Cedex, France
e-mail: veronique.minard@gustaveroussy.fr

J.C. Gray, A. Marabelle (eds.), *Immunotherapy for Pediatric Malignancies*,
https://doi.org/10.1007/978-3-319-43486-5_7

Scientific advances during the past decades have demonstrated the critical role of immune system in the elimination of cancer [1–3]. Better knowledge of immune cancer evasion has enabled the development of new cancer immunotherapy targeted to host immune system and in particular, to inhibitory immune checkpoints [4–6]: PD-1 (programmed cell death protein-1), PD-L1 (programmed death ligand1) and CTLA-4 (cytotoxic T lymphocyte antigen-4). Dramatic results were obtained in advanced melanoma (34% survival at 5 years with anti-PD-1) [7] and non-small cell lung cancer and proof of efficacy has been demonstrated with PD-1/PD-L1 antibodies in more than 20 cancer types in adults. By contrast, there are still limited clinical trials focusing on immunotherapies targeting the host immune system in pediatric oncology [8] but some outstanding results have been reported in specific tumor histology [9–12]/genetic predisposition syndrome [13, 14].

Tumor immunogenicity results from a combination of antigenicity and adjuvanticity, in which a theoretical "signal 1" links to the antigenicity of cancers, and "signal 2" links to their adjuvanticity (Fig. 7.1). In the case of T cells, the ultimate amplitude and quality of the response, which is initiated through antigen recognition by the T cell receptor (TCR) (signal 1), is regulated by a balance between co-stimulatory and inhibitory signals (that is, immune checkpoints) and "bystander activation" of tumor antigen specific T lymphocytes (signal 2). Under normal physiological conditions, immune checkpoints are crucial for the maintenance of self-tolerance, and also to protect tissues from damage when the immune system is responding to pathogenic infection. The expression of immune-checkpoint proteins

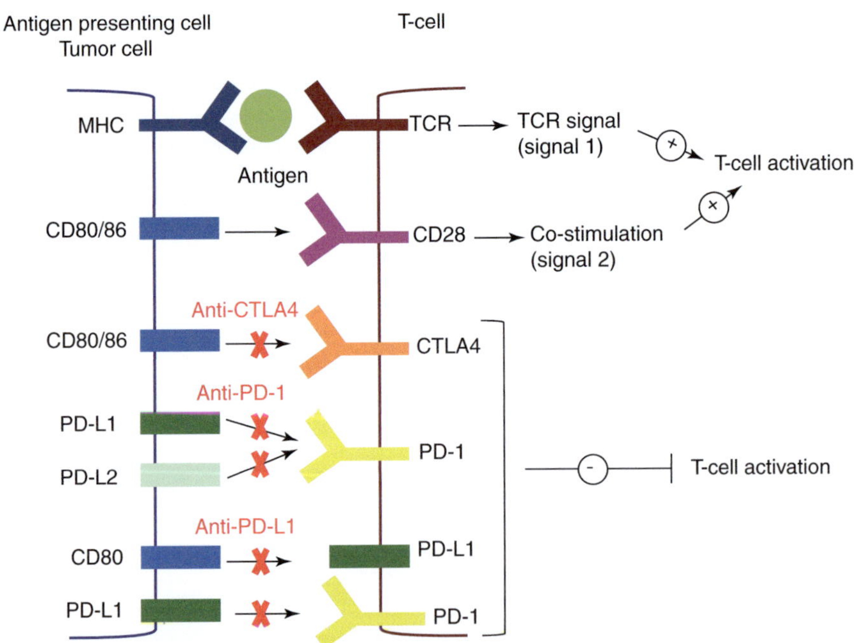

Fig. 7.1 Immunological synapse and Immune checkpoint blockers

can be deregulated by tumors as an important immune resistance mechanism [15]. T cells have been the major focus of efforts to therapeutically manipulate endogenous anti-tumor immunity but, as we will discuss herein, other immune therapies should also be considered in pediatric oncology such as NK and myeloid cells-directed therapies.

In this chapter, we will briefly review the known specificity of pediatric tumor immunology and examine immune targets, preclinical data, and pediatric clinical trials with monoclonal antibodies targeting the immune system.

7.1 Specific Features of Pediatric Tumor Immunology

The immune system plays a major role in the control of tumor growth and progression, a process known as cancer immunoediting [1, 3]. Since the formalized introduction of the cancer immunosurveillance concept by Paul Ehrlich, the idea that the immune system may have a protective role in tumor development has been subjected to debate. Recent work, however, has lent new support that the immune system can indeed prevent tumor formation. At the same time, this work has shown that the immune system also functions to promote or select tumor variants with reduced immunogenicity, thereby providing developing tumors with a mechanism to escape immunologic detection and elimination. These findings have led to the development of the cancer immunoediting hypothesis, a refinement of cancer immunosurveillance that takes a broader view of immune system–tumor interactions by acknowledging both the host-protecting and tumor-sculpting actions of the immune system on developing tumors. The host immune system can also contribute to the efficacy of some cancer therapies where the tumor death induced may be "immunogenic" [16]. These two major recent concepts, *i.e.*, cancer immunoediting and immunogenic cell death, have largely been defined in mice with tumors, and have now been demonstrated in humans and adults but very few is still known in pediatric immuno-oncology. Some specific features should be highlighted before to address development of immunotherapies targeting the immune system in children/adolescents with tumors:

Immunity varies with age [17], reflecting unique age-dependent challenges including the neonatal phase, infancy and age-related thymic involution. First, newborns and infants have relatively fewer effector memory T-cells ($CD45RA^{-}$, CD45 RO^{+}) and effector memory B-cells ($CD27^{+}$). Additionally, neonatal $CD4^{+}$T cells are epigenetically biased towards T helper (Th) 2 cytokine production and demonstrate higher susceptibility to apoptosis of Th1 cells and large numbers of $CD4^{+}$, $CD25^{+}$, $Foxp3^{+}$ Regulatory T-cells (Tregs) are preferentially present in fetal and neonatal lymph nodes possibly residing in *secondary lymphoid organs for years after birth* [18]. Moreover, various immuno-suppressive cytokines (IL-4, IL-10 IL-13, TGF-β) are expressed at high concentrations early in life. Age-related changes of innate immunity including natural killer (NK), dendritic cell (DC), monocyte (MC) and neutrophil populations have been also noted from childhood through old age

[19, 20]. Overall, ontogeny of early life immunity may reduce protective adaptive immunity against cancer and contribute to specific/early tumor immunoediting in children.

Microbiota, which influence immune checkpoint blockers (ICB) activity [21, 22], **varies with environmental factors and age** [23, 24]. Zitvogel's group showed the mandatory role of microbiota (*Bacteroidales* and *Burkholderiales*) for anti-CTLA4 monoclonal antibody (mAb) efficacy and its prophylactic role against subclinical colitis in mice [22]. In parallel, Gajewski's group demonstrated the role of *Bifidobacterium* in maturing DC allowing the expansion of anti-cancer T cells in the tumor beds and their activation with anti-PDL1 mAb [25]. Several interrelated factors could disrupt normal gut microbiota: (a) poor maternal nutritional status, (b) enteropathogen invasion (also induced by therapy such as chemotherapy and/or radiotherapy), (c) history of consumption of antibiotics, (d) disturbances in gut mucosal immune system development, and/or (e) history of breastfeeding. In children, gut microbiota has been predominantly studied in brain disorders and especially in autism spectrum disorder in which the emerging idea of the microbiota as a modulator of neural physiology has recently been investigated through the concept of the "microbiota-gut-brain axis" [26], and in malnutrition [27]. Future research should evaluate how the gut microbiota impacts natural cancer immunosurveillance and ICB efficacy in children.

The majority of pediatric cancers are characterized by low mutational burden and few recurrently mutated genes [28]. Mutation frequencies as low as 0.1/Mb (~one change across the entire exome) have been reported in pediatric cancers, while at the opposite extreme, melanoma and lung cancer exceed 100/Mb (high mutation frequencies attributable, at least in part, to extensive exposure to carcinogens, such as ultraviolet radiation and tobacco smoke) [28]. Even within the same tumor type, mutation profiles in pediatric samples are distinct from their adult counterpart. For example, in rhabdomyosarcoma (RMS), which can occur in pediatric and adult age with similar histologic subtypes (i.e. embryonal or alveolar), both the *PAX* gene fusion-negative and *PAX* gene fusion-positive genotypes have a distinct relationship between mutational frequency and age, with an increasing number of somatic mutations with older age of diagnosis and a steeper slope of curve in *PAX* gene fusion-positive tumors [29]. Amazingly, for example, one remarkable *PAX* gene fusion-positive RMS from a 3-month-old patient had no protein-coding somatic alterations with the exception of the *PAX3–FOXO1* fusion and copy neutral loss of heterozygosity (LOH) on chromosome 11p. Patient-mutated epitopes, known as neoantigens, play an important role in the T cell response driven by checkpoint blockade [30–32]. This was first assessed by van Rooij and colleagues who published a case report of a patient with metastatic melanoma (MM) who derived clinical benefit from ipilimumab treatment. They performed tumor whole-exome sequencing which revealed high level of somatic mutations and using a bioinformatics platform, they derived 448 potential CD8 T cell epitopes that were analyzed for reactivity against the patient's tumor-infiltrating lymphocytes (TIL)s. This hypothetical relationship between mutation load and clinical benefit from immunotherapy was explored further in patients with MM and metastatic non-small cell lung cancers (NSCLC) with ipilimumab and pembrolizumab (anti-PD1 mAb).

A higher somatic non-synonymous mutation burden was associated with ICB efficacy. Recent technological innovations have made it possible to dissect the immune response to patient-specific neoantigens that arise as a consequence of tumor-specific mutations [32]. Thus, neoantigen load may form a biomarker in cancer immunotherapy (threshold of mutation load to define) and provide an incentive for the development of novel therapeutic approaches that selectively enhance T-cell reactivity against this class of antigens [34].

In contrast to adult malignancies (apart from some breast and colorectal cancers), a significant proportion of childhood tumors occur in the context of cancer predisposition syndromes (~8–10%) [33]. One of these predisposition syndromes, so-called biallelic or congenital mismatch repair (MMR) deficiency syndrome (bMMRD) is of particular interest because of its unique mutation load and potent antigenicity [34, 35]. bMMRD is caused by homozygous germline mutations in one of the four MMR genes (PMS2, MLH1, MSH2, and MSH6) and is the most penetrant cancer predisposition syndrome, with 100% of biallelic mutation carriers developing cancers in the first two decades of life. While the incidence of cancers in those patients is quite well described, the prevalence of bMMRD is not well known in pediatric cancers. Because of their unique degree of ultra/hypermutation, bMMRD associated cancers have a higher chance of harboring neoantigens, especially when additional somatic mutations in DNA polymerase are present [35]. Moreover, each bMMRD tumor lacks replication repair in every cell cycle, and therefore, all replicating tumor cells will inevitably accumulate new mutations per cell division, exponentially increasing the number of non-synonymous mutations available to encode novel neoantigens. While specific tumor histology and immune contexture of bMMRD have not been well described yet, outstanding responses to anti-PD1 immunotherapy have been reported in recurrent high-grade gliomas associated with bMMRD [13].

Thus, immune contexture of pediatric cancers is extremely variable and depends on many factors including age, genetic prediction syndrome, microbiota, tumor mutation load and neoantigen, and tumor type. However, data from studies in several types of pediatric cancers have demonstrated that the majority of tumors are immunologically “cold tumors” with few tumor-infiltrating lymphocytes (TILs). In a cohort of 53 pediatric solid tumors [36], counts of tumor-infiltrating CD8+ T-cells/high-power field (HPF) revealed low level of TILs in the majority of tumors (mean CD8+ T-cells/HPF < 10) except for germinomas (mean CD8+ T-cells/HPF = 34) and NBL (mean CD8+ T-cells/HPF = 15). As previously described in many adult tumors including lymphomas, marked infiltration of tumors by cytotoxic T lymphocytes (including (but not limited to) $CD3^+$, $CD8^+$ cytotoxic T lymphocytes) as well as high $CD8^+$/FOXP3 ratio, appear to be associated with a good prognosis in pediatric cancers such as NBL [37], osteosarcoma (OST) [38] and Ewing sarcoma (ES) [39]. Interestingly, excluding patients with primary brain tumors, patients with distant metastases have also higher numbers of tumor-infiltrating CD8+ T-cells when compared with localized disease [36]. In OST, density of $CD3^+$ T-cells has also been reported as higher in metastases than in primary tumors and local relapses [40]. Moreover, in metastatic NBL, the abundance of infiltrating $CD3^+$, $CD8^+$, and $CD4^+$ T-cells is significantly higher in both tumor nest and septa in stage 4 s when compared with stage 4 tumors [37].

One of the most widely reported mechanisms by which solid tumor cells evade immune T lymphocytes effectors is the down-regulation of major histocompatibility complex (MHC) Class I antigen. Many pediatric cancers, such as NBL, ES, RMS, acute myeloblastic leukemia (AML) show low or negative HLA-I surface expression [41]. By contrast, other tumors such as OST have strongly positive or heterogeneous HLA class I expression [40]. A role for NK-cells may be particularly significant in tumor cells that express low levels of HLA-I and cannot efficiently stimulate T-cells. For example, both *in vitro* and *in vivo* in mice, among pediatric solid tumors, ES and RMS are exquisitely sensitive to expanded NK cells cytotoxicity [42].

The role of tumor-associated macrophages (TAM) has been extensively studied in OST and is still subject of debate. Indeed, In contrast to most other tumor types, Tumour associated macrophages (TAMs) ($CD14^+$) have been first associated with reduced metastasis and improved survival in OST [43]. An additional work reported that deregulation of macrophage polarization is associated with metastatic extension in OST, with M2- ($CD163^+$) TAMs correlated with $CD146^+$ vascular cells and M1- ($INOS^+$) TAMs higher in localized/metastatic OST [44]. In metastatic NBL, higher infiltration with $CD163^+$ and $AIF1^+$ TAMs has been observed when compared with localized disease [45]. Moreover, infiltrating suppressive CSF-1R myeloid cells predicts poor survival in NBL [46]. Finally, in murine model of RMS, tumor progression has been demonstrated with preferential expansion of myeloid-derived suppressor cells, required CXCR2 axis mediation, and is associated with reduced anti-PD1 treatment efficiency (see below) [47].

Thus, while infiltration of the tumor with lymphocytes may be one factor associated with a favorable outcome in pediatric cancers, the milieu required for optimal functioning of the immune system is also defined by the presence of potent antigen presenting cells (APC), immunostimulatory cytokines, and optimal surface molecule expression by both the tumor cells and the infiltrating lymphocytes. The complexities of these interactions are just beginning to be defined; a further difficulty that must be addressed in the development of cancer immunotherapy regimens is that various forms of pediatric cancers appear to have different TILs mobilizations and immune system requirements.

7.2 Immune Targets in Pediatric Malignancies

7.2.1 T-Cell Checkpoints

The ultimate T-cell immune response, which is initiated through antigen recognition by the TCR, is regulated by a balance between co-stimulatory and inhibitory signals (that is, immune checkpoints) (Fig. 7.1). Under normal physiological conditions, immune checkpoints are crucial for the maintenance of self-tolerance (prevention of autoimmunity) and also to protect tissues from damage when the immune system is responding to pathogenic infection. The expression of immune-checkpoint proteins can be deregulated by tumors as an important immune escape mechanism.

7.2.1.1 CTLA-4

Cytotoxic T-lymphocyte-associated antigen 4 (CTLA-4; also known as CD152), the first immune-checkpoint receptor to be clinically targeted, is expressed exclusively on T-cells where it primarily regulates the amplitude of the early stage of T-cell activation ("priming"). CTLA-4 is a cell surface receptor belonging to the human immunoglobulin gene superfamily found on $CD4^+$ and $CD8^+$ T cells, as well as Tregs. First, CTLA-4 counteracts the activity of the T-cell co-stimulatory receptor, CD28. Once antigen recognition occurs by TCR, CD28 signaling strongly amplifies TCR signaling to activate T-cells. CD28 and CTLA-4 share identical ligands: CD80 (also known as B7.1) and CD86 (also known as B7.2). CTLA-4 binds CD80 and CD86 with greater affinity and avidity than CD28 thus enabling it to outcompete CD28 for its ligands. Second, CTLA4 also confers 'signaling-independent' T-cell inhibition through the active removal of CD80 and CD86 from the APC surface. Third, CTLA-4 blocks T-cell activation through different signaling pathways activation of the protein phosphatases, SHP2 (also known as PTPN11) and PP2A, which are important in counteracting kinase signals that are induced by TCR and CD28. Thus, CTLA-4 has a central role for keeping T-cell activation in check.

Inherited CTLA-4 gene polymorphisms have been shown to influence T-cell activation, susceptibility to autoimmunity (such as type 1 diabetes in children) and malignancies. In particular, CTLA-4 single nucleotide polymorphism +49A/G, which results in greater affinity of CTLA-4 to bind the CD80 molecule leading to increased inhibition of T-cell activation, is associated with increased risk of malignant bone tumors, including OST [48] and ES [49]. Data are very limited regarding CTLA4 expression in pediatric malignancies. Patients with newly diagnosed or relapsed OST and ES had increased expression of peripheral blood CTLA-4 on both $CD4^+$ and $CD8^+$ T-cells compared with healthy controls [50]. Furthermore, cell surface CTL4-A expression has been reported in different pediatric tumor cell lines such as NBL, RMS and OST, but to our knowledge, it has not been evaluated on human samples. In the K7 M2 mouse model of pulmonary metastatic OST, T-cells infiltrating anti-PD-L1-resistant tumors up regulate additional inhibitory receptors, notably CTLA-4, which impair their ability to mediate tumor rejection. Combination immunotherapy with anti-CTLA-4 and anti-PDL-1 in this mouse model interestingly showed complete control of tumors in a majority of mice as well as immunity to further tumor inoculation [51].

7.2.1.2 PD-1/PD-L1

Programmed cell death-1 (PD-1) is an immune receptor belonging to the CD28/CTLA-4 family of T-cell immune-checkpoints. In contrast to CTLA-4, the major role of PD1 is to limit the activity of *effector T-cells in peripheral tissues* at the time of an inflammatory response to infection and to limit autoimmunity [52, 53]. This translates into a major immune resistance mechanism within the tumor microenvironment [15]. PD-1 expression is induced when T-cells become activated. The engagement of PD-1 by one of its ligands inhibits kinases that are involved in T-cell activation mostly through the phosphatase SHP2. The two ligands for PD-1 are PD-1 ligand 1 (PD-L1; also known as B7-H1 and CD274) and PD-L2 (also known as B7-DC and CD273) [54]. These B7 family members share sequence homology and arose through gene duplication, which has positioned them within 100 kb of each other in the genome (on 9p24.1). Importantly, PD-L1 not only binds to PD-1, but also to CD80 (ligand for CD28 and CTLA4), and CD80/PD-L1 interaction also induces inhibitory signals in T-cells. PD1 is much more broadly expressed than CTLA4. PD-1 is expressed on $CD4^+$ and $CD8^+$ T-cells, B cells, NK cells, monocytes and dendritic cells. Resting T cells do not express PD1. PD-1 expression is induced after TCR ligation and augmented by TNF stimulation. Therefore, although PD1 blockade is typically viewed as enhancing the activity of effector T-cells in tissues and in the tumor microenvironment, it also enhances NK-cell activity and also enhances antibody production or modulates regulatory B-cells function. PD-L1 is detected in virtually all tissues and cell types, is mostly induced by type I and II IFNs and can vary over time in response to different factors in the microenvironment. PD-L2 is expressed on activated T-cells, myeloid dendritic cells, macrophages and by epithelial cells.

PD-L1 expression has been assessed in a variety of childhood cancers, and in the majority of cases, a low frequency of PDL1 expression has been observed [36, 55]. In a series of 91 whole slides sections and 365 tissue microarray of different pediatric solid tumors including lymphoma, 40 cases (9%) were considered positive. Tumour types with the highest frequency of expression comprised non-Hodgkin lymphoma (8/10), high-grade glioma (6/20), and NBL (17/118). No PD-L1 staining was observed in ES (0/20) or medulloblastoma (0/40). Despite a relatively low frequency of PD-L1+ pediatric cancers, the majority contained immune cells (73%, 334/456). Of these immune cells infiltrated tumors, 73% of samples contained lymphocytes only, 25% contained lymphocytes and macrophages and 3% contained macrophages only. Twenty-one percent of tumor-infiltrating cells demonstrated PD-L1 expression, mostly comprising PDL1 expression on macrophages (65%, 60/92), while lymphocytes expressed PD-L1 in only 7% (22/324). Taken together, PD-L1 was expressed in tumor and/or tumor-infiltrating cells in 20% of samples (90/456) [55]. Other series reported negative to moderate PD1, PDL1 and PDL2 expression by both immunochemistry and mRNA expression in >500 children cancer samples (including ES, OST, RMS, medulloblastoma, high grade glioma, Wilms tumor [56] and NBL [57]). Of note, germinoma exhibit unique high level of PDL1 expression on tumor infiltrating cells [36]. In adult tumors, PD-L1 is expressed by a wide variety of tumors and expression is often associated with poor prognosis. The same observation has been reported in Wilms tumor (PDL1 expression correlates with poorer outcome but also anaplastic subtype [56]) and in OST [58]. In contrast, Chowdhury et al. [59] reported membranous PDL1 expression in 66 (57%) of 115 pediatric solid tumors, including high-risk NBL, RMS, bone sarcomas, without evident explanation for such discrepancy. However, PDL1 molecular level analyzed (mRNA, protein), thresholds to consider its positivity (1, 5 or 50%), techniques used (antibodies staining and procedure) and cells (tumor and tumor-infiltrating immune cells) on which this biomarker should be assessed are not yet universally agreed. Although the positivity of the PDL1 status is significantly correlated with response to anti-PD-1 in malignant melanoma and NSCLC, therapeutic benefit has also consistently been reported in PDL1-negative patients.

For some tumors, it has been demonstrated that PD-L1 expression is driven by constitutive oncogenic signaling pathways in the tumor cell ("intrinsic" immune resistance). In classical Hodgkin lymphoma, chromosome 9p24.1/PDL1/PDL2 alterations (i.e. disomy, polysomy, copy gain, amplification, translocation) have been shown be a "hallmark" of the disease with amplification of 9p24.1 more common in patients with advanced disease and associated with shorter progression free survival [60]. Similarly, constitutive anaplastic lymphoma kinase (ALK) signaling, which is observed in >95% of pediatric anaplastic large cell lymphoma but also inflammatory myofibroblastic tumors and neuroblastoma, has been reported to drive PD-L1 expression through signal transducer and activator of transcription 3 (STAT3) signaling [61].

In a TH-NMYC murine NBL model, targeting PD-1/PD-L1 with blocking antibodies was insufficient to control tumor growth alone; however, combining PD-1/PD-L1 blockade with a selective colony-stimulating factor-1 receptor (CSF1R) inhibitor that blocks induction of suppressive MDSCs resulted in significant tumor responses [46]. In mice inoculated with different RMS cell lines, treatment with anti-PD1 plus anti-CXCR2 antibodies, which prevent trafficking of MDSCs into the tumor bed was more effective than treatment with anti-PD1 alone [47]. Together, these results implicate myeloid derived suppressor cells in tumor immune escape in RMS and suggest that a future clinical approach that combined immunotherapy with anti-PD1 holds promise.

7.2.1.3 B7-H3

B7-H3 (also known as CD276), is an immune checkpoint molecule belonging to the B7-CD28 pathways. B7-H3 is constitutively found on non-immune resting fibroblasts, endothelial cells, osteoblasts, and amniotic fluid stem cells. Moreover, B7-H3 expression is induced on immune cells, specifically APCs. In particular, coculture with regulatory T cells, IFNg, lipopolysaccharide, or anti-CD40 *in vitro* stimulation all induce the expression of B7-H3 on DC. B7-H3 is also detected on natural killer (NK) cells, B cells, and a minor population of T cells following PMA/ionomycin stimulation. The precise role of B7-H3, its binding partner, and regulating function of tumor-infiltrating immune cells and its activity in cancer cells has yet to be fully elucidated. The B7-H3 pathway has a dual role in contributing to the regulation of innate immune responses. One study found that NBL cells express B7-H3 on their cell surface, which protects them from NK cell-mediated lysis [62]. In OST, high expression of B7-H3 is associated with a shorter survival and inversely correlated with the number of $CD8^+$ TILs [63]. Thus, B7-H3 is largely overexpressed in several human tumor tissues and needs to be assessed in pediatric cancers. Since no blocking mAb against B7-H3 is yet available, additional strategies in screening antibodies for neutralization capacity need to be developed.

7.2.2 *NK-Cell Checkpoints*

NK cells are cytotoxic lymphocytes specialized in early defense against virus-infected and transformed cells. To prevent the killing of normal healthy cells, NK cells primarily use inhibitory receptors that bind to major MHC class I molecules on target cells. In addition, NK cells require combined signals from multiple activating receptors to elicit effective cytotoxicity against cancer cells. Thus, the decision of an NK cell to kill target cells is determined by a signaling balance between activating and inhibitory receptors. In this context, cancer cells can be sensed and killed by NK cells through the loss of MHC class I molecules, which are constitutively present on normal healthy cells. NK cells express multiple inhibitory receptors, such as killer cell immunoglobulin-like receptors (KIRs), CD94/NKG2A specific for HLA-E, and leukocyte immunoglobulin-like receptor-1 (LILRB1) which recognizes a broad spectrum of HLA-I molecules, T-cell immunoglobulin- and mucin-domain-containing molecule 3 (TIM-3), and T-cell immunoreceptor with Ig and immunoreceptor tyrosine-based inhibition motif domains (TIGIT) (CD96, TIM-3 and TIGIT are as well expressed on cytotoxic T-cells). KIRs constitute a polygenic and polymorphic family including 6 inhibitory receptors that recognize shared epitopes defining allelic variants of HLA-I molecules, and six activating receptors, whose ligand specificity remains elusive. Particularly important are KIR2DL1 and KIR2DL2/3 which recognize subsets of HLA-C alleles and KIR3DL1 specific for a shared epitope in some HLA-B and HLA-A alleles. The role of KIRs has been well established in acute myeloblastic leukemia and neuroblastoma. The 'missing self' hypothesis is that NK cells recognize target cells by the absence of self-MHC class I molecules, in which receptors on NK cells are inhibitory KIRs in humans. In neuroblastoma children treated with GD2 mAb, patients with KIR3DL1 and HLA-B subtype combinations that were predictive of weak interaction had superior outcomes compared with those that were predictive of strong interaction and both groups were inferior to those with non-interacting subtype combinations [64]. An anti-KIR Ab (IPH2101 by Innate Pharma, Marseille, France) has been proven to be safe without toxicity and autoimmunity in multiple myeloma and AML patients. However, the efficacy was different; IPH2101 enhances *ex vivo* NK cytotoxicity in multiple myeloma patients, but in AML patients, there were no significant differences in NK cell number and cytotoxicity. CD94/NKG2A is a C-type lectin receptor, in which the ligand is HLA-E. The first phase I/II clinical trial is on-going and employs an anti-NKG2A Ab (IPH2201 by Innate Pharma) since 2015. No trial is developed in children/adolescents. A better understand of the receptors/common pathways and mechanisms governing NK cell activities are warranted for optimal design of NK-directed immunotherapy in combination with other therapies in pediatric cancers.

7.3 Clinical Trials in Children Malignancies

In 2013, Science magazine declared that, all sciences considered, cancer immunotherapy had been the major breakthrough of the year based on promising results with three immunotherapies: anti-CTLA-4 ipilimumab phase 3 study, phase 1 clinical trials with anti-PD-1, and Chimeric Antigen Receptor (CAR) T-cells biotherapy. There are still limited clinical trials focusing on immunotherapies targeting the host immune system in pediatric oncology (see Table 7.1 for summary) but some outstanding results have been reported in specific tumor histology/genetic predisposition syndrome. Immune checkpoints functions are dependents of ligand-receptor interactions and the idea to use monoclonal antibodies to block this interaction became attractive at the end of the 90's. Indeed, in contrast to most currently approved antibodies for cancer therapy, antibodies that block immune checkpoints do not target tumor cells directly; instead they target lymphocyte receptors or their ligands in order to enhance endogenous anti-tumor activity.

Table 7.1 Summary of ongoing/suspended/terminated (unpublished) studies with monoclonal antibodies targeting the immune system in pediatric oncology (studies recruiting adolescents only are not listed)

Molecule	Indication	Trial modalities	Sites	Status	NCI reference
Ipilimumab (anti-CTLA4)					
	Non-Hodgkin Lymphoma ALL	Ph. 1 CD19 CAR + ipilimumab, unique dose	USA	Suspended	NCT00586391
	Melanoma	Ph. 1 + tumor vaccine (gp100 and MART-1)	USA	Ongoing	NCT00025181
Nivolumab (anti-PD-1)					
	All solid tumors	Ph. 1/2 +/− ipilimumab	USA	Ongoing	NCT02304458
	Glioblastoma	Ph. 2	Spain	Ongoing	NCT02550249
	All tumors	Proof of concept trial +cyclophosphamide +/− radiation therapy or ablation	Europa	Ongoing	NCT02813135
Pembrolizumab (anti-PD-1)					
	Malignant glioma – DIPG	Ph. 1	USA	Suspended	NCT02359565
	Melanoma, Lymphoma Solid tumors PDL-1+	Ph. 1/2	USA Europa Israel	Ongoing	NCT02332668
	Neuroblastoma	Ph. 1 + CAR GD2	USA	Ongoing	NCT01822652
Atezolizumab (MPDL3280A) (anti-PD-L1)					
	All solid tumors	Ph. 1	International	Ongoing	NCT02541604

From https://clinicaltrials.gov

7.3.1 Anti-CTLA-4

First clinical trials with CTLA4 mAb have been developed in the 2000's in metastatic melanoma with ipilimumab (Yervoy®, Bristol-Meyers Squibb) and tremelimumab (AstraZeneca). Ipilimumab is a fully engineered human monoclonal antibody (IgG1) that blocks CTLA4 binding to its ligands CD80/CD86, allowing binding of co-stimulatory receptor CD28 to its ligands and T-cell activation. Tremelimumab is a human IgG2 monoclonal antibody binding to CTLA-4 and blocking the interaction with CD80/CD86. By unbalancing the immune system, CTLA-4 immunotherapies also generate dysimmune toxicities, called immune-related adverse events (IRAEs) [65, 66]. In adult trials with CTLA-4 mAb, 90% of patients experienced any IRAEs, with 15–35% of grade 3–4. Clinical spectrum of Immune Related Adverse Events (IRAEs) is large involving the skin (pruritus, rash, vitiligo), gastrointestinal tract (diarrhea up to severe colitis), endocrine glands (hypophysitis, thyroid dysfunction), liver, and lung and can potentially affect any tissue. Most IRAEs occur within 3–6 months of the initiation of CTLA4 mAb and IRAEs risk appears to be dose-dependent. Most of these adverse events can be managed by symptomatic treatment, immunotherapy suspension or termination, counteracting lymphocyte activation with steroids, and rarely with anti-TNF or mycophenolate mofetil. Importantly, physicians should be aware of this new family of immune toxicities, to be able to prevent, anticipate, and manage appropriately before they can become life-threatening, and teams with significant experiences report “learning-curve” in this [66].

The first pediatric checkpoint inhibitor study was a phase 1 trial of ipilimumab in patients (2–21 years) with recurrent or refractory solid tumors [8]. Thirty-three patients (28 months–21 years of age) with melanoma (n = 12), sarcoma (n = 17 including 8 OST), renal or bladder carcinoma (n = 3), or neuroblastoma (n = 1) received ipilimumab 1, 3, 5, or 10 mg/kg intravenously (dose escalation 3 + 3 fashion followed by expansion cohort in two age groups (1–11 years and 12–21 years)). Induction therapy comprised 4 cycles of ipilimumab IV every 3 weeks. If there was no evidence of progressive disease or dose limiting toxicity (DLT), maintenance therapy was initiated 3 weeks following induction with infusions of the same dose every 12 weeks. The serum half-life of ipilimumab ranged from 8–15 days with a mean that is lower than the 15 day mean half-life identified in the phase 1/2 study of ipilimumab in adults with melanoma. The first two dose levels (1 mg/kg and 3 mg/kg) accrued three patients each without any DLT, but DLT occurred at 5 mg/kg- and 10 mg/kg-dose levels (all in children <12 years). Overall, 18 (55%) of subjects developed any grade IRAEs and 9 (27%) developed grade 3 or 4 IRAEs with gastrointestinal and liver toxicities being most common. The incidence of IRAEs is within the range observed on adult studies, except for skin manifestations, which occurred at a lower frequency in pediatric and adolescent patients. Although no fatal events occurred, one patient developed hypophysitis and subsequent panhypopituitarism, and two other patients developed colitis (one colonic perforation requiring surgical management and one requiring anti-TNF therapy). There was no objective response to ipilimumab, but stable disease was seen in six subjects for 4–10 cycles (melanoma = 1, OST = 2, synovialosarcoma = 1, clear cell sarcoma = 1 and renal cell carcinoma = 1). As reported in adult tumors, an increased overall survival in patients who developed grade 2 or greater IRAEs was observed, compared to patients who did not have any immune toxicity. An ongoing phase I/II pediatric trial through the Children's Oncology Group (COG) is investigating the safety of the PD-1 mAb nivolumab, with and without ipilimumab in patients with recurrent or refractory solid tumors (NCT02304458).

7.3.2 Anti-PD1/PD-L1

Anti-PD-1 antibodies include pembrolizumab (Keytruda®, Merck Sharp & Dohme), a humanized IgG4 mAb, and nivolumab (Opdivo®, Bristol-Meyers Squibb), a fully human IgG4 mAb. Pidilizumab (Pfizer), a humanized IgG1 mAb exclusively developed in lymphoma, was originally thought to bind PD-1, but this is currently uncertain. These PD-1 antibodies can prevent the binding of PD-1 to its ligands PDL1 and PDL2, resulting in the disruption of inhibitory mechanisms and restoring T-cell effector phase function. Both pembrolizumab and nivolumab were evaluated in many clinical trials in adult solid tumors and hematologic malignancies. A common observation from these trials was that nivolumab and pembrolizumab were equally effective in inducing long-term durable responses, which was accompanied by significantly far less toxicity (~10% Grade 3–4 IRAEs) when compared with ipilimumab. In a recent meta-analysis of the risk of IRAEs with anti-CTLA4 and anti-PD1 mAb, including 21 studies and 11,144 adult patients, anti-CTLA4 therapy was associated with a significantly higher risk of overall IRAEs, diarrhea, immune-related colitis, pruritus and rash compared to control therapies (relative risk (RR) = 2.43, 2.10, 11.39, 3.88, 3.87; $p < 0.001$ for all outcomes) while anti-PD1 therapy was associated with a significantly higher risk of pruritus only (RR = 4.01, $p < 0.001$) [67]. However, pediatric physician should also be aware of clinical spectrum of IRAEs induced by anti-PD1: (a) because the risk is still unknown in children/adolescents, (b) long term side effects of anti PD-1 are unknown, and (c) because most the trial in progress and in the near future will include combination therapy with anti-PD1 in children which has been shown to increase toxicity and IRAEs in adults (for example, Grade 3–4 IRAEs rate of 55% when ipilimumab is combined with nivolumab) [68].

Beyond melanoma (overall response rate (ORR) 22–33%) and NSCLC (ORR 20–30%), anti-PD-1 are showing promising responses across many different cancer subtypes including small-cell lung cancer (15% ORR), renal cell carcinoma (25% ORR), urothelial cancer (25% ORR), head and neck squamous cell carcinoma (12–25% ORR), gastric cancer (20% ORR), hepatocellular carcinoma (20% ORR), ovarian cancer (15% ORR), and triple negative breast cancer (20% ORR). Importantly, these responses are durable with 5-years survivals in malignant melanoma and NSCLC of 34% and 16%, respectively.

Although no completed pediatric studies have been reported yet with anti-PD1, several studies are ongoing and summarized in Table 7.1. However, in our experience, disappointing results were observed with anti-PD1 monotherapy in the majority of pediatric malignancies, although some remarkable responses have been reported in particular tumor subtypes, such as desmoplastic small round cells tumor, epithelioid sarcoma, and pleomorphic RMS (personal communication) [69], highlighting the need to establish predictive biomarkers of response to immunotherapy. The first-reported biomarker for predicting the efficacy of anti-PD1 therapy was the expression level of PD-L1 on tumor cells. However, there is still no consensus on how a PD-L1-positive tumor should be defined, since each pharmaceutical company has used different antibodies clones for its immunohistochemical staining, different scoring algorithms, and different positivity thresholds. Other biomarkers said to be predictive of the efficacy of immune checkpoint blockade therapy include peripheral blood cell counts, markers of T-cell activation, factors in the tumor's inflammatory microenvironment, a high frequency of T-cell receptor clonotypes, and a high mutational burden in the tumor.

In a recent publication, authors reported a dramatic response to nivolumab in two young siblings with recurrent glioblastoma multiforme and bMMRD [13, 14]. Indeed, as discussed above, malignant tumors associated with bMMRD exhibit unique level of mutation load among human cancers and a particularity of non-bMMRD cancers exhibiting high mutation loads -subsets of malignant melanomas and lung, bladder, and microsatellite-unstable gastro-intestinal cancers—is responsiveness to immune checkpoint inhibitors. While patients with Lynch syndrome (heterozygous monoallelic germline mutation in MMR genes) usually do not develop cancers in childhood, it is crucial for pediatric physician to be able to diagnose bMMRD for therapeutic decision (MMR-deficient tumors do not respond to cytotoxic chemotherapy as these agents may require intact DNA mismatch repair to be effective). Thus, PD-1 blockade is now considered of "the Achilles heel for MMR-deficient tumors" [14].

In classical Hodgkin's lymphoma, in which chromosome 9p24.1/PDL1/PDL2 alterations have been shown to be a "hallmark" of the disease, an ORR of 87% (20/23 pts) and a CR rate of 17% (4/23 pts) have been reported in phase 1 [9]. The responses obtained were durable with a 6-month progression-free survival (PFS) of 86% and no significant difference in the ORR in the subset of 18 participants who had previously failed brentuximab vedotin. This was confirmed further in a Phase 2 registration national study in heavily pretreated patients who had failed autologous stem cell transplantation and brentuximab vedotin: nivolumab demonstrated investigator-assessed ORR of 73%, the potential to produce durable responses including durable partial responses, with ongoing responses in 62% of patients at data cut-off [10, 70]. FDA and EMA recently approved single-agent nivolumab for the treatment of adults with relapsing or refractory classical Hodgkin Lymphoma following failure of autologous stem cell transplantation and brentuximab vedotin. A phase 2 is ongoing in children/adolescents evaluating nivolumab + brentuximab vendotin followed by brentuximab + bendamustine, for patients with relapsed/refractory classic Hodgkin's lymphoma who have failed first-line therapy. In ALK+

anaplastic large cell lymphoma, we and others reported dramatic response to anti-PD1 therapy in patients in refractory disease (including failures after ALK inhibitors and/or brentuximab vendotin and/or allogeneic hematologic stem cell transplantation) (personal communication) [12].

Anti-PD-L1 mAb include atezolizumab (Roche), a human monoclonal IgG1 with an engineered Fc domain, BMS-936559 (Bristol-Meyers Squibb), a fully human IgG4, and Durvalumab (AstraZeneca), a fully human IgG1. PD-L1 mAb have a distinct mechanism of action from PD-1 mAb. Indeed, in addition to block PD-L1 and PD-1 interaction, which can reinvigorate suppressed immune cells to eliminate cancer cells; it blocks PD-L1 and CD80 binding, which might further enhance immune responses. In 2016, the FDA approved atezolizumab for the treatment of patients with locally advanced or metastatic urothelial carcinoma whose disease progressed during or following platinum-containing chemotherapy based on results of a single-arm trial in 310 patients with a confirmed ORR of 14.8% [71]. Importantly, of the 46 responders, 37 patients had an ongoing response for ≥6 months. Toxicity profile was quite similar to anti-PD-1 mAb. Moreover, similar antitumor activity was reported for other PD-1 or PD-L1 targeted products in advanced urothelial carcinoma with response rates were approximately 18–30%. More studies are needed to compare efficacy and toxicity profiles of anti-PD1 and PDL1 mAb. Several studies with anti-PD-L1 are ongoing in children malignancies.

7.4 Future Challenge and Directions

In adults with cancer, dramatic and durable results were obtained with immune checkpoint blockers in advanced melanoma and non-small cell lung cancer and proofs of efficacy have been demonstrated with PD-1/PD-L1 antibodies in more than 20 cancer types. However, there are still limited clinical trials focusing on immunotherapies targeting the host immune system in pediatric oncology but some outstanding results have been reported in specific tumor histology (such as Hodgkin lymphoma and some soft tissue sarcoma subtypes)/genetic predisposition syndrome (such as MMR deficiency). In particular, low to moderate PD-L1 expression and mutation load/neoantigen repertoire is reported in the majority of pediatric cancers and may translate in future trial results with anti-PD1 monotherapy in disappointing response rates. In addition to common challenge with adult immuno-oncology (including but not limited to, safety and maximum tolerated dose definition, responses and efficacy assessment, and biomarker for predicting the efficacy), some specific questions/challenges should be considered in pediatric immunotherapy development. First, how to modulate tumor microenvironment to reverse immune ignorance/tolerance of pediatric cancers? Indeed, many different combination can be considered to increase tumor immunogenicity including chemotherapy and radiotherapy (so-called "immunogenic cell death" which in turn induces $CD8^+$ T-cells, NK-cells, and macrophages activation, antigen release and pro-inflammatory cytokines), toll-like receptors agonists, tumor vaccines or oncolytic viruses, and combination of immune checkpoints blockers. Thus, rather than administered alone, blocking mAbs are more likely to achieve synergistic antitumor effects if they are combined with a chemotherapeutic regimen or other checkpoint inhibitors. These combination therapies are largely developed in adult oncology with promising and attractive results. For example, in a randomized phase 3 trial in advanced melanoma, patients treated with nivolumab and ipilimumab achieved a median PFS of 11.5 months *vs* 2.9 and 6.9 months with ipilimumab and nivolumab alone, respectively. Importantly, grade 3–4 toxicity was higher in the combination arm (55%) *vs* 27 and 16% in the ipilimumab and nivolumab arms, respectively. Second, because several lines of evidence support the role of NK-cells as well tumor-associated myeloid cells in governing immunosurveillance of different pediatric cancers, it seems promising to develop specific NK and myeloid-directed therapies also in combination with other immune or conventional therapies. Third, by contrast to adult malignancies, the majority of pediatric cancers are chemosensitive disease but, especially for metastatic sarcoma, not curable by chemotherapy. However, patients need potent immune system to achieve maximum therapeutic benefit from immune therapies. Thus, the optimal design to develop immune therapies should be defined: either at diagnosis, with bulky disease and combined with myelosuppressive chemotherapy or as consolidative immunotherapy in minimal residual disease status. We are also just at the beginning of this existing research area but pediatric physicians should be aware of immune related toxicities and unknown long term consequences of immune checkpoints blockers in children/adolescents. These toxicities should be evaluated in large trials and registered in international database. Finally, a better understanding of pediatric tumor microenvironment including tumor–host interaction and immune escape mechanisms, as well as collaboration with industry and early drug development is warranted to allow rapid clinical progress in pediatric immune-oncology.

References

1. Schreiber RD, Old LJ, Smyth MJ. Cancer immunoediting: integrating immunity's roles in cancer suppression and promotion. Science. 2011;331(6024):1565–70.
2. Dunn GP, Bruce AT, Ikeda H, Old LJ, Schreiber RD. Cancer immunoediting: from immunosurveillance to tumor escape. Nat Immunol nov. 2002;3(11):991–8.
3. Teng MWL, Galon J, Fridman W-H, Smyth MJ. From mice to humans: developments in cancer immunoediting. J Clin Invest. 2015;125(9):3338–46.
4. Pardoll DM. The blockade of immune checkpoints in cancer immunotherapy. Nat Rev Cancer. 2012;12(4):252–64.
5. Postel-Vinay S, Aspeslagh S, Lanoy E, Robert C, Soria J-C, Marabelle A. Challenges of phase 1 clinical trials evaluating immune checkpoint-targeted antibodies. Ann Oncol. 2016;27(2):214–24.
6. Menon S, Shin S, Dy G. Advances in cancer immunotherapy in solid tumors. Cancers. 2016;8(12):106.
7. OASIS [Internet]. (cité 29 avr 2017). Disponible sur: http://www.abstractsonline.com/Plan/ViewAbstract.aspx?mID=4017&sKey=371fa616-a0cf-4bf8-993d-ce424853b52c&cKey=616f965e-a236-4bd2-9f7a-6399bd6f3f6c&mKey=1d10d749-4b6a-4ab3-bcd4-f80fb1922267

8. Merchant MS, Wright M, Baird K, Wexler LH, Rodriguez-Galindo C, Bernstein D, et al. Phase I clinical trial of ipilimumab in pediatric patients with advanced solid tumors. Clin Cancer Res Off J Am Assoc Cancer Res. 2016;22(6):1364–70.
9. Ansell SM, Lesokhin AM, Borrello I, Halwani A, Scott EC, Gutierrez M, et al. PD-1 blockade with nivolumab in relapsed or refractory Hodgkin's lymphoma. N Engl J Med. 2015;372(4):311–9.
10. Chen R, Zinzani PL, Fanale MA, Armand P, Johnson NA, Brice P, et al. Phase II study of the efficacy and safety of pembrolizumab for relapsed/refractory classic hodgkin lymphoma. J Clin Oncol. 2017;35(19):2125–32. doi:10.1200/JCO.2016.72.1316.
11. Foran AE, Nadel HR, Lee AF, Savage KJ, Deyell RJ. Nivolumab in the treatment of refractory pediatric hodgkin lymphoma. J Pediatr Hematol Oncol. 2017;39(5):e263–e266.
12. Hebart H, Lang P, Woessmann W. Nivolumab for refractory anaplastic large cell lymphoma: a case report. Ann Intern Med. 2016;165(8):607–8.
13. Bouffet E, Larouche V, Campbell BB, Merico D, de Borja R, Aronson M, et al. Immune checkpoint inhibition for hypermutant glioblastoma multiforme resulting from germline biallelic mismatch repair deficiency. J Clin Oncol. 2016;34(19):2206–11.
14. Lin AY, Lin E. Programmed death 1 blockade, an Achilles heel for MMR-deficient tumors? J Hematol Oncol J Hematol Oncol. 2015;8:124.
15. Dong H, Strome SE, Salomao DR, Tamura H, Hirano F, Flies DB, et al. Tumor-associated B7-H1 promotes T-cell apoptosis: a potential mechanism of immune evasion. Nat Med. 2002;8(8):793–800.
16. Galluzzi L, Buqué A, Kepp O, Zitvogel L, Kroemer G. Immunogenic cell death in cancer and infectious disease. Nat Rev Immunol. 2017;17(2):97–111.
17. Dowling DJ, Levy O. Ontogeny of early life immunity. Trends Immunol. 2014;35(7):299–310.
18. Mold JE, Michaëlsson J, Burt TD, Muench MO, Beckerman KP, Busch MP, et al. Maternal alloantigens promote the development of tolerogenic fetal regulatory T cells in utero. Science. 2008;322(5907):1562–5.
19. Levy O. Innate immunity of the newborn: basic mechanisms and clinical correlates. Nat Rev Immunol. 2007;7(5):379–90.
20. Kollmann TR, Levy O, Montgomery RR, Goriely S. Innate immune function by Toll-like receptors: distinct responses in newborns and the elderly. Immunity. 2012;37(5):771–83.
21. Zitvogel L, Ayyoub M, Routy B, Kroemer G. Microbiome and anticancer immunosurveillance. Cell. 2016;165(2):276–87.
22. Vétizou M, Pitt JM, Daillère R, Lepage P, Waldschmitt N, Flament C, et al. Anticancer immunotherapy by CTLA-4 blockade relies on the gut microbiota. Science. 2015;350(6264):1079–84.
23. Korpela K, de Vos WM. Antibiotic use in childhood alters the gut microbiota and predisposes to overweight. Microb Cell Graz Austria. 2016;3(7):296–8.
24. Tun HM, Konya T, Takaro TK, Brook JR, Chari R, Field CJ, et al. Exposure to household furry pets influences the gut microbiota of infant at 3–4 months following various birth scenarios. Microbiome. 2017;5(1):40.
25. Sivan A, Corrales L, Hubert N, Williams JB, Aquino-Michaels K, Earley ZM, et al. Commensal Bifidobacterium promotes antitumor immunity and facilitates anti-PD-L1 efficacy. Science. 2015;350(6264):1084–9.
26. Umbrello G, Esposito S. Microbiota and neurologic diseases: potential effects of probiotics. J Transl Med. 2016;14(1):298.
27. Blanton LV, Barratt MJ, Charbonneau MR, Ahmed T, Gordon JI. Childhood undernutrition, the gut microbiota, and microbiota-directed therapeutics. Science. 2016;352(6293):1533.
28. Downing JR, Wilson RK, Zhang J, Mardis ER, Pui C-H, Ding L, et al. The pediatric cancer genome project. Nat Genet. 2012;44(6):619–22.
29. Shern JF, Chen L, Chmielecki J, Wei JS, Patidar R, Rosenberg M, et al. Comprehensive genomic analysis of rhabdomyosarcoma reveals a landscape of alterations affecting a common genetic axis in fusion-positive and fusion-negative tumors. Cancer Discov. 2014;4(2):216–31.
30. van Rooij N, van Buuren MM, Philips D, Velds A, Toebes M, Heemskerk B, et al. Tumor exome analysis reveals neoantigen-specific T-cell reactivity in an ipilimumab-responsive melanoma. J Clin Oncol. 2013;31(32):e439–42.

31. Schumacher TN, Schreiber RD. Neoantigens in cancer immunotherapy. Science. 2015;348(6230):69–74.
32. Strønen E, Toebes M, Kelderman S, van Buuren MM, Yang W, van Rooij N, et al. Targeting of cancer neoantigens with donor-derived T cell receptor repertoires. Science. 2016;352(6291):1337–41.
33. Zhang J, Walsh MF, Wu G, Edmonson MN, Gruber TA, Easton J, et al. Germline mutations in predisposition genes in pediatric cancer. N Engl J Med. 2015;373(24):2336–46.
34. Lavoine N, Colas C, Muleris M, Bodo S, Duval A, Entz-Werle N, et al. Constitutional mismatch repair deficiency syndrome: clinical description in a French cohort. J Med Genet. 2015;52(11):770–8.
35. Shlien A, Campbell BB, de Borja R, Alexandrov LB, Merico D, Wedge D, et al. Combined hereditary and somatic mutations of replication error repair genes result in rapid onset of ultra-hypermutated cancers. Nat Genet. 2015;47(3):257–62.
36. Aoki T, Hino M, Koh K, Kyushiki M, Kishimoto H, Arakawa Y, et al. Low frequency of programmed death ligand 1 expression in pediatric cancers. Pediatr Blood Cancer. 2016;63(8):1461–4.
37. Mina M, Boldrini R, Citti A, Romania P, D'Alicandro V, De Ioris M, et al. Tumor-infiltrating T lymphocytes improve clinical outcome of therapy-resistant neuroblastoma. Oncoimmunology. 2015;4(9):e1019981.
38. Fritzsching B, Fellenberg J, Moskovszky L, Sápi Z, Krenacs T, Machado I, et al. CD8(+)/FOXP3(+)-ratio in osteosarcoma microenvironment separates survivors from non-survivors: a multicenter validated retrospective study. Oncoimmunology. 2015;4(3):e990800.
39. Yabe H, Tsukahara T, Kawaguchi S, Wada T, Torigoe T, Sato N, et al. Prognostic significance of HLA class I expression in Ewing's sarcoma family of tumors. J Surg Oncol. 2011;103(5):380–5.
40. Sundara YT, Kostine M, Cleven AHG, Bovée JVMG, Schilham MW, Cleton-Jansen A-M. Increased PD-L1 and T-cell infiltration in the presence of HLA class I expression in metastatic high-grade osteosarcoma: a rationale for T-cell-based immunotherapy. Cancer Immunol Immunother. 2017;66(1):119–28.
41. Haworth KB, Leddon JL, Chen C-Y, Horwitz EM, Mackall CL, Cripe TP. Going back to class I: MHC and immunotherapies for childhood cancer. Pediatr Blood Cancer. 2015;62(4):571–6.
42. Cho D, Shook DR, Shimasaki N, Chang Y-H, Fujisaki H, Campana D. Cytotoxicity of activated natural killer cells against pediatric solid tumors. Clin Cancer Res Off J Am Assoc Cancer Res. 2010;16(15):3901–9.
43. Buddingh EP, Kuijjer ML, Duim RAJ, Bürger H, Agelopoulos K, Myklebost O, et al. Tumor-infiltrating macrophages are associated with metastasis suppression in high-grade osteosarcoma: a rationale for treatment with macrophage activating agents. Clin Cancer Res Off J Am Assoc Cancer Res. 2011;17(8):2110–9.
44. Dumars C, Ngyuen J-M, Gaultier A, Lanel R, Corradini N, Gouin F, et al. Dysregulation of macrophage polarization is associated with the metastatic process in osteosarcoma. Oncotarget. 2016;7(48):78343–54.
45. Asgharzadeh S, Salo JA, Ji L, Oberthuer A, Fischer M, Berthold F, et al. Clinical significance of tumor associated inflammatory cells in metastatic neuroblastoma. J Clin Oncol. 2012;30(28):3525–32.
46. Mao Y, Eissler N, Blanc KL, Johnsen JI, Kogner P, Kiessling R. Targeting suppressive myeloid cells potentiates checkpoint inhibitors to control spontaneous neuroblastoma. Clin Cancer Res Off J Am Assoc Cancer Res. 2016;22(15):3849–59.
47. Highfill SL, Cui Y, Giles AJ, Smith JP, Zhang H, Morse E, et al. Disruption of CXCR2-mediated MDSC tumor trafficking enhances anti-PD1 efficacy. Sci Transl Med. 2014;6(237):237ra67.
48. Bilbao-Aldaiturriaga N, Patino-Garcia A, Martin-Guerrero I, Garcia-Orad A. Cytotoxic T lymphocyte-associated antigen 4 rs231775 polymorphism and osteosarcoma. Neoplasma. 2017;64(2):299–304.
49. Feng D, Yang X, Li S, Liu T, Wu Z, Song Y, et al. Cytotoxic T-lymphocyte antigen-4 genetic variants and risk of Ewing's sarcoma. Genet Test Mol Biomark. 2013;17(6):458–63.

50. Hingorani P, Maas ML, Gustafson MP, Dickman P, Adams RH, Watanabe M, et al. Increased CTLA-4(+) T cells and an increased ratio of monocytes with loss of class II (CD14(+) HLA-DR(lo/neg)) found in aggressive pediatric sarcoma patients. J Immunother Cancer. 2015;3:35.
51. Lussier DM, Johnson JL, Hingorani P, Blattman JN. Combination immunotherapy with α-CTLA-4 and α-PD-L1 antibody blockade prevents immune escape and leads to complete control of metastatic osteosarcoma. J Immunother Cancer. 2015;3:21.
52. Nishimura H, Nose M, Hiai H, Minato N, Honjo T. Development of lupus-like autoimmune diseases by disruption of the PD-1 gene encoding an ITIM motif-carrying immunoreceptor. Immunity. 1999;11(2):141–51.
53. Nishimura H, Okazaki T, Tanaka Y, Nakatani K, Hara M, Matsumori A, et al. Autoimmune dilated cardiomyopathy in PD-1 receptor-deficient mice. Science. 2001;291(5502):319–22.
54. Freeman GJ, Long AJ, Iwai Y, Bourque K, Chernova T, Nishimura H, et al. Engagement of the PD-1 immunoinhibitory receptor by a novel B7 family member leads to negative regulation of lymphocyte activation. J Exp Med. 2000;192(7):1027–34.
55. Assessment of PD-L1 expression and tumor associated immune cells in pediatric cancer tissues. | 2016 ASCO Annual Meeting | Abstracts | Meeting Library [Internet]. (cité 29 avr 2017) Disponible sur: http://meetinglibrary.asco.org/content/167514-176
56. Routh JC, Ashley RA, Sebo TJ, Lohse CM, Husmann DA, Kramer SA, et al. B7-H1 expression in Wilms tumor: correlation with tumor biology and disease recurrence. J Urol. 2008;179(5):1954–9. discussion 1959-1960
57. The PD-L1 Expression Increases After Consecutive Multimodal Therapies In Neuroblastoma: P-392 [Internet]. (cité 29 avr 2017). Disponible sur: https://insights.ovid.com/pediatric-blood-cancer/pedbc/2015/11/004/pd-l1-expression-increases-consecutive-multimodal/769/01445489
58. Shen JK, Cote GM, Choy E, Yang P, Harmon D, Schwab J, et al. Programmed cell death ligand 1 expression in osteosarcoma. Cancer Immunol Res. 2014;2(7):690–8.
59. Chowdhury F, et al. PD-L1 and CD8+PD1+ lymphocytes exist as targets in the pediatric tumor microenvironment for immunomodulatory therapy. OncoImmunology. 2015;4(10) doi:10.1080/2162402X.2015.1029701. [Internet]. (cité 29 avr 2017)
60. Roemer MGM, Advani RH, Ligon AH, Natkunam Y, Redd RA, Homer H, et al. PD-L1 and PD-L2 genetic alterations define classical Hodgkin lymphoma and predict outcome. J Clin Oncol. 2016;34(23):2690–7.
61. Marzec M, Zhang Q, Goradia A, Raghunath PN, Liu X, Paessler M, et al. Oncogenic kinase NPM/ALK induces through STAT3 expression of immunosuppressive protein CD274 (PD-L1, B7-H1). Proc Natl Acad Sci U S A. 2008;105(52):20852–7.
62. Castriconi R, Dondero A, Augugliaro R, Cantoni C, Carnemolla B, Sementa AR, et al. Identification of 4Ig-B7-H3 as a neuroblastoma-associated molecule that exerts a protective role from an NK cell-mediated lysis. Proc Natl Acad Sci U S A. 2004;101(34):12640–5.
63. Wang L, Zhang Q, Chen W, Shan B, Ding Y, Zhang G, et al. B7-H3 is overexpressed in patients suffering osteosarcoma and associated with tumor aggressiveness and metastasis. PLoS One. 2013;8(8):e70689.
64. Forlenza CJ, Boudreau JE, Zheng J, Le Luduec J-B, Chamberlain E, Heller G, et al. KIR3DL1 allelic polymorphism and HLA-B epitopes modulate response to anti-GD2 monoclonal antibody in patients with neuroblastoma. J Clin Oncol. 2016;34(21):2443–51.
65. Michot JM, Bigenwald C, Champiat S, Collins M, Carbonnel F, Postel-Vinay S, et al. Immune-related adverse events with immune checkpoint blockade: a comprehensive review. Eur J Cancer Oxf Engl 1990. 2016;54:139–48.
66. Champiat S, Lambotte O, Barreau E, Belkhir R, Berdelou A, Carbonnel F, et al. Management of immune checkpoint blockade dysimmune toxicities: a collaborative position paper. Ann Oncol Off J Eur Soc Med Oncol. 2016;27(4):559–74.
67. Komaki Y, Komaki F, Yamada A, Micic D, Ido A, Sakuraba A. Meta-analysis of the risk of immune-related adverse events with anti-cytotoxic T-lymphocyte-associated antigen 4 and anti-programmed death 1 therapies. Clin Pharmacol Ther. 2017; doi:10.1002/cpt.633.

68. Larkin J, Chiarion-Sileni V, Gonzalez R, Grob JJ, Cowey CL, Lao CD, et al. Combined Nivolumab and Ipilimumab or Monotherapy in Untreated Melanoma. N Engl J Med. 2015;373(1):23–34.
69. Paoluzzi L, Cacavio A, Ghesani M, Karambelkar A, Rapkiewicz A, Weber J, et al. Response to anti-PD1 therapy with nivolumab in metastatic sarcomas. Clin Sarcoma Res. 2016;6:24.
70. Armand P, Shipp MA, Ribrag V, Michot J-M, Zinzani PL, Kuruvilla J, et al. Programmed death-1 blockade with pembrolizumab in patients with classical hodgkin lymphoma after brentuximab vedotin failure. J Clin Oncol. 2016;34(31):3733–9.
71. Rosenberg JE, Hoffman-Censits J, Powles T, van der Heijden MS, Balar AV, Necchi A, et al. Atezolizumab in patients with locally advanced and metastatic urothelial carcinoma who have progressed following treatment with platinum-based chemotherapy: a single-arm, multicentre, phase 2 trial. Lancet Lond Engl. 2016;387(10031):1909–20.

Chapter 8
Adoptive T Cell Therapies for Children's Cancers

Jonathan Fisher and John Anderson

Abstract Adoptive T-cell therapies involve generation and administration of large numbers of cancer-specific cytotoxic T-cells. Early proof of concept for efficacy of T cells in paediatric cancer was seen in the "graft-versus-leukaemia" effects following allogeneic bone marrow transplantation. Subsequently, the approach has been trialled in solid tumours following genetic modification of T-cells to retarget them against cancer. Optimised T-cell products can be derived from tumour-infiltrating lymphocytes, or bulk populations of T-cells can be engineered by gene therapy techniques to express tumour antigen-specific recognition receptors that redirect T cell to tumour. Engineered T-cell stimulating receptors lead to activation in the presence of the tumour with subsequent inflammatory response and amplification of the T cell clones. Following clinical success of chimeric antigen receptors modified T cells in acute lymphoblastic leukaemia, T cell immunotherapeutics are now a preclinical growth area in the field of childhood cancer immunotherapeutics.

Keywords Immunotherapy • Adoptive transfer • Chimeric antigen receptor • T-cell • TCR-transfer

The concept of infusing large numbers of T cells into a patient with cancer, with a view to effecting long term disease control is not novel. Increasingly it is recognized that the clinical benefits of allogeneic bone marrow transplantation for some forms of leukaemia depend on detection and destruction of cancer cells by T cells within the graft. A further development; to infuse purified populations of the donor's T lymphocytes following engraftment, has resulted in the direct demonstration of this *graft versus leukaemia* effect [1, 2]. Subsequent refinements have used selected or engineered T cells in both the allogeneic and autologous settings. In this chapter

J. Fisher
Cancer Section, UCL Great Ormond Street Insitute of Child Health, London, UK

J. Anderson (✉)
Department of Paediatric Oncology, Great Ormond Street Hospital
and Institute of Child Health, University College London, London, UK
e-mail: j.anderson@ucl.ac.uk

J.C. Gray, A. Marabelle (eds.), *Immunotherapy for Pediatric Malignancies*,
https://doi.org/10.1007/978-3-319-43486-5_8

we will review the historical development of T cell therapies for cancer and describe current and potential applications in paediatric cancers.

8.1 T Cell Biology

A brief overview of some aspects of mechanism of action of T cells is required to appreciate key factors determining clinical utility of T cell adoptive transfer.

8.1.1 The Generation of Diversity

T lymphocytes are one of the major effector cells of the adaptive immune system. Like B lymphocytes, T cells undergo a rearrangement of their immune receptor genes to create a vast degree of diversity. In the case of B cells, the diversity is generated by rearrangement of the immunoglobulin gene locus during haematopoiesis. T cells undergo an analogous rearrangement of the T cell receptor (TCR) gene locus during early thymic development. In both cases diversity is generated through multiple mechanisms including the random pairing of two chains (heavy and light in the case of immunoglobulins and alpha and beta in the case of the majority of T cells), and the random selection of variable genes, which are joined to constant regions through random incorporation of joining (J) and diversity (D) segments. The pairing of alpha and beta chains is achieved through association of the constant regions to create an antigen recognition region comprising the variable regions of the alpha and beta chains respectively (Fig. 8.1). It is estimated that through random rearrangement of the αβTCR gene loci, up to 10^{16} potential different antigenic specificities can be generated. It is this remarkable degree of diversity within the T cell receptor repertoire that affords T cells their ability to respond to non-self, for example in the form of infectious agents.

8.1.2 T Cell Receptors Recognize a Surface of Self-MHC and Non-self Peptide Antigen

The primary purpose of T cell development within the thymus is the generation of a vast repertoire of unique clones each with a unique antigenic specificity determined by the TCR. Each clone has the capacity to respond to danger when stimulated by the target ligands, displayed on the surface of a target cell, that bind the TCR. αβTCRs that have binding affinity for MHC molecules undergo selection

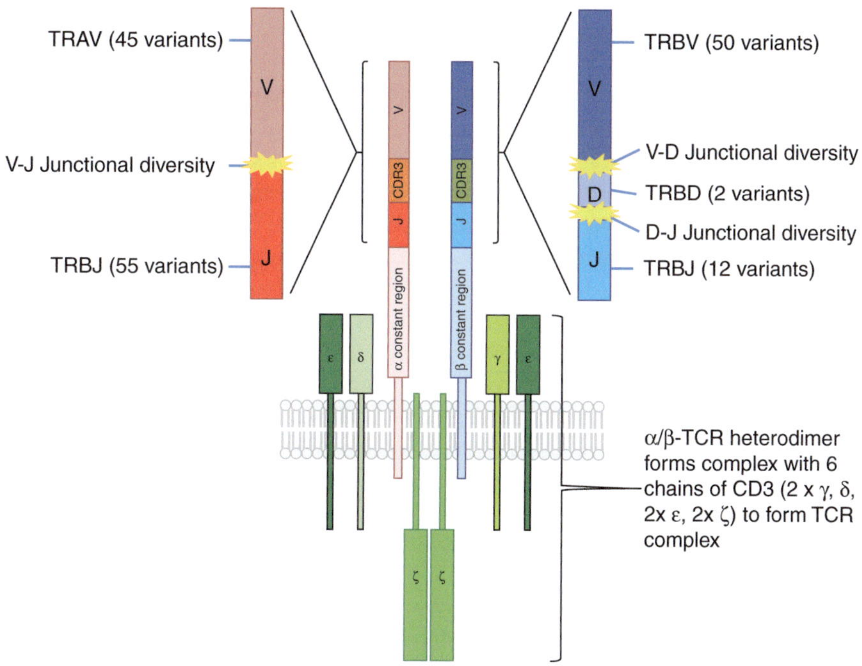

Fig. 8.1 The αβTCR, showing the areas of potential diversity

within the thymus. MHC molecules are highly polymorphic and therefore afford the immune system a fundamental mechanism of distinguishing self from non-self. The actual ligand for the T cell receptor in the context of an adaptive immune response is a self MHC molecule bound to (presenting) a peptide fragment of a protein antigen. In the face of a high antigen load, for example in the context of viral infection, there is a huge expansion of a limited repertoire of T cells with specificities for viral peptides presented on self-MHC molecules (class I for CD8 positive cytotoxic T cells and class II for CD4 T helper cells). Exceptions to this general principle include gamma delta T cells and invariant NKT cells which recognize a non-peptide antigen in the context of non-MHC presenting molecules. Cancer can also be recognised as foreign by the immune system. This occurs because cancer presents a wide range of potential danger signals and "foreign" antigens. This can be in the form of mutated "neo-antigens" arising as a result of genomic mutation causing activation of oncogenes. In addition, over expression of non-mutated proteins by cancer cells can result in a sufficiently high density of peptide/MHC complexes to engage and cause signalling in T cells bearing positively selected TCR with intermediate affinity.

8.2 Approaches to Adoptive Immunotherapy in Leukaemia

Early compelling evidence that cancer-reactive T cells have the potential to effect disease regression came from the analysis of trial results of allogeneic bone marrow transplantation (BMT) for leukaemia in which a donor's T cells were included within the therapeutic graft [1, 3]. Whilst most allogeneic grafts are depleted of donor T cells before or after infusion, subsequent infusions of cryopreserved donor's T cells can be used following engraftment at the time of reduced immunosuppression to effect specific anti-leukaemia effects; so called donor lymphocyte infusions (DLI) to effect graft versus leukaemia (GVL) effect. Monitoring of low levels of leukaemia cells has established correlations between DLI and reductions in leukaemia burden, especially in acute myeloid leukaemia [4, 5]. Clinical data correlating the degree of MHC mismatch, the degree of graft vs. host disease (GVHD) and incidence of leukaemia progression have confirmed the hypothesis that a graft versus leukaemia response is a component of the therapeutic efficacy of allogeneic BMT for leukaemia.

Whilst unequivocally established as effective modalities of adoptive T cell immunotherapy for leukaemia, allogeneic BMT and DLI are also exemplars of the major drawback of this the adoptive transfer field, namely the high risk of off-target toxicity. Despite optimal matching of MHC types between donor and recipient, T cell mediated GVHD occurs as a result of grafted T cells recognizing tissues within the recipient as foreign. The greater the degree of mismatch between graft and recipient, the higher the likelihood of the GVL effect but the higher the risk of morbid GVHD. The likely higher antigen density of the residual leukaemia cells suggests that the leukaemia cells themselves similarly have as much or even greater capacity to be attacked by the graft, but this must be balanced against clinically challenging toxicity. Hence allogeneic BMT for leukaemia has become a balancing act of optimizing the degree and time for donor T cells to mediate anti leukaemia effects, titrated against the degree of GVHD through the judicious use of immunosuppressive drugs.

8.3 Expansion and Adoptive Transfer of Tumour Infiltrating Lymphocytes

The dilemma for adoptive T cell therapies is that allogeneic cells cause toxicity whilst autologous T cells are tolerised for self antigens. Cancers however are potentially rich in non-self antigen as a result of large numbers of genomic mutations (so called neo-antigens). Cancers that develop on epithelial surfaces as a result of environmental damage (e.g. melanoma and lung cancer) have the highest incidence of neo-antigen formation [6, 7]. Interestingly, analysis of tumour infiltrating lymphocytes (TILs) has revealed the highest incidence of tumour reactive TILs in tumours with the highest mutation rate [7]. In melanoma the presence of tumour reactive

TILs has been exploited therapeutically by several groups, but most comprehensively by the NCI group [8]. In a series of sequential clinical trials using adoptive transfer of autologous ex vivo expanded TILs, the following key finding have been clearly observed: (1) Infusion of TIL has the capacity to effect sustained clinical remissions in patients even with solid, vacularised, chemotherapy-resistant tumour deposits, (2) optimal T cell therapy employs a mixture of CD4 and CD8 T cells, (3) prior lymphodepletion of the patient greatly improves both clinical response rate and survival [9].

Although patients are self selecting on the basis of successful TIL expansion, and while the process has not thus far been successfully replicated for other cancers, impressive clinical response rates of around 50% are achievable in melanoma patients following full lymphodepleting conditioning [8]. The reasons for the requirement of lymphodepletion prior to adoptive transfer are not completely clear but most likely involve several mechanisms, including loss of competition for homeostatic cytokines, depletion of regulatory T cells-especially in the tumour microenvironment, and the upregulation of proinflammatory danger signals in damaged normal tissues or the tumour site.

It remains uncertain if TIL therapy approaches can be translated to other cancer types. In childhood cancers the mutation rate is much lower than adult epithelial cancers and the predicted neo-antigen density is correspondingly lower [6]. This suggests that the TIL approach is unlikely to be useful for many childhood cancers although the higher mutation rate at relapse [8] may warrant investigation of TIL derived immunotherapies in this context.

8.4 Approaches Involving Engineered Autologous T Cells

Allogeneic T cell transfer has some benefits in leukaemia though this is offset by graft versus host toxicity. There is very little evidence however of a graft versus tumour effect in childhood solid cancers. In general there has been a reluctance to explore allogeneic transplant in childhood solid cancers due to lack of preclinical evidence of efficacy and the risk of morbid GVHD. Thus, in the absence of evidence of natural T cell immunity against many childhood solid cancers, attention has turned to engineering of autologous T cells to retarget them against the cancer. This approach is attractive because it has the potential to be directed against a very specific tumour antigen, avoiding off target toxicity and alloreactivity.

8.5 Engineering T Cell for Tumour Antigen Specificity

T cells are amenable to genetic manipulation with viral or non viral vector systems to transfer genes of interest, leading to expression of a new receptor to alter antigenic specificity. Viral vectors (e.g. gamma retroviruses or lentiviruses) can facilitate introduction of a gene of interest into the germline DNA, resulting in a cell population with the capacity for engineered immunological memory. The two approaches that have been translated into clinical studies are gene transfer of T cell receptors and gene transfer of chimeric antigen receptors.

8.6 T Cell Receptor Gene Transfer

The limitation of the autologous T cell repertoire in terms of anti cancer immunity is tolerance, either because tumour antigens are self antigens and high affinity TCRs have been clonally deleted, or because tumour specific neo-antigens fail to induce T cell immune responses due to the immunoinhibitory nature of the tumour micro-environment. One approach to break this tolerance is to introduce very high affinity T cell receptors for tumour specific antigens into a patient's T cell population and to return these redirected cells back into the patient [11]. Lymphodepletion is usually required to create space for expansion of the infused cells. Various technical hurdles must be overcome to make this approach a reality. For example, the introduced alpha and beta chains need to avoid mis-pairing with the endogenous TCR chains, which could potentially create autoreactive cells, the introduced TCR has to out-compete endogenous TCR for access to CD3, and the introduced alpha and beta chains need to be expressed at approximately equimolar levels. By and large most of these limitations have been overcome through approaches such as co-expressing both chains from a single transcript under the control of a strong promoter, and mutation of constant regions with cysteines that allow pairing disulphide bridges to form only between the introduced alpha and beta chains.

The first reported successful transfer of TCR engineered T cells into a human came when Dudley and co-workers treated melanoma patients with autologous T cells engineered to express a high affinity T cell receptor recognizing a class I (HLA-A0201)-restricted 9 amino acid peptide from the MART1 tumour associated antigen [9, 12]. One area of particular research interest is the requirement and role of CD4 helper cells engineered to engage targets in an MHC class I restricted manner, normally a property observed only in CD8 cytotoxic cells. There is emerging evidence both that CD4 helper cells are important to effect anti tumour efficacy, and that CD4 targeted to an MHC class I restricted tumour associated antigen can provide this help [10]. Phase I studies have now been completed in adult cancers for a number of TCRs targeting a range of tumour associated antigens [11]. Morgan et al. modified autologous normal lymphocytes to express a TCR which was highly reactive against the melanoma antigen MART-1. 2/15 patients who received the modified cells experienced regression of lung and liver metastases and remained disease-free at 2 years of follow-up [9]. Unfortunately, antigen selection remains an issue—a trial of adoptively transferred cells expressing an anti-MAGE-A3 TCR led to clinical responses in 5/9 patients (4 melanoma, 1 synovial sarcoma) but 4/9 (including 2 of the responders) suffered severe neurological toxicity due to rare

MAGE-A occurring CNS neurons [12]. TCR gene transfer therapies have not yet been translated into paediatric malignancy although the range of target antigens that have been tested in adults are expressed in many childhood cancers; for example WT1 expressed in AML and Wilms' tumour.

8.7 Chimeric Antigen Receptors

One reason for the relatively slow growth of the TCR gene transfer field has been the MHC-restriction of inserted TCRs, which lead to the requirement for a patient population to possess a particular HLA type. For example, the most abundant targeted MHC class I allele is HLA-A0201, which is present in only 40% of Caucasians and is rare in other racial groups. TCRs recognising antigen presented on HLA-A0201 will not recognise the same antigen presented on a different MHC-1 haplotype. The emergence of chimeric antigen receptor (CAR) technology, which bypasses the requirement for MHC restriction, has offered an alternative.

Adoptive immunotherapy of T cells engineered to express CARs is an exciting type of cancer immunotherapy which has recently led to unprecedented clinical responses in acute lymphoblastic leukaemia [13]. CAR T cell approaches are undergoing development in many more cancer settings. CARs are recombinant receptors that consist of an ectodomain that provides strong and specific antigen binding and endodomains that are made up of cytoplasmic portions of immune receptors that provide strong T-cell signalling, expressed within a single polypeptide chain (Fig. 8.2). When expressed in a T-cell, CARs allow activatory signals to be provided in the presence of a specific surface antigen.

CARs were first described as T bodies over 20 years ago [14] and the first iterations of the design incorporated antigen binding components of immunoglobulins in the ectodomain fused with most commonly the zeta chain of the TCR/CD3 complex, and less commonly, the gamma chains of Fc-epsilon immunoglobulin receptor

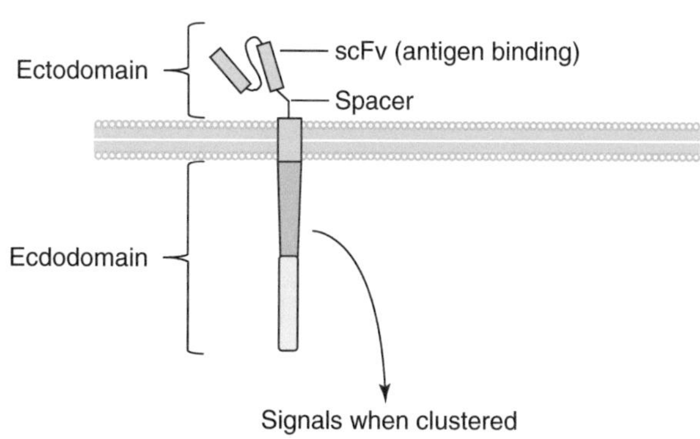

Fig. 8.2 Schematic layout of a chimeric antigen receptor (CAR). Upon encountering a cell expressing the target antigen, CAR clustering brings endodomains from multiple CARs into close proximity inducing signal transduction

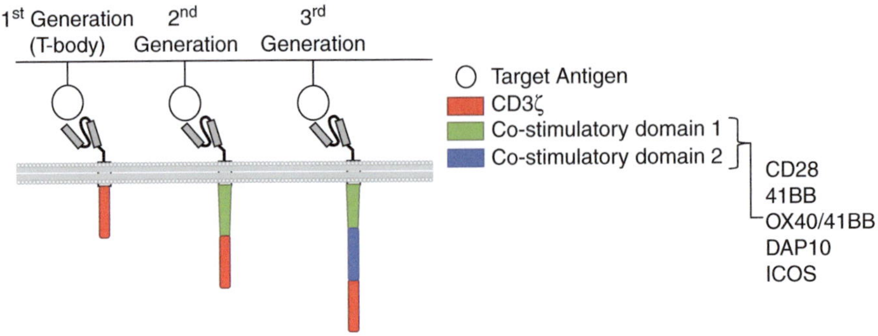

Fig. 8.3 Evolution of chimeric antigen receptors from 1st to 3rd generations

or the gamma chain of CD3 [15]. As CAR design evolved, one or more co-stimulatory endodomains were added in series to CD3ζ (Fig. 8.3).

CARs typically have four components:

1. Antigen recognition motif. This is most commonly a single chain variable fragment (scFv) derived from the variable portion of an antibody.
2. Spacer/linker. The spacer anchors the scFv to the membrane. Sapcers can be of different lengths and levels of flexibility, influencing their effect on CAR clustering and antigen access.
3. Trans-membrane domain. Typically, but not exclusively this will be derived from the linker or the membrane-proximal endodomain.
4. Stimulatory endodomain. In first generation CARs, the endodomain CD3ζ was used. Second generation CARs combined this with co-stimulatory endodomains such as CD28 or 41BB, and third generation CARs contain two co-stimulatory endodomains in addition to CD3ζ.

8.8 Evolution of CAR Generations

Following the demonstration that cross-linking CD3ζ was sufficient to produce T-cell activation [16] at a sufficient level to induce cytotoxicity, the first fusion constructs were developed using an scFv derived from immunoglobulin targeting haptens (small immunogenic molecules attached to larger non-immunogenic species). T-cells expressing these constructs were able to lyse hapten coated target cells [14]. Having demonstrated that combining an scFv with the endodomain of CD3ζ led to focused cytotoxicity against antigen bearing cells, a series of phase 1 trials of first generation CARs were undertaken. Whilst encouraging responses were observed in some settings, a frequently reported difficulty was the failure of CAR expressing T-cells to persist in the recipient, most likely due to an inadequate signal strength provided by the CD3ζ endodomain alone [17]. The signal strength required to induce cytotoxicity is lower than that which is required for other T-cell functions including a robust cytokine response to support proliferation of the activated T cells and secondary expansion upon re-exposure to the target antigen.

Thus, additional signals are required to produce a response of sufficient magnitude. Fusing the CD3ζ chain and the cytoplasmic potions of costimulatory receptors including CD28, 4-1BB, DAP10, OX40 and ICOS led to the creation of second generation CARs, which are now undergoing clinical trials and have shown unprecendented success against lymphoid malignancies [17].

8.9 The Importance of Other CAR Parts

As mentioned above, CARs are composed of four to six components, depending on the identity and number of the endodomains present. Because they are synthetic molecules, there is opportunity for optimisation of all of these components.

The antigen binding scFv used in a CAR can be of varying affinity. When generating scFv libraries against a tumour antigen it is common to have a number of possible clones which will have subtly different characteristics, recognising slightly different epitopes. This can lead to marked differences in the immunological properties of a CAR carrying the scFv. For example, anti ROR1 scFvs with higher affinity have been shown to produce superior anti-tumour reactivity in terms of cytotoxicity, cytokine production and the ability to control ROR1+ *in vivo* models of leukaemia compared to scFvs with lower affinity [18].

The length and flexibility of the spacer which connects the scFv to the rest of the CAR has implications for antigen engagement and CAR clustering. Longer spacers may allow access to membrane proximal epitopes, which are not accessible to shorter linkers. If the spacers are too long however, then CAR clustering may not be tight enough; reducing the possibility for trans-phosphorylation events required for the signaling of some endodomains. A controlled comparison of different spacer lengths was performed by Hudecek and colleagues [18, 19] who demonstrated that spacer length influences anti-tumour efficacy, secondary expansion and cytokine production in response to antigen exposure. In CAR using spacers derived from immunoglobulin constant sequences, the ability of the spacer to bind Fc receptors on immune effector cells can limit on tumour efficacy and lead to off tumour toxicity [19–21].

An additional factor affecting CAR design is "leakiness", which is signalling associated with the ectodomain in the absence of antigen ligation. In the context of an anti-GD2 scFv, leakiness was shown to be mediated by associations between adjacent scFv molecules in CARs leading to immune complex formation and antigen-independent signalling. This led to, early T cell exhaustion and correlated with lack of in vivo efficacy [22]. Tonic signalling has also been described in an anti-CD19-41BB-CD3ζ CAR and, in this context, might be important for physiological function analogous to tonic 41BB signalling during T cell activation [23].

One key factor determining CAR efficacy is the nature and arrangements of the endodomains within second and third generation CARs. For example, in the context of CD19 targeting, the 41BB endodomain has been shown to be superior to CD28 in terms of T cell persistence of the CAR T cells and correlating with enhanced function [23]. In the clinic, CD19 targeting CARs with different scFv and evaluated in a number of clinical trials have demonstrated clinical efficacy. This indicates some of the difficulty in determining the optimal variables in CAR design especially within the early phase clinical trial setting where randomization between different variables is challenging due to cost and complexity.

8.10 Engineered T Cells in Paediatric Clinical Trials

Compared to the number of engineered T cell therapy trials in adult patients, there is a relative paucity of reported experience in paediatric oncology. Following the successes shown in the treatment of lymphoid malignancy, there is increasing enthusiasm for extending these strategies to the paediatric setting. At present, paediatric T cell immunotherapy trials mainly focus on haematological disease, though some success has been made in bringing anti-neuroblastoma immunotherapy to the clinic. A summary of currently active clinical trials from the United States Europe and Asia is provided in Table 8.1.

So far there have been very few reports of clinical studies of CAR-T cell therapy against solid cancers. Insufficient patients have been reported to determine whether the potency of second generation CARs targeting CD19 in B cell disease will also be observed in solid cancers. One major factor predicted to limit effectiveness is the requirement for the T cells to enter the tumour and overcome its immunosuppressive microenvironment [24]. There is encouraging data however from preclinical models; for example in a mesothelioma model, both local and systemic administration of T cells expressing second generation CARs (CD28ζ and/or 4-1BBζ) targeting mesothelin lead to engraftment and tumour regression [25]. Neuroblastoma, one of the commonest extra-cranial solid tumours in children, has been subject to notable success in antibody mediated immunotherapy [26]. It is perhaps unsurprising therefore that this tumour has been targeted with T cell immunotherapy. In 2007, Jensen et al. re-targeted cytolytic T cells against CD171 (LCAM), an antigen overexpressed on neuroblastoma, showing complete response in 1/6 patients [27]. A more commonly targeted neuroblastoma antigen—GD2, was the subject of CAR T cell trials by Pule et al. [28, 29] using a first generation anti-GD2-CD3ζ CAR expressed in EBV specific CTLs. A follow up study is now open in the UK using a second generation CAR (aGD2-28ζ) expressed in bulk-expanded T cells. American studies are testing third generation CAR systems against neuroblastoma, and as GD2 is also expressed on some types of sarcoma, Crystal Mackall's NCI group have opened their trial of a 3rd generation anti-GD2 CAR to include sarcoma patients as well.

Paediatric trials of T cell receptor gene transfer are rarer, though a recent Chinese study using a HLA-A201 restricted TCR against NY-ESO-1 is open to children with a wide range of solid and haematological malignancies including neuroblastoma, melanoma, synovial sarcoma and other metastatic solid cancers.

Table 8.1 Overview of selected recent clinical trials

Sponsor	Disease	Treatment	Design	Trial ID
Seattle Children's Hospital	Relapsed CD19+ ALL	anti-CD19-41BBζ CAR T cells	Phase I	NCT02028455
Memorial Sloan Kettering Cancer Center (NYC)	Relapsed B-ALL	anti-CD19-28ζ CAR T cells	Phase I	NCT01860937
National Cancer Institute	CD22+ B cell malignancies (Follicular lymphoma, ALL, NHL, Large cell lymphoma)	anti-CD22-41BBζ CAR T cells	Phase I	NCT02315612
Seattle Children's Hospital	Relapsed/refractory CD19+ leukaemia	anti-CD19-41BBζ CAR T cells	Phase I/II	NCT02028455
Novartis (Europe)	ALL	CTL019 (anti-CD19-41BBζ CAR T cells)	Phase II	NCT02228096
National Cancer Institute	GD2+ malignancies (neuroblastoma, sarcoma)	Anti-GD2-OX40-41BBζ	Phase I	NCT02107963
Baylor College of Medicine	Neuroblastoma	Anti-GD2-CD28-OX40ζ	Phase I	NCT01822652
University College London (CARPALL)	ALL, Burkitt Lymphoma	anti-CD19-41BBζ CAR T cells	Phase I	NCT02443831
Shanghaii Tongji Hospital, Tongji University	Leukaemia, Lymphoma	Anti-CD19 CAR, endodomain unspecified	Phase I/II	NCT02537977
Shenzen Second People's Hospital (China)	NY-ESO-1 expressing tumour including neuroblastoma	HLA-A2 restricted anti-NY-ESO-1 TCR	Phase I	NCT02457650
Seattle Children's Hospital	Neuroblastoma, ganlioneuroblastoma	Anti-CD171-41BBζ CAR T cells	Phase I {Park:2007gk}	NCT02311621
Fred Hutchinson Cancer Research Centre	CD20+ leukaemia or lymhoma	Anti-CD20-CD28-41BBζ CAR T cells	Phase I Completed	NCT00621452
University College London	ALL	EBV specific CTLs expressing anti-CD19-ζ	Phase I/II	NCT01195480
National Cancer Institute	B-cell leukaemia or lymphoma	Anti-CD19-28ζ CAR T cells	Phase I {Lee:2015 bp}	NCT01593696
Seattle Children's Hospital	B-cell leukaemia	Anti-CD19 CAR T cells, endodomain unspecified	Phase I	NCT01683279
Baylor College of Medicine	Sarcoma	Anti-HER2-CD28ζ CAR T cells	Phase I {Ahmed:2015ik}	NCT00902044

The most marked clinical successes of CAR-T cell therapy in children have been in lymphoid malignancy. There are a number of small phase I and phase I/II studies in children [13, 30] using a range of receptors and conditioning regimens; the common factor being the use of CD19 as a target antigen. Through these studies, the potential to improve clinical response rates in chemotherapy refractory patients has been unequivocally demonstrated. Due to the different conditioning regimens used and the fact that in most cases, CD19-CAR-T have been used as a bridge to transplant, future studies are needed to identify optimal combinations of regimen and receptor [31].

In contrast with the spectacular results seen against ALL, there have been relatively few even preclinical studies evaluating a similar approach for AML. AML is the second most common type of leukaemia in children, and still has an unacceptably high treatment failure rate. One major impediment to development of engineered T cell therapies in AML is the lack of tumour-associated antigens that are not components of normal myelopoietic cells. Preclinical models have focused attention on CD33 and CD123 [32, 33]. Whilst some specific killing of AML blasts has been demonstrated using CD33 and/or CD123 directed second or third generation CARs, the expression of these antigens on normal myeloid cell as well as on Kupfer cells of the liver in the case of CD33 remain concerning for clinical translation. Anecdotal reported clinical studies have not yet contributed significantly to addressing these safety concerns [34].

8.11 The Future; Universal T Cells?

A potential limitation of the adoptive transfer of autologous genetically modified T cells is the cost and complexity of manufacture of a bespoke product on a patient-by-patient basis. If gene modified T cells are to become established first line treatments for common high risk malignancies then either huge investment in cell therapy manufacturing resources, or alternative sources of T cells will be required. One possible future development is the use of third party gene modified T cell products manufactured in bulk in a pharmacological GMP setting and shipped out as a cryopreserved drug product to treatment centres. Several technical hurdles need to be overcome to make this a reality; firstly, adequate numbers of QC tested cells need to be generated. Although T cells can be expanded, they have finite replicative capacity and the variation between donors would mean that rigid QC criteria including functional testing would be needed; Secondly, gene editing, for example deletion of endogenous T cell receptor and MHC molecules would be required to generate off the shelf T cell therapies that will not cause GVHD or be subject to rejection by the host. Although gene editing is likely to become more widely available through technologies such as TALENs and CrispR/CAS, the generation of sufficient T cells for a viable commercial therapeutic product seems a long way off. It is likely however that gene edited T cells might have a role in patients for example with heavily pretreated blood malignancies, for whom autologous T cell product cannot be produced. In this context, use of resources such as cord blood banks is an attractive and intriguing prospect.

References

1. Porter DL, et al. Adoptive immunotherapy with donor mononuclear cell infusions to treat relapse of acute leukemia or myelodysplasia after allogeneic bone marrow transplantation. Bone Marrow Transplant. 1996;18:975–80.
2. Sprangers B, Van Wijmeersch B, Fevery S, Waer M, Billiau AD. Experimental and clinical approaches for optimization of the graft-versus-leukemia effect. Nat Clin Pract Oncol. 2007;4:404–14.
3. Collins RH, et al. Donor leukocyte infusions in 140 patients with relapsed malignancy after allogeneic bone marrow transplantation. J Clin Oncol. 1997;15:433–44.
4. Kröger N, Miyamura K, Bishop MR. Minimal residual disease following allogeneic hematopoietic stem cell transplantation. Biol Blood Marrow Transplant. 2011;17:S94–100.
5. Kolb H-J. Graft-versus-leukemia effects of transplantation and donor lymphocytes. Blood. 2008;112:4371–83.
6. Alexandrov LB, et al. Signatures of mutational processes in human cancer. Nature. 2013;500:415–21.
7. Heemskerk B, Kvistborg P, Schumacher TNM. The cancer antigenome. EMBO J. 2013;32:194–203.
8. Eleveld TF, et al. Relapsed neuroblastomas show frequent RAS-MAPK pathway mutations. Nat Genet. 2015;47:864–71.
9. Morgan RA, et al. Cancer regression in patients after transfer of genetically engineered lymphocytes. Science. 2006;314:126–9.
10. Xue S-A, et al. Human MHC Class I-restricted high avidity CD4(+) T cells generated by co-transfer of TCR and CD8 mediate efficient tumor rejection in vivo. Oncoimmunology. 2013;2:e22590.
11. Engels B, Uckert W. Redirecting T lymphocyte specificity by T cell receptor gene transfer--a new era for immunotherapy. Mol Asp Med. 2007;28:115–42.
12. Morgan RA, et al. Cancer regression and neurological toxicity following anti-MAGE-A3 TCR gene therapy. J Immunother. 2013;36:133–51.
13. Lee DW, et al. T cells expressing CD19 chimeric antigen receptors for acute lymphoblastic leukaemia in children and young adults: a phase 1 dose-escalation trial. Lancet. 2015;385:517–28.
14. Eshhar Z, Waks T, Gross G, Schindler DG. Specific activation and targeting of cytotoxic lymphocytes through chimeric single chains consisting of antibody-binding domains and the gamma or zeta subunits of the immunoglobulin and T-cell receptors. Proc Natl Acad Sci U S A. 1993;90:720–4.
15. Ramos CA, Dotti G. Chimeric antigen receptor (CAR)-engineered lymphocytes for cancer therapy. Expert Opin Biol Ther. 2011;11:855–73.
16. Irving BA, Weiss A. The cytoplasmic domain of the T cell receptor zeta chain is sufficient to couple to receptor-associated signal transduction pathways. Cell. 1991;64:891–901.
17. Brocker T, Karjalainen K. Signals through T cell receptor-zeta chain alone are insufficient to prime resting T lymphocytes. J Exp Med. 1995;181:1653–9.
18. Hudecek M, et al. Receptor affinity and extracellular domain modifications affect tumor recognition by ROR1-specific chimeric antigen receptor T cells. Clin Cancer Res. 2013;19:3153–64.
19. Hudecek M, et al. The nonsignaling extracellular spacer domain of chimeric antigen receptors is decisive for in vivo antitumor activity. Cancer Immunol Res. 2015;3:125–35.
20. Guest RD, et al. The role of extracellular spacer regions in the optimal design of chimeric immune receptors: evaluation of four different scFvs and antigens. J Immunother. 2005;28:203–11.
21. Jonnalagadda M, et al. Chimeric antigen receptors with mutated IgG4 Fc spacer avoid fc receptor binding and improve T cell persistence and antitumor efficacy. Mol Ther. 2015;23:757–68.
22. Long AH, et al. 4-1BB costimulation ameliorates T cell exhaustion induced by tonic signaling of chimeric antigen receptors. Nat Med. 2015;21:581–90.
23. Milone MC, et al. Chimeric receptors containing CD137 signal transduction domains mediate enhanced survival of T cells and increased antileukemic efficacy in vivo. Mol Ther. 2009;17:1453–64.

24. Mussai F, et al. Neuroblastoma arginase activity creates an immunosuppressive microenvironment that impairs autologous and engineered immunity. Can Res. 2015; doi:10.1158/0008–5472.CAN-14-3443.
25. Carpenito C, et al. Control of large, established tumor xenografts with genetically retargeted human T cells containing CD28 and CD137 domains. Proc Natl Acad Sci U S A. 2009;106:3360–5.
26. Yu AL, et al. Anti-GD2 antibody with GM-CSF, interleukin-2, and isotretinoin for neuroblastoma. N Engl J Med. 2010;363:1324–34.
27. Park JR, et al. Adoptive transfer of chimeric antigen receptor re-directed cytolytic T lymphocyte clones in patients with neuroblastoma. Mol Ther. 2007;15:825–33.
28. Pule MA, et al. Virus-specific T cells engineered to coexpress tumor-specific receptors: persistence and antitumor activity in individuals with neuroblastoma. Nat Med. 2008;14:1264–70.
29. Louis CU, et al. Antitumor activity and long-term fate of chimeric antigen receptor-positive T cells in patients with neuroblastoma. Blood. 2011;118:6050–6.
30. Grupp SA, et al. Chimeric antigen receptor–modified T cells for acute lymphoid leukemia. N Engl J Med. 2013;368:1509–1518 doi:10.1056/NEJMoa1215134.
31. Amrolia PJ, Pule M. Chimeric antigen receptor T cells for ALL. Lancet. 2015;385:488–90.
32. Pizzitola I, et al. Chimeric antigen receptors against CD33/CD123 antigens efficiently target primary acute myeloid leukemia cells in vivo. Leukemia. 2014;28:1596–605.
33. Pizzitola I, et al. In vitro comparison of three different chimeric receptor-modified effector T-cell populations for leukemia cell therapy. J Immunother. 2011;34:469–79.
34. Wang Q-S, et al. Treatment of CD33-directed chimeric antigen receptor-modified T cells in one patient with relapsed and refractory acute myeloid leukemia. Mol Ther. 2015;23:184–91.

Chapter 9
NK Cell and NKT Cell Immunotherapy

Kenneth DeSantes and Kimberly McDowell

Abstract NK cells are a vital component of our innate immune system and serve a variety of biologic functions, including the eradication of tumor. Their importance in preventing leukemic relapse after stem cell transplantation is well documented. The cytotoxic activity of NK cells is regulated by activating and inhibitory signals resulting from interactions between their cell surface receptors and ligands expressed on potential targets. NK cells may destroy tumors directly, or may participate in antibody dependent cellular cytotoxicity (ADCC). The function of NK cells can be augmented by the use of drugs, cytokines, or through genetic modifications. NK cells may also be expanded, ex vivo, for use in adoptive immunotherapy. NKT cells possess features of both the innate and adaptive immune system, and express an invariant T cell receptor (iNKT cells) that recognizes glycolipid antigens in the context of the MHC class-I-like CD1d molecule. iNKT cells are also being utilized for cancer immunotherapy.

Keywords NK cell • NKT cell • ADCC • Adoptive immunotherapy • KIR • BiKE • TriKe

9.1 NK Cell Biology

Natural killer (NK) cells are lymphocytes that are able to recognize and naturally lyse tumor cells without prior sensitization and thus, NK cells are considered to be a part of the innate immune system. NK cells distinguish abnormal cells from healthy cells by means of a repertoire of germ line-encoded cell surface receptors that do not undergo somatic recombination. The maturation of NK cells occurs in the bone

K. DeSantes, M.D. (✉)
Department of Pediatrics, University of Wisconsin, American Family Children's Hospital, Madison, WI, USA
e-mail: kbdesantes@wisc.edu

K. McDowell, M.D., Ph.D.
Division of Pediatric Hematology, Oncology and Bone Marrow Transplant, University of Wisconsin, American Family Children's Hospital, Madison, WI, USA

J.C. Gray, A. Marabelle (eds.), *Immunotherapy for Pediatric Malignancies*,
https://doi.org/10.1007/978-3-319-43486-5_9

marrow and likely multiple extramedullary tissues, since NK cell developmental intermediates circulate through peripheral blood and are routinely found in secondary lymphoid tissue, liver, mucosa-associated lymphoid tissue and the gravid uterus [1].

NK cells are defined phenotypically as CD3-CD56+ lymphocytes and can generally be divided into two subsets based on the density of CD56 (neural cell adhesion molecule) cell surface expression. $CD56^{bright}$ cells are found mainly in secondary lymphoid tissues, are proliferative, produce immunoregulatory cytokines in response to monokine (cytokines produced by monocytes or macrophages) stimulation, but are poorly cytotoxic at rest. Based on their location, this subset is able to interact with other immune cells, and through secretion of soluble factors can influence adaptive immune responses. $CD56^{dim}$ cells are found in bone marrow, spleen, sites of acute inflammation [2], and comprise 90% of NK cells circulating in peripheral blood. These cells have potent cytotoxic capabilities and secrete cytokines in response to target cell recognition [3, 4]. Importantly, these NK cells express FcγRIIIa receptors (CD16) and are capable of facilitating antibody-dependent cellular cytotoxicity (ADCC).

9.2 Functions of NK Cells

NK cells have four key biological roles of which the latter is the focus of this chapter. NK cells are critical for the (1) maintenance of lymphoid system homeostasis, (2) maintenance of a balance between placental function and fetal requirements during pregnancy, (3) control of infections and (4) control of malignancies. When an NK cell engages a target (e.g. virally infected or malignant cell), it may be activated or inhibited based on integrated stimuli resulting from a network of interactions between receptors expressed on the surface of the NK cell and ligands expressed by the target, as will be discussed in more detail below. If activation signals predominate, then the NK cell will destroy its target by implementing effector functions such as cytokine production and cellular cytotoxicity (Fig. 9.1).

9.3 Cytokine Production

Cytokine production by NK cells occurs in response to soluble signals from other cells and in response to signals generated from cell-to-cell contact. NK cells respond to monokines (e.g., IL-1, IL-10, IL-12, IL-15, IL-18) secreted by other immune cells, such as macrophages and dendritic cells, through constitutively expressed receptors on their cell surface. Upon stimulation by monokines, NK cells secrete immunomodulatory cytokines, predominantly IFNγ and TNFα, as well as IL-5, IL-10, IL-13, GM-CSF and chemokines CCL2 (MCP-1), CCL3 (MIP1α), CCL4 (MIP1β), and CCL5 (RANTES). Alternately, NK cells can produce cytokines in response to target cell contact. The $CD56^{bright}$ subset is most efficient at cytokine production in response to monokine stimulation while the $CD56^{dim}$ subset is

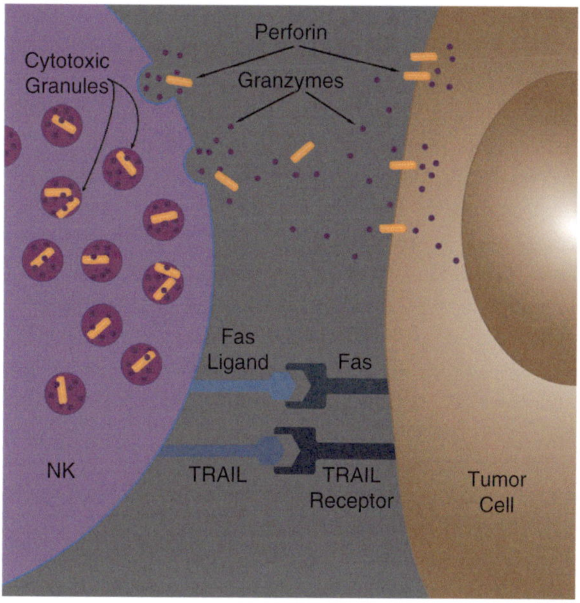

Fig. 9.1 Cytotoxic Mechanisms of NK Cells. NK cells use two mechanisms to kill tumor cells: (1) cellular lysis and (2) apoptosis. The exocytosis of lytic granule contents causes cellular lysis through the action of perforin, which induces pore formation and the disruption of osmotic balance, and granzymes that induce apoptosis. In addition, death receptor ligands on NK cells bind tumor cell death receptors resulting in tumor cell apoptosis

dramatically more efficient at target cell-induced cytokine production. The time course of cytokine release is different between the two NK cell subsets, where CD56^{dim} NK cells produce INFγ as early as two hours after stimulation while CD56^{bright} NK cells release INFγ later (>16 h after stimulation) [5].

Cytokines produced by NK cells influence other immune cells and may directly affect target cells such as virally infected or malignant cells. Interferon-γ causes the up-regulation of major histocompatibility (MHC) class I expression by antigen presenting cells, activates macrophages and influences naïve CD4+ cell differentiation toward a Th1 phenotype. In addition, IFNγ has a direct antiproliferative effect on tumor cells. TNFα also activates macrophages and is pro-inflammatory, recruiting other immune cells, in part, by stimulating endothelial cells to produce adhesion molecules and chemokines that are chemotactic to neutrophils and macrophages.

The NK cell secretion of IFNγ and TNFα promotes the maturation and activation of dendritic cells (DC), which contributes to the antitumor function of NK cells. Cell-to-cell contact between NK cells and DCs is also required for NK-cell-mediated DC activation and involves NKp30 receptors on NK cells [6].

9.4 Cytotoxicity

A critical function of NK cells is the ability to recognize and destroy unhealthy cells either by means of cellular lysis or through the initiation of apoptosis. Cellular lysis occurs relatively quickly, within minutes to hours, while death triggered by apoptosis transpires in hours to days. Both of these cellular cytotoxic mechanisms involve cell-to-cell contact between the NK cell and its target. NK cells routinely patrol lymphoid and non-lymphoid tissues, making exploratory cell-to-cell contacts in order to distinguish healthy cells from those that require elimination. Approximately 10% of lymphocytes in peripheral blood are NK cells and thus, ample circulating NK cells are available to extravasate from the circulation into tissues under inflammatory conditions (e.g., infection, malignancy).

NK cell lysis of target cells involves the secretion of lytic granule contents (degranulation) into the intercellular space between the NK cell and its target at a zone of cell-to-cell contact, a type of immune synapse called the NK cell lytic synapse (NK-LS). The NK-LS is a highly organized supra-molecular structure comprised of cytoskeletal elements, adhesion molecules, receptors, signaling molecules, and co-stimulatory ligands. Several steps are involved in the formation of the NK-LS [7], the first of which is establishment of a close association between the NK cell and its target, presumably by 'tethering' that occurs between molecules on the surface of NK cells (e.g., selectin and CD2) and molecules on the target cell (various carbohydrates and Lewis X molecules, respectively). Based on transient initial contact, firm adhesion may occur via interactions of higher affinity receptors such as the NK cell integrins, LFA1 and MAC1, to their respective ligands on target cells. Following target cell recognition and NK-LS initiation, reorganization of cellular elements at the point of contact between cells occurs. Receptor clustering and lipid-raft aggregation begin at the NK-LS and appear to require actin polymerization and the ERM (ezrin, radixin and moesin) family of proteins. Receptor clustering is important for the production of robust integrated intracellular signaling in response to ligand binding of various NK cell activating and inhibitory receptors. For efficient cellular lysis, lytic granules distributed throughout the cell must polarize to the NK-LS. Actin reorganization produces "conduits" within the NK cell cortex through which lytic granules pass and accumulate at the synaptic cleft region of the NK-LS. The lytic granules dock at the synaptic cleft membrane with subsequent priming, fusion and secretion. Each intracellular event in the process of NK-LS formation is highly regulated and enables NK cells to carefully direct their potent cytotoxic capabilities.

Lytic granules contain a collection of lysosomal enzymes as well as proteins specific to lytic granules, including perforin, granzymes, cathelicidin and defensins. Of these, perforin and granzymes have been most thoroughly studied. Perforin is a protein that forms pores in the target cell membrane allowing the entry of ions and small molecules, which disrupts osmotic equilibrium and causes cell death. The gene for perforin is constitutively transcribed in NK cells, with $CD56^{dim}$ cells having the highest levels of perforin.

Granzymes are a family of serine proteases (Granzymes -A, -K, -B, -H, and –M) that are also constitutively transcribed in NK cells. Within lytic granules, granzymes are packed tightly by forming complexes with serglycin and are processed to an active form by cathepsin C or H. When released into the synaptic cleft, granzymes can enter the target cell through the perforin-induced pores or by endocytosis after granzyme-binding of mannose 6-phosphate receptors on the surface of the target cell. Interestingly, endocytosis in the target cell is increased due to cellular wound healing in the region of membrane disruption caused by perforin-induced pores.

Granzymes entering the cell via endocytotic vesicles then gain access to the cytoplasm via perforin-induced pores in the endocytotic vesicle membrane. In general, granzymes induce cell death through apoptotic mechanisms. Granzyme A induces cell death by indirectly generating single-stranded DNA nicks through the cleavage of numerous cellular substrates including (1) SET, an inhibitor of the endonuclease NM23-H1 allowing this molecule to nick DNA, (2) Ku70 and PARP-1, DNA repair molecules, (3) linker histone H1, which opens up chromatin allowing any nuclease to access DNA, and (4) lamins which disrupt the nuclear envelope [8]. Granzyme B activates caspases, specifically the executioner caspase, caspase-3 and thus produces rapid induction of caspase-dependent apoptosis [9]. The cellular substrates for Granzyme C and H have not yet having been identified. However, it has been shown that Granzyme C disrupts mitochondrial ultrastructure and results in DNA destruction via single-stranded nicks not involving caspase-activated DNase. Granzyme H has been shown to cleave two adenoviral proteins, DBP (DNA-binding protein) and the adenovirus 100 K assembly protein [8] and thus, may play a unique role in the immune defense against this pathogen.

NK cell-induced apoptosis of target cells occurs through the action of granzymes released into the synaptic cleft of the NK-LS (described above) or by interaction of target cell surface death receptors with death receptor ligands expressed on NK cells, such as the TNF-superfamily ligands, TRAIL (TNF-related apoptosis-inducing ligand) and FasL (ligand for the apoptosis antigen 1 receptor, or Fas). When NK cell FasL or TRAIL bind their respective receptors on target cells, apoptosis of the target cell ensues through the activation of caspases 8 and 9 of the extrinsic pathway [10, 11].

9.5 Regulation of Function Through Activating and Inhibitory Receptors

9.5.1 Activating Receptors

The ability of NK cells to recognize and become activated to kill transformed or infected cells is through a repertoire of germ-line encoded, activating and inhibitory receptors (Fig. 9.2). Whether an NK cell is activated to produce cytokines or secrete the contents of lytic granules depends on the balance of positive and negative signals received through these receptors (Fig. 9.3). The clustering of receptors and signal molecules at the NK-LS enables integration of signals to yield a net activation or inhibition switch ("to kill" or "not to kill"). Notably, negative signals from inhibitory receptors tend to be dominant.

Healthy somatic cells do not generally express ligands for NK cell activating receptors. However, cells experiencing genotoxic stress, heat shock or infection, do. Activating receptors include C-type lectin-like receptors (e.g., NKG2D, NKG2C, NKG2E), natural cytotoxicity receptors (e.g., NKp30, NKp44, NKp46), FcγRIIIa

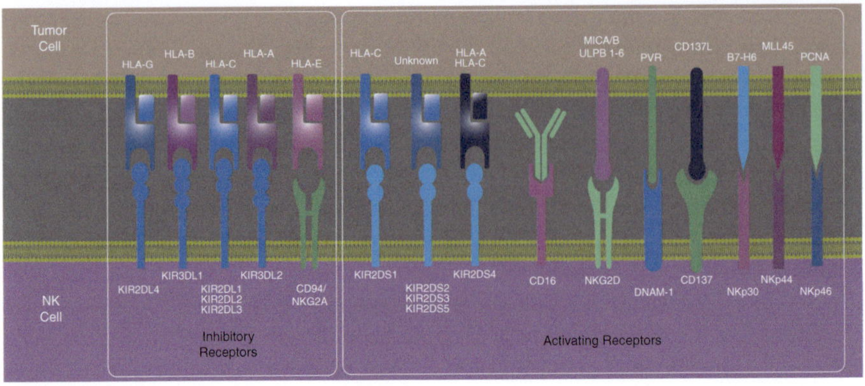

Fig. 9.2 NK Cell Receptors. Selected NK cell inhibitory and activating receptors and their known ligands are shown

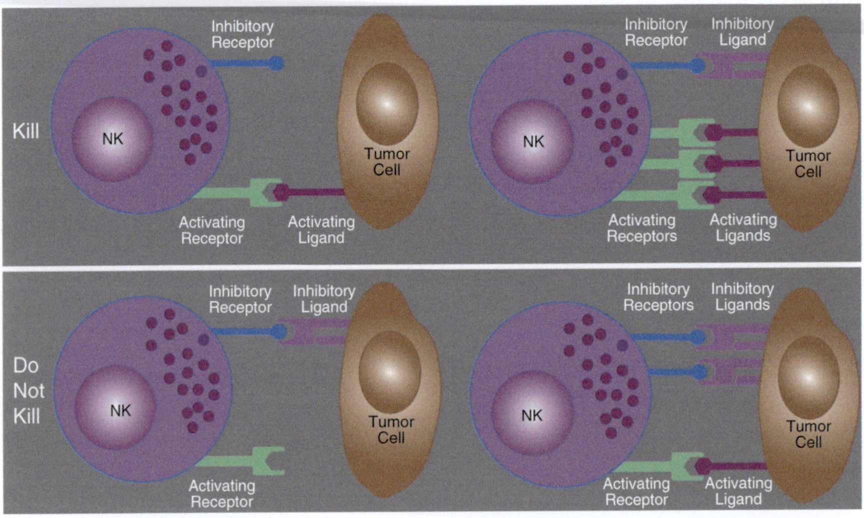

Fig. 9.3 Regulation of NK Cell Cytotoxicity. NK cell activity is regulated through the integration of inhibitory and activating signals. Killing of tumor cells may occur following binding of NK cell activating receptors by their ligands provided inhibitory signals are absent or minimized

(CD16), SLAM family receptors (2B4, CRACC), receptors for nectin or nectin-like molecules (e.g., DNAM-1), and several members of the Killer-cell Immunoglobulin-like Receptor family (KIR2DL5, KIR2DS1, KIR2DS2, KIR2DS3, KIR2DS5, KIR3DS, KIR2DL4). In addition, a small percentage of NK cells express surface Toll-like receptors 2 and 4 at low density.

An activating receptor that is particularly important in the context of immunotherapy is FcγRIIIa (CD16). Most resting CD56^{dim} NK cells possess a high density of CD16, while resting CD56^{bright} NK cells express limited CD16, which can be upregulated with cytokine stimulation. The ligand for CD16 is the Fc domain of IgG antibody. Antibody bound to target cell surface antigens via the antibody F_v domain, produces a lattice of antibody molecules with exposed Fc domains that "tag" the tumor cell for destruction by NK cells employing a mechanism called antibody-dependent cellular cytotoxicity (ADCC). Interestingly, the only activating receptor that is sufficient to produce degranulation without co-stimulation from another activating receptor is CD16. All other activating receptors require co-stimulation by at least one other activating receptor in order to trigger NK cell degranulation, which contributes to this process being under tight control to prevent the destruction of healthy tissue. Degranulation in response to antibody binding CD16 may be more permissive in light of the fact that specificity has already been determined through the production of antibodies by B cells of the adaptive immune system.

The activating receptor NKG2D is encoded by a single gene with limited polymorphism, but this receptor recognizes a wide variety of ligands encoded by numerous genes, some possessing considerable allelic polymorphism. Expression of NKG2D is constitutive on NK cells but can be modulated by cytokine-induced effects on transcription and posttranscriptional processing of NKG2D and DAP10 (an adapter transmembrane protein necessary for signaling). Ligands for NKG2D are induced on cells undergoing cellular or genotoxic stress, and include MICA, MICB (major histocompatibility complex class I-related chain glycoprotein A and B), and ULBP-1, -2, -3, -4, -5, -6 (cytomegalovirus UL-16 binding proteins 1-6). Numerous pediatric malignancies express NKG2D ligands including AML, lymphoma, Ewings' sarcoma, glioma and neuroblastoma. Unfortunately, some tumor cells (e.g., neuroblastoma) evade NKG2D-facilitated NK cell killing by proteolytic shedding of NKG2D ligands, via the action of ADAM 10 and 17 proteases. High levels of soluble NKG2D ligands can interact with NKG2D receptors on NK cells preventing their interaction with NKG2D ligands on the surface of tumor cells.

Natural cytotoxicity receptors (NCR), NKp30, NKp46 and NKp44, recognize ligands on malignant and virally infected cells. NKp30 is constitutively expressed on NK cells and binds B7-H6, a B7 family member that appears to be expressed exclusively on tumor cells [12], including neuroblastoma [13]. Similar to soluble NKG2D ligands, soluble B7-H6 may play a role in the ability of cancer cells to evade NK cell immune destruction. Soluble B7-H6 contained in the serum of high-risk neuroblastoma patients was correlated with down-regulation of NKp30 expressed on NK cells and inhibited NK cell function *in vitro* [13]. Although the ligands for NKp46 are currently unknown, pre-clinical studies indicate that NKp46 inhibits the growth of tumor metastases [14]. NKp44 is expressed only on activated NK cells (except for a specialized subset of resting NK cells in the decidua). Despite tumor associated ligand(s) not yet being identified, NKp44 is implicated in the recognition and killing of numerous malignant cell types, including neuroblastoma.

It has been recently suggested that NCRs may participate in pattern recognition of DAMPs (damage-associated molecular pattern molecules) [15]. DAMP molecules are proteins that normally function intracellularly but are released from the cell (or sequestered to the cell surface) in response to cellular injury, such as ischemia, hypoxia, transformation, chemotherapy-induced DNA damage, or other trauma. Bat3 (NKp30 ligand), MLL5 (NKp44 ligand), and PCNA (NKp46 ligand) are molecules involved in regulating cell cycle and DNA repair mechanisms and whose presence on the cell surface likely indicate intracellular stress related to DNA damage and/or improper cell cycle control. However, further work is needed to clarify the role of these ligands in the normal function of NK cells.

Another activating receptor that plays a role in the NK cell response to transformed cells, is DNAM-1 (DNAX Accessory Molecule 1). Ligands for DNAM-1 are PVR (Poliovirus Receptor) and Nectin-2, which are present on some tumor cells, including freshly isolated neuroblastoma cells [12] and neuroblastoma cell lines [16]. Preclinical work has shown that DNAM-1 plays an important role in preventing spontaneous tumor formation and in controlling tumor growth [17, 18]. Specifically, the susceptibility of freshly isolated neuroblastoma cells to NK cell killing has been shown to directly correlate with the surface expression of the DNAM-l ligand, PVR [6].

Some members of the KIR and CD94/NKG2A family of receptors are activating, rather than inhibitory, owing to their association with DAP12. These receptors participate in NK cell education and licensing, as do inhibitory KIR receptors, as discussed below. However, the clearest role for activating KIRs in tumor recognition is in leukemia patients undergoing hematopoietic stem cell transplant (HSCT) [19–21].

9.5.2 *Inhibitory Receptors*

Of the NK cell receptors reported to transmit an inhibitory signal (2B4, PD1, KLRG1, LAIR1, SIGLEC-3,-7,-9, KLRB1, TIGIT, Tactile, CD94/NKG2A, LIR1, KIR2DL-1,-2,-3, KIR2DL5-A,-B, KIR3DL-1,-2, KIR3DL3) (Fig. 9.1), the most well studied are members of the KIR family and CD94/NKG2A. Ligands for these receptors are MHC class I molecules (classical and non-classical, respectively), which are expressed on all nucleated cells. Through the recognition of these molecules, NK cells are rendered tolerant of self. NK cells become "licensed (to kill)" through an educational process [22] that is flexible based on the adaptation of NK cells to the MHC-class I environment, in effect making the license to kill revocable. In order to be licensed, an NK cell must express at least one inhibitory receptor that recognizes a self-MHC class I molecule [23, 24], otherwise it is functionally hyporesponsive. In this way, NK cell-mediated destruction of "self" is usually avoided unless self-cells have reduced expression of MHC class I molecules. In fact, many tumor cells have diminished MHC class I expression, likely through selective pressure to avoid recognition by T cells. For example, many pediatric tumors express very low levels of MHC class I molecules including neuroblastoma, Ewing sarcoma/PNET and poorly differentiated rhabdomyosarcoma [25–28]. It is important to note that cells expressing MHC class I molecules may still be killed if the activating signals are sufficiently strong.

9.6 Natural Cytotoxicity Versus ADCC

In the absence of antibody binding the target cell, NK cell-induced killing is called "natural cytotoxicity" (i.e., antibody-independent cellular cytotoxicity). Natural cytotoxicity results from all activating and inhibitory receptor inputs except for CD16. However, the cumulative signal is not a simple mathematical summation, but a complex integration of signals from numerous intracellular pathways. In the presence of antibody binding the target cell, ADCC results from all activating and inhibitory receptor inputs including CD16.

9.7 Evidence Supporting Clinically Significant NK Cell – Mediated Anti-Tumor Activity

There is ample data suggesting that NK cells play an important role in preventing relapse for patients who have undergone hematopoietic stem cell transplantation. In a landmark study, Ruggeri et al. reported that adult AML patients who received T cell depleted haploidentical grafts had a markedly reduced risk of post-transplant relapse if the donor and recipient were KIR ligand mismatched, compared to KIR ligand matched donor/recipient pairs (0% vs. 75%, $P < .0008$), suggesting an important role for NK cell alloreactivity in eradicating residual leukemia after HSCT [29]. Interestingly, the benefit of utilizing a KIR ligand mismatched donor was not evident in adult patients transplanted for ALL. Leung et al. analyzed the outcome of 36 pediatric patients with hematologic malignancies treated by haploidentical HSCT [30]. Donors and recipients were categorized as being KIR—KIR ligand mismatched (i.e. the donor expressed at least 1 KIR for which the recipient lacked the corresponding inhibitory ligand), or KIR—KIR ligand matched. The relapse risk for patients with KIR matched donors, whose NK cells would be expected to display reduced cytotoxicity was 54%, compared to 13% for patients transplanted with NK cell alloreactive (i.e. KIR—KIR ligand mismatched) donors. This difference was even more striking when the investigators analyzed only those patients transplanted for lymphoid malignancies (relapse risk 75% vs. 15%, $p = 0.01$), demonstrating that the anti-leukemic effect mediated by NK cells is not limited to patients with AML, at least in children. The survival advantage gained from utilizing donors whose NK cells would be predicted to have increased alloreactivity against the recipient's leukemia due to reduced inhibitory signaling is not limited to the setting of haploidentical HSCT, but has also been observed in unrelated donor and HLA matched sibling transplants [31–33].

Other HSCT data have demonstrated a reduced risk of relapse if donors manifest an activating KIR genotype. Cooley et al. analyzed the results of 448 AML patients transplanted with grafts from unrelated donors who did or did not possess at least one activating KIR haplotype (KIR B/x vs. KIR A/A) [19]. The 3 year overall survival was significantly higher if patients were transplanted with KIR B/x donors

(31% vs. 20%, p = 0.007). In fact, it is now routine practice to evaluate prospective unrelated donors for the presence of activating KIR as part of the donor selection algorithm when transplanting patients with AML. A similar observation was made in patients treated by haploidentical HSCT for advanced hematologic malignancies [34].

Collectively, these data strongly support a role for NK cells in mitigating the risk of leukemic relapse following HSCT. Importantly, data also exist suggesting that NK cells play a role in preventing relapse for children undergoing HSCT for solid tumors. Venstrom et al. evaluated the outcome of 169 children with high-risk neuroblastoma treated by autologous stem cell transplantation, based on patient KIR and HLA typing [35]. Since HLA haplotypes present on chromosome 6 segregate independently from KIR genes located on chromosome 19, it is possible for individuals to be KIR—KIR ligand mismatched with themselves. In other words, patients can express specific KIR, but lack the corresponding inhibitory KIR ligand(s). In this study, children missing any of the inhibitory HLA class I KIR ligands demonstrated significantly better post-transplant survival compared to those possessing all inhibitory ligands (median survival 9.5 years vs. 3.8 years, p = 0.007). Similarly, Delgado et al. evaluated the response patterns of relapsed neuroblastoma patients treated with hu14.18-IL2, an anti-GD2 immunocytokine [36]. No responses were observed in the 14 children who were KIR-KIR ligand matched with themselves, whereas 7 of 28 children who were KIR—KIR ligand incompatible achieved a CR or showed significant clinical improvement (p = 0.03).

9.8 Sources of NK Cells for Cancer Immunotherapy

From the information presented thus far, it should be evident that NK cells are capable of mediating potent, clinically important anti-tumor activity. With a better understanding of NK cell biology, gained in recent years, it is now feasible to consider utilizing NK cells for cancer immunotherapy. However, one of the factors limiting the implementation of adoptively transferred NK cells as a treatment for cancer is the ability to obtain sufficient effector cells to mediate meaningful antitumor activity. To address this issue, a number of techniques have been established to expand and activate NK cells, ex-vivo. Methodologies typically involve culturing peripheral blood mononuclear cells or purified NK cells with cytokines (e.g. IL-2, IL-15) alone, or more commonly with an irradiated feeder cell line that promotes selective growth of NK cells. Feeder cell lines have included K562 cells transfected to express membrane bound IL-15 and 41BBL, Jurkat T-lymphoblast subline KL-1, EBV transformed lymphoblastoid cells, and K562 cells genetically modified to express membrane bound IL-21 and other co-stimulatory molecules [37–42]. This latter approach has resulted in a particularly robust NK cell expansion (>47,000 fold) through avoidance of telomere shortening and cell senescence [43]. To obtain clinical grade reagents, NK cells are grown in a good manufacturing practices (GMP)-compliant facility utilizing gas permeable bags or a bioreactor, such as the

WAVE or Gas-permeable Rapid Expansion (GRex) Flask system. However, a methodology was recently established to expand NK cells utilizing the CliniMACS Prodigy immunomagnetic cell processing device [44]. This is a closed system and the procedure, which resulted in a mean NK cell expansion of 850 fold, could therefore be performed in most clinical HSCT laboratories, making this a more easily exportable technology.

While the exact phenotype of the cultured NK cells depends on the conditions employed during the expansion process, the expanded cells typically upregulate functionally important molecules, such as TRAIL, FasL and CD16, as well as most activating NK cell receptors including DNAM-1, NKp46, NKp44, NKp30 and NKG2D [38, 39, 45–47]. Upregulation of chemokine receptors, CXCR3, CXCR4 and CXCR6, has also been reported [45, 47], which may enhance localization to the tumor microenvironment. In addition, ex-vivo expanded NK cells have shown increased expression of adhesion molecules CD54 and CD56, which facilitates adherence to target cells, the first stage of immune synapse formation [45, 47]. Furthermore, expanded NK cells demonstrate equivalent or superior killing of target cell lines when compared to freshly isolated NK cells [39, 45–49]. Consequently, these ex-vivo expanded NK cell products may be ideally suited for clinical use.

NK cells may be derived from sources other than peripheral blood. Spanholtz et al. established a technique for the logarithmic expansion of NK cells from CD34+ progenitor cells obtained from umbilical cord blood [50]. NK cells were expanded >15,000 fold, showed high expression of NKG2D and other activating receptors, and demonstrated efficient cytolytic activity against a number of tumor cell lines. Another novel approach involves generating NK cells from human embryonic stem cells (hESC). NK cells differentiated from hESC were found to be uniformly $CD94^{+}/CD117^{low/-}$, a phenotype associated with high cytolytic activity, and were able to eradicate K562 xenografts in NOD/SCID mice [51, 52]. Sufficient numbers of hESC derived NK cells can be produced for clinical use [53]. Human NK cell lines may also be employed for cancer immunotherapy. The utilization of such an "off the shelf" product is attractive because of its uniform phenotype, economic efficiency, ready availability, and is particularly appealing for testing in a multi-center trial. The NK cell line NK-92, established in 1994 from a patient with non-Hodgkin lymphoma [54], has undergone extensive pre-clinical evaluation in SCID tumor xenograft models and was found to be safe in phase 1 clinical trials [55–57]. The NK-92 cells lack almost all inhibitory KIR, possess the normal array of activating receptors, and can be expanded under GMP-compliant conditions [58, 59].

9.9 Exploiting NK Cell Anti-Tumor Activity for Clinical Use

NK cells may be recruited for the treatment of cancer in a variety of ways including the utilization of NK cell alloreactive donors for HSCT, as previously discussed, the administration of cytokines (e.g. IL-2, IL-15) or drugs (e.g. lenalidomide, bortezomib) that enhance NK cell function, the administration of monoclonal antibodies (mAbs) which work, at least in part, by ADCC (e.g. rituximab, dinutuximab), and the adoptive transfer of autologous or allogeneic ex vivo activated and/or expanded NK cells. Additionally, NK cells may be genetically modified for clinical use in order to increase their target specificity and/or function.

9.9.1 Cytokines that Enhance NK cell Activity

A number of cytokines activate NK cells and promote proliferation and/or enhance function, including IL-2, IL-12, IL-15, IL-18, and IL-21. The bulk of clinical experience utilizing cytokines to enhance NK cell effector function is with the gamma-cytokines, IL-2 and IL-15.

Interleukin-2 (IL-2) stimulates the proliferation and maturation of $CD56^{bright}$ NK cells. IL-2 also increases the surface expression of CD16, NCRs, and NKG2D, and increases the production of perforin [60–62]. In $CD56^{dim}$ NK cells, IL-2 upregulates surface expression of NCRs [63–65], NKG2D [62, 63, 66] and DNAM-1 [63–65] and increases the production of perforin and granzymes [66, 67], enhancing both antibody-independent (natural) cytotoxicity and ADCC. Moreover, the production of IFN-γ is augmented in IL-2-stimulated NK cells [66, 68–76].

A number of early clinical trials administered IL-2 to adult patients with advanced cancer, and although anti-tumor activity was documented, complete responses were infrequent and few responses were durable [77]. IL-2 is however, FDA approved to treat renal cell carcinoma and melanoma in adults. The use of IL-2 as monotherapy for pediatric malignancies has yielded unimpressive results [78–80]. Nonetheless, IL-2 may still function in an adjuvant capacity to augment immune responses against pediatric tumors. A phase 1 trial was conducted to determine the maximum tolerated dose (MTD) of subcutaneous IL-2 administered in the outpatient setting to children with stage 4 neuroblastoma after autologous HSCT [81]. The study defined the MTD of IL-2 to be 6×10^6 U/m^2/day given in 5 day cycles every 2 weeks. NK cell numbers were increased a median of 711% above baseline, and this trial helped establish a dose of IL-2 that could be used in combination with other immunotherapeutic agents. A phase 1/2 trial for children with neuroblastoma administered IL-2 together with an anti-GD2 mAb [82]. Anti-tumor activity was documented in this study and IL-2 was therefore included in an adjuvant regimen to treat children with high-risk neuroblastoma in a large Children's Oncology Group (COG) phase 3 trial, as will be discussed below.

IL-15 is a pivotal cytokine for the development [83], survival [84], and proliferation [85] of NK cells. IL-15 upregulates perforin [86, 87] and granzymes [83], enhances ADCC [85, 88–93], and like IL-2, can be administered to prolong the survival of adoptively transferred NK cells. An important advantage of IL-15 over IL-2 is that IL-15 does not recruit and activate regulatory T cells; an immune cell subset that has been shown to diminish the survival of adoptively transferred haploidentical NK cells [94]. A clinical trial using IL-15 to support adoptively transferred allogeneic NK cells to treat to adults with AML has recently been completed

(NCT01385423) but results have not yet been published. A phase 1 trial utilizing IL-15 monotherapy in adult patients with metastatic melanoma or renal cell cancer defined the MTD to be 0.3 mcg/kg/day given as an IV bolus over 12 consecutive days [95]. A 10 fold expansion of NK cells was observed, as was markedly increase levels of inflammatory cytokines including IFN-α and IL-6. Two patients demonstrated clearing of pulmonary metastases. There are several ongoing clinical trials in adults with cancer, in which IL-15 is administered, alone (NCT01727076, NCT01021059, NCT02452268), or in conjunction with a tumor specific mAb (NCT0268943). A phase I clinical trial treating children and young adults with advanced solid tumors (NCT01875601) with *ex vivo* expanded autologous NK cells, followed by at least 12 daily doses of IL-15, was recently completed though results are not yet available.

IL-21 is a type I cytokine that shares homology with IL-2 and IL-15, and is thought to regulate the proliferation and maturation of NK cells. A phase 1 trial of IL-21 was conducted in 26 adult patients with metastatic melanoma or renal cell carcinoma [96]. The MTD was determined to be 200 mcg/kg given s.c. 3 days a week. At this dose level, significant increases in granzyme B expression was seen in NK and CD8+ T cells. Serum soluble CD25, a marker of immune activation, was also found to increase in a dose-dependent manner. Three patients experienced a partial response.

9.9.2 *Drugs that Enhance NK Cell Function*

Lenalidomide and pomalidomide are structural analogs of thalidomide that have been shown to augment NK cell function [97, 98]. A phase 1 study, conducted by the COG, administered once daily lenalidomide for 21 consecutive days every 28 days to children with solid tumors [99]. No dose limiting toxicities were seen at the highest dose level evaluated (70 mg/m^2/dose). After 21 days of treatment, increases in the percentage and absolute number of circulating NK cells was observed, and cytotoxicity against K562 and Daudi tumor targets by NK cells from patients receiving lenalidomide was significantly increased compared to baseline. A phase 1 trial using pomalidomide to treat children with relapsed/refractory CNS malignancies is currently underway (NCT02415153).

Several drugs have been shown to upregulate tumor ligands for activating NK cell receptors and/or downregulate inhibitory receptor ligands, potentially contributing to their antitumor activity. Bortezomib is an ubiquitin-proteasome pathway inhibitor that has been shown to upregulate surface expression of the death receptor TRAIL-R2 (DR5) on tumor cells, and decrease expression of MHC class 1 [100–102]. Pediatric phase I trials of bortezomib alone [103, 104] and in combination with chemotherapy [105] or vorinostat [106] demonstrated safety and tolerability, and numerous pediatric studies that include bortezomib or a similar drug, carfilzomib, are ongoing. In a phase 2 trial conducted by the COG, bortezomib was administered in combination with ifosfamide and vinorelbine to patients with relapsed or refractory Hodgkin disease [107]. There was a suggestion of improvement in the overall response rate compared to historical controls treated with ifosfamide and vinorelbine alone. No immunologic parameters were assessed in that trial. Another phase 2 COG study explored the addition of bortezomib to combination chemotherapy with idarubicin/cytarabine or cytarabine/etoposide, for patients with relapsed or refractory AML [15]. The study was closed early because it failed to meet predetermined efficacy thresholds. The Therapeutic Advances in Childhood Leukemia and Lymphoma (TACL) consortium treated 22 children with relapsed ALL, who had failed 2–3 prior therapies, with bortezomib combined with a standard 4- drug reinduction regimen. The CR and CRp (complete response with incomplete platelet recovery) rate was 80% in patients with B ALL, suggesting that bortezomib synergized with chemotherapy to promote eradication of the leukemia.

Histone deacetylase (HDAC) inhibitors, such as romidepsin, suberoylanilide hydroxamic acid (SAHA, vorinostat), and valproic acid, have been shown to upregulate expression of NKG2D ligands on tumors, thereby increasing their sensitivity to NK cell mediated killing [108, 109], and this effect may be augmented by radiation [110]. Pediatric phase 1 studies of valproic acid [111] and romidepsin [112, 113] demonstrated safety and tolerability of these agents which are undergoing further evaluation, in combination with chemotherapy, for the treatment of pediatric leukemia and solid tumors, including CNS malignancies.

Demethylating agents, such as 5-azacytidine and 5-aza-2'-deoxycytidine (decitabine), have also been demonstrated to increase NKG2D ligand expression on B-ALL and myeloid leukemia cells [114, 115]. In a COG trial, decitabine was administered to 8 pediatric and young adult relapsed/refractory AML patients who had failed multiple prior regimens. Three patients achieved a CR or CR with incomplete count recovery [116].

9.10 Utilizing mAbs to Facilitate NK Cell Mediated Anti-Tumor Activity

9.10.1 Conventional ADCC

Monoclonal antibodies have become an important therapeutic tool for the treatment of both adult and pediatric malignancies. Many of these mAbs work by engagement of the activating receptor, FcγRIIIa (CD16), present on NK and other immune effector cells, enabling the formation of an immune synapse with the tumor. The importance of this interaction has been demonstrated in studies correlating FcγRIIIa polymorphisms with clinical outcome. The "V/V" polymorphism (homozygous for valine at position 158) results in an FcγRIIIa that binds to IgG1 antibodies with high affinity, while the "F/F" polymorphism (homozygous for phyenylalanine at position 158) results in low affinity binding. The "V/F" genotype leads to an FcγRIIIa with intermediate affinity to antibody. In a landmark study, Weng et al. reported that patients with follicular lymphoma bearing the V/V FcγRIIIa genotype had a significantly better response to rituximab (an anti-CD20 mAb) compared to patients bearing the F/F FcγRIIIa genotype [117]. Rituximab has also been combined with chemotherapy to treat pediatric patients with Burkitt leukemia/lymphoma, resulting in a 3 year EFS and OS of 90% [118]. These encouraging results prompted a phase 3 study randomizing patients to receive rituximab + chemotherapy vs. chemotherapy alone. The study has been completed, though results have not yet been published.

Perhaps the most intriguing data supporting the efficacy of mAb therapy for pediatric cancer stems from work utilizing anti-GD2 mAbs for patients with high-risk neuroblastoma. In a phase 3 COG trial, neuroblastoma patients were randomized to receive ch14.18 + cis retinoic acid vs. retinoic acid alone, following recovery from autologous stem cell transplantation [119]. The ch14.18 mAb was administered with either IL-2 or GM-CSF to stimulate NK cells and neutrophils/monocytes/macrophages, respectively, thereby augmenting ADCC. Children randomized to the immunotherapy arm of the study had a 2 year EFS of 66%, compared to 46% in the control arm ($p = 0.01$). The Memorial Sloan Kettering team reported their results using 3F8, another anti-GD2 mAb, administered with GM-CSF, to treat children with high-risk neuroblastoma [120]. This study demonstrated that patients missing any of the MHC class I ligands for their inhibitory KIR (i.e. KIR–KIR ligand mismatched with themselves) had better progression-free and overall survival compared to patients possessing all KIR ligands, suggesting an important role for NK cell mediated ADCC in preventing relapse.

9.10.2 Checkpoint Blockade

Another means by which monoclonal antibodies may recruit the antitumor activity of NK cells is through checkpoint blockade. Immune checkpoints refer to inhibitory pathways incorporated into the immune system that maintain self-tolerance and limit the duration and amplitude of the immune response, which avoids damage to healthy tissue. The prototypical checkpoint pathways that have gained considerable recent attention involve the T cell inhibitory receptors, CTLA-4 and PD-1. The expression of these inhibitory receptors increases upon T cell activation and their ligation attenuates (or "checks") the T cell immune response. Monoclonal antibodies specific for CTLA-4 or PD-1, or their ligands, prevents the interaction of receptor with ligand and thus blocks the negative feedback loop ("checkpoint blockade"). Many tumor cells express ligands for these receptors and essentially usurp these inhibitory pathways to avoid elimination. Checkpoint blockade is a means to "release the brakes" from suppressed T cells, recovering their antitumor activity.

Expression of the inhibitory receptor, PD-1 has also been demonstrated on activated NK cells and freshly isolated NK cells from patients with cancer [121]. This suggests a potential role for checkpoint blockade to restore NK cell mediated antitumor activity. Caligiuri and colleagues [121] showed in vitro that blockade of PD-1 increased NK mediated cytotoxicity against PD-L1 expressing autologous tumor cells, but not against PD-L1 negative autologous healthy cells. The effect of CTLA-4 blockade on NK cells is not clear. However, since the anti-CTLA-4 mAb, ipilimumab, is an IgG1, NK cell mediated ADCC of ipilimumab bound cells could potentially be involved in the overall response. For instance, CTLA-4 is constitutively expressed on some tumor cells, including neuroblastoma, rhabdomyosarcoma, osteosarcoma and neoplastic lymphoid and myeloid cells [122, 123]. Thus, ipilimumab may opsonize tumor cells and lead to NK cell mediated lysis. Moreover, there is evidence that NK cell- [124] and macrophage/monocyte- [125, 126] mediated ADCC of intratumoral regulatory T cells, which contribute to the immunosuppressive tumor microenvironment, may be involved in the antitumor responses of ipilimumab [124, 127]. A phase 1 trial of 33 pediatric patients with advanced solid tumors showed that ipilimumab was safely administered when immune-related toxicity management algorithms were used [128]. In the subset of patients demonstrating immune-related toxicities, overall survival was improved compared to patients without these toxicities. A number of clinical trials using checkpoint blockers to treat children or young adults with cancer, alone and in combination with other treatments, are ongoing.

9.10.3 mAbs Engineered to Have Increased Affinity for NK Cells

Therapeutic mAbs can be engineered in a number of ways to increase their clinical utility by optimizing interactions with NK cells. First, mAbs can be "glycoengineered" to increase binding affinity to CD16 by optimizing the glycosylation pattern of Fc-linked oligosaccharides [129, 130]. Specifically, afucosylation of IgG1 antibodies increases affinity for CD16 by removal of steric hindrance caused by core-fucosylation [129]. An example of such a mAb used in a pediatric trial to treat non-Hodgkin lymphoma is obinutuzumab (GA101), which is specific against CD20, with increased CD16 binding affinity and augmented ADCC activity [131] (NCT02393157). Second, introduction of point mutations can modify the affinity of an antibody for specific Fcγ receptors, of which there are three stimulatory (FcγRI, FcγRIIa, FcγRIIIa) and one inhibitory (FcγRIIb). For instance, a triple mutation (S239D/I332E/A330L) in the Fc region of an IgG1 mAb results in higher affinity for FcγRIIIa (CD16), lower affinity for FcγRIIb, and augments ADCC [132]. MGA271 is an anti-B7-H3 mAb engineered to have increased binding affinity to FcγRIIIa and decreased affinity for FcγRIIb [133]. B7-H3 is a cell surface antigen overexpressed in many pediatric malignancies including Ewing's sarcoma, rhabdomyosarcoma, osteogenic sarcoma, Wilms' tumor, neuroblastoma and desmoplastic small round cell tumors [49, 91, 129, 134, 135]. A phase 1 clinical trial utilizing MGA271 to treat children with relapsed/refractory B7-H3 positive tumors is underway (NCT02982941).

9.10.4 mAbs that Bind to Activating or Inhibitory NK Cell Receptors

Monoclonal antibodies can contribute to the antitumor activity of NK cells by agonistic binding to co-activating NK cell receptors, such as CD137. Ligation of CD16 by tumor-bound mAb upregulates CD137 expression on NK cells. Preclinical studies have demonstrated that agonistic anti-CD137 mAbs increase NK cell proliferation, cytokine section, and ADCC of tumor cells [136]. In a mouse model of sarcoma, agonistic anti-CD137 mAb amplified the antitumor effect of a therapeutic mAb [137] and this effect was shown to be mediated by NK cells [138]. The synergistic effect of agonistic anti-CD137 mAb has also been demonstrated in mouse models of lymphoma [139], breast cancer [140] and EGFR-expressing tumors [141] when administered with the therapeutic mAbs, rituximab, trastuzumab and Cetuximab, respectively. This approach is now being pursued in three clinical trials for adult patients with cancer (NCT02110082, NCT01775631, NCT01307267) using urelumab (IgG4 isotype) and PF-05082566 (IgG2 isotype).

Monoclonal antibodies can also enhance antitumor activity of NK cells by antagonistic binding of inhibitory receptors thereby blocking interactions with their ligands. Tumor cells that express MHC class I molecules can avoid NK cell killing through the engagement of MHC class I ligands with their cognate inhibitory KIRs on NK cells. Employing anti-KIR mAbs could tip the balance of NK cell signals toward activation. Preclinical work with anti-KIR mAbs suggests that they do not cause autoimmunity [142–144] and augment in-vitro ADCC when tumor cells are opsonized with tumor specific mAbs [141, 145]. Of note, these mAbs were developed using the IgG4 isotype, which does not activate complement and is bound by CD16 with very low affinity. Thus, anti-inhibitory KIR mAbs bound to NK cells do not result in NK cell mediated cytotoxicity against NK cells [143]. Based on the efficacy of anti-inhibitory KIR mAbs in murine tumor xenograft models alone, and in combination with tumor specific mAbs [141, 144, 146], this approach has moved into clinical testing. Safety was demonstrated in a phase 1 trial using the fully humanized, anti-inhibitory KIR mAb, IPH2101, to treat elderly patients with AML in first CR [147]. A modification of IPH2101, lirilumab (IH2102), is being tested in 7 adult phase 1 or 2 clinical trials, alone or in combination with other therapeutic mAbs and/or chemotherapy (NCT02399917, NCT01592370, NCT02252263, NCT02599649, NCT02481297, NCT01687387, NCT01714739).

Importantly, lirilumab and its predecessor, IPH2101, block all inhibitory KIRs (KIR2DL1, KIR2DL2, KIR2DL3) that recognize virtually all HLA-C allotypes. Since all individuals possess a subset of NK cells that are inhibited by only one MHC class I allotype (e.g., HLA-C), blocking the binding of any HLA-C ligand to any inhibitory KIR recognizing HLA-C, will essentially blind that subset to MHC class I on tumor cells, tipping the balance toward activation and the generation of a "kill" signal. Thus, lirilumab should enhance antitumor NK cell cytotoxicity in all individuals eliminating the need for prior HLA or KIR typing.

9.10.5 Conjugated mAbs

A number of bispecific fusion proteins have been developed in an attempt to direct NK cell cytotoxicity toward tumor cells by conjugating a ligand for an NK cell activating receptor to a mAb (or mAb fragment) specific for a tumor antigen. Recombinant MICA has been conjugated to mAb Fabs specific for CD20, CEA and HER2, and these reagents elicited NK cell induced tumor lysis in vitro [148]. Recombinant ULBP2 has been conjugated to the mAb Fab specific for CD138 (overexpressed on multiple myeloma cells). Preclinical studies showed this reagent induced release of IFNγ from NK cells and resulted in NK-mediated lysis of CD138+ tumor targets. In a nude mouse model, the combination of human PBMCs and the ULB2/anti-CD138 conjugate abrogated growth of CD138+ tumor cells [149].

Therapeutic mAbs can also be conjugated to cytokines, creating molecules known as immunocytokines (ICs), by fusing the human gene for the cytokine to the mAb gene. Through the use of ICs, the immunomodulatory effect of cytokines can be more efficiently localized to the tumor microenvironment. ICs bind to tumor cell antigens via their Fab arm while binding the NK cell through both: (1) the IC Fc arm which recognizes CD16 and (2) the cytokine moiety which recognizes the NK cell cytokine receptor [150, 151]. The immunocytokine, hu14.18-IL2 has been used safely in children with neuroblastoma in phase 1 and 2 clinical trials and demonstrated antitumor activity in patients with a relatively low disease burden [152–154].

9.10.6 Bispecific and Trispecific Killer Engagers (BiKEs and TriKEs)

Bispecific and trispecific killer engagers are engineered molecules that contain two (bispecific) or three (trispecific) different monoclonal antibody single-chain antibody fragments (scFvs), which crosslink epitopes on tumor cells to an epitope of an effector cell activating receptor (Fig. 9.4). For NK cells, the immune effector activating receptor scFv is specific for CD16. Since subsets of TCRγδ+ T cells also possess CD16, these reagents may elicit antitumor responses through their action on TCRγδ+ T cells in addition to NK cells. BiKEs and TriKEs opsonize tumor cells via their tumor-specific scFv and elicit ADCC and cytokine release through binding of the anti-CD16 scFv to NK cell CD16. Gleason and colleagues showed that the ADCC resulting from BiKE- and TriKE- CD16 ligation is more potent compared to CD16 ligation by a conventional mAb [118]. This is because the anti-CD16 scFv of BiKEs and TriKEs binds to a different epitope of the CD16 molecule [155]. Thus, the benefit of these reagents should be equivalent regardless of CD16 receptor polymorphism possessed by the patient and may be particularly useful for individuals with low (Fcγ158-F/F) or intermediate (Fcγ158-F/V) affinity CD16.

Tumor cell antigens targeted by anti-CD16 containing BiKEs and TriKEs include CD33 (AML, MDS), CD19 (B cell malignancies), HLA class II (lymphoma), CD30 (Hodgkin lymphoma), EGFR (epithelial cancers), HER2 (breast, osteosarcoma),

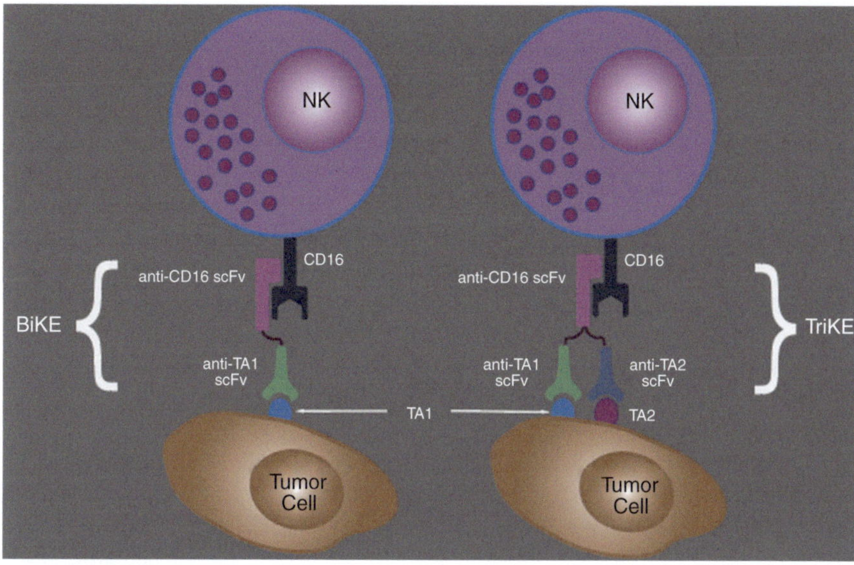

Fig. 9.4 BiKEs and TriKEs. BiKEs are bispecific engineered molecules that contain two monoclonal antibody single-chain fragments (scFvs) which crosslink a tumor associated antigen (TA1) with an NK cell activating receptor, such as CD16. TriKEs are trispecific engineered molecules that crosslink an activating receptor on the NK cell with a tumor associated antigen, but have additional specificity for a second tumor associated antigen (TA2) or another activating molecule, such as IL-15

EPCAM (carcinomas), and CEA (colon). One promising new TriKE developed and tested preclinically at the University of Minnesota [156] is designated 161533. TriKE 161533 contains scFvs for CD33 and CD16 together with a modified human IL-15 crosslinker. The addition of the IL15 crosslinking component imparts enhanced cytotoxicity and cytokine release in response to CD33+ targets compared to a BiKE containing the scFvs for CD33 and CD16 alone. A mouse xenogeneic model showed significant antitumor activity without toxicity when TriKE 161533 was given daily to NSG mice following NK cell adoptive therapy. Importantly, TriKE 161533 supported the in vivo persistence and expansion of NK cells while the analogous BiKE did not.

9.11 Adoptive Therapy with Allogeneic NK Cells

Adoptive therapy with allogeneic NK cells has been performed in both the transplant and non-transplant settings. Utilizing donor derived NK cells following HSCT is appealing since NK cells: (1) may mediate anti-tumor activity due to lack of inhibition by self class I HLA antigens, (2) are thought not to cause graft versus host disease (GVHD), and (3) would not face immunologic rejection by the host. In the non-transplant setting, this approach requires that patients receive lymphodepletive chemotherapy prior to adoptive NK cell transfer in order to create an immunologic environment permissive for allogeneic cell expansion and survival. Miller et al. administered haploidentical NK cells to adults with poor prognosis AML. Two different pre-infusion lymphodepletion regimens were used to prevent immunologic rejection and remove endogenous "cytokine sinks" thereby increasing the availability of growth factors for the newly infused cells [90]. The more aggressive lymphodepletion regimen, which consisted of 1–2 doses of cyclophosphamide 60 mg/kg/dose and fludarabine 25 mg/m^2/dose for 5 consecutive days (Flu/Cy), resulted in significantly greater in vivo expansion of the haploidentical NK cells with 8 of 15 patients demonstrating ≥1% donor engraftment at day 7 or later. Complete remissions were achieved in 5 of 19 AML patients on this trial. Factors that correlated with improved outcomes were donor-recipient KIR ligand mismatch and greater numbers of circulating donor NK cells detected in the patients. A similar approach was reported by Curti et al., who treated 13 elderly AML patients with Flu/Cy, followed by haploidentical NK cell infusion and administration of s.c. IL-2 (10×10^6 U/day 3 days/week for 2 weeks) [157]. Patients with active disease did not respond to this approach, but 3 of 6 individuals treated in CR remained disease-free 18–34 months post-NK cell infusion. Rubnitz et al., treated 10 pediatric AML patients, who had achieved CR with a standard chemotherapy regimen, with KIR-KIR ligand mismatched haploidentical NK cells after preconditioning with Flu/Cy [85]. All patients demonstrated persistence of NK cells for 2–189 days (median 10 days) post-infusion and remain in CR with a median follow up of 964 days. GVHD was not observed in any of these trials.

Haploidentical NK cells infusions have also been used to treat adult solid tumors including breast cancer, ovarian cancer and non-small cell lung cancer, but minimal clinical activity was observed [40, 158]. The poor efficacy may be secondary to lack of persistence of donor NK cells and reconstitution of host regulatory T cells. It is also possible that these malignancies are inherently resistant to NK cell mediated cytotoxicity. Little data exists on the use of haploidentical NK cell infusions to treat pediatric solid tumors. The University of Wisconsin has obtained an IND (IND 16865) to treat children with relapsed or refractory neuroblastoma with ex-vivo activated and expanded haploidentical NK cells, in combination with hu14.18-IL-2 (an anti-GD2 immunocytokine). Trial activation is anticipated in 2017.

A number of studies have evaluated the use of NK cell-selected donor lymphocyte infusions following HSCT [159–164]. Rizzieri et al., isolated NK cells from HLA matched and mismatched family donors using the CliniMACS device and performed 51 NK cell infusions in 30 patients with hematologic malignancies starting at 6–8 weeks post-transplant [161]. Patients were allowed to receive up to 3 NK cell infusions 8 weeks apart. The infusions were well tolerated, though 2 patients developed ≥ grade 3 (severe) GVHD, possibly a consequence of T cells contaminating the NK cell product. Some of the patients showed improved NK cell function, as measured by in vitro cytotoxicity assays, following the NK cell infusions. Stern et al., reported infusing haploidentical NK cells, purified with the CliniMACS device, to 16 children and adults with high risk hematologic malignancies or solid tumors at day +3, +40 and +100 post-transplant [163]. The NK cell infusions were well tolerated, though no clinical benefit could be discerned. Four patients developed ≥ grade 2 GVHD, all of whom received a T cell dose > 0.5 × 10^5/kg, a level of contamination known to be capable of inducing GVHD in haploidentical transplant recipients. Choi et al. conducted a dose escalation trial in which patients with hematologic malignancies treated by haploidentical transplantation were infused with donor NK cells at 2 and 3 weeks post-transplant [165]. The NK cells were purified with the CliniMACS device and then cultured with IL-15 and IL-21 for 13–20 days. The dose of NK cells ranged from 2 × 10^7/kg to >1 × 10^8/kg. No dose limiting toxicities were observed and the NK cell infusions were felt to reduce the risk of leukemia progression from 74% (in historic controls) to 46%. NK cells obtained from haploidentical donors have also been used to treat patients with relapsed or persistent AML/MDS following HLA matched sibling or unrelated donor HSCT [162]. Patients received cyclophosphamide +/− fludarabine followed by freshly isolated haploidentical NK cells and a short course of subcutaneous IL-2. The median NK cell dose administered was 10.6 × 10^6/kg. The third party NK cells were not detected in any patient following infusion, though 1 AML and 1 MDS patient achieved a transient CR.

In a trial for children and young adults with very high-risk solid tumors treated by T cell depleted matched sibling or unrelated donor HSCT, donor derived NK cells were cultured with a feeder cell line (KT32.A2.41BBL.64) + IL15 for 9–11 days and then infused on days 7 and 35 post-transplant [166]. A high incidence of acute GVHD was observed (5 of 9 patients), with three patients developing grade 4 GVHD. Since the transplanted T cell dose was low in this study (1–2 × 10^4/kg), the investigators concluded that the ex vivo activated and expanded NK cells contributed to the development of GVHD. In another trial for pediatric solid tumors, six children received donor NK cells that had been incubated overnight with IL-15, 30 days after haploidentical HSCT. The mean number of NK cells infused was 11 × 10^6/kg (range 3–27 × 10^6/kg). No toxicity was associated with the NK cell infusions and 4 of 6 patients had a clinical response, though all patients ultimately died of disease progression [167] or transplant-related toxicity [168].

The NK cell line, NK-92, has also been utilized for cancer immunotherapy [167, 169]. Tonn et al. treated 15 adult and pediatric patients suffering from a broad range of refractory cancers, with two NK-92 infusions given 48 hours apart. The cell dose started at 1 × $10^9/m^2$ and was escalated to 1 × $10^{10}/m^2$. The infusions were well tolerated; 2 patients achieved mixed responses and 1 patient experienced disease stabilization for 2 years.

In summary, allogeneic NK cell infusions are generally thought to be safe and have been associated with clear anti-tumor activity, especially in patients with myeloid malignancies. When administered in the setting of HSCT, activated donor NK cells have the potential to induce GVHD, the risk likely related to the method of NK cell activation, level of T cell contamination, and timing of the infusion in relation to the transplant. For NK cell adoptive immunotherapy to be effective against pediatric solid tumors, further optimization will be required, potentially involving use of multiple NK cell infusions, combined therapy with other agents such as mAbs to facilitate tumor targeting, or through the utilization of genetically modified NK cells to improve tumor specificity, expansion and survival.

9.12 Genetically Modified NK Cells

NK cells may be genetically modified to alter their function and/or specificity in order to augment tumor cytotoxicity. While gene delivery into NK cells has historically been difficult, recent advances in viral transduction methodologies and the utilization of electroporation have improved the efficiency of transgene delivery and decreased the deleterious effects on cell viability. Viral transduction results in stable transgene expression, although transduction efficiencies are variable and multiple cycles of transduction may be required. Transfection of NK cells using electroporation has been shown to be an effective alternative strategy involving a short electric pulse that temporarily induces small pores in the cell membrane, allowing charged molecules (e.g., DNA, RNA) to move into the cell. This approach avoids the necessity of viral vectors and thus, requires lower-level biosafety laboratories, which dramatically reduces the cost of production and the number of regulatory hurdles associated with development and production. Transfection efficiencies are typically high, especially when mRNA is used rather than cDNA. A drawback to this approach is that transgene expression is transient. However, since NK cells are relatively short-lived, this may be less important than transient transgene expression in other cell types (e.g., T cells).

9.12.1 NK Cell CARs (Chimeric Antigen Receptors)

A chimeric antigen receptor (CAR) is a genetically engineered "hybrid" receptor comprised of an extracellular single-chain antibody fragment (scFv), which recognizes a tumor associated antigen, linked by a transmembrane domain to an intracellular signaling moiety. The earliest constructs used the CD3ζ signaling moiety and are called "first generation" CARs. Second and third generation CARs possess the CD3ζ signaling moiety in addition to one or two costimulatory activating motifs (e.g., 2B4, CD28, 4-1BB, OX-40), respectively.

Preclinical testing of NK cells transduced to express CARs demonstrated efficient in vitro and in vivo killing of tumor cells. In fact, CARs mediate a more potent NK cell cytotoxic response than CD16 ligation of antibody to the same target, in part since CARs have been engineered to maximize intracellular signaling.

Primary human NK cells have been transduced to express CARs specific for mesothelin (ovarian, mesothelioma), CS1 (multiple myeloma), CD19 and CD20 (lymphoid malignancies), HER2 (breast, osteosarcoma, head and neck, ovarian, glioblastoma) and GD2 (neuroblastoma, melanoma) [168, 170–176]. The NK leukemia cell line, NK-92, has been transduced to express CARs for CD19, CD20, CD138 (multiple myeloma), HER2, GD2, EpCAM (breast, pancreatic), EBNA3C (EBV infected cells), CS1 (multiple myeloma), LMAN1 (neuroblastoma, melanoma) and PSCA (prostate) [177–190]. An advantage of using CAR expressing NK-92 cells over autologous, primary NK cells expressing CARs includes their convenience and rapid "off-the-shelf" availability. However a disadvantage is that NK-92 cells are a tumor cell line infected with EBV and they must be irradiated before administration thus shortening their longevity.

Interestingly, the use of NK cell CARs may hold several advantages over the use of T cell CARs. First, mature NK cells are relatively short lived and therefore, a suicide switch may not be necessary if the cells mediated undesirable on or off -target toxicities. Second, cytokine release syndrome and other deleterious side effects may be less likely since NK cells do not possess an autocrine, positive feedback loop, such as IL-2 functions for T cells. Lastly, even if targeted tumor cells stop expressing the CAR-specific antigen due to selective pressure, CAR expressing NK cells could still function to eliminate tumor cells through engagement of their endogenous activating receptors. However, the latter advantage may be less prominent in CAR expressing NK-92 cells since they no longer express NCRs or CD16 receptors.

At the time of this writing, there are two clinical trials currently open using CAR expressing NK cells (NCT 00995137, NCT 01974479). Both of these trials utilize haploidentical donor NK cells that are first expanded by co-culture with feeder cells (K562-41BBL-mbIL15) and then transduced to express the CAR, anti-CD19-BB-zeta. Both clinical trials involve treating children with B-cell ALL.

9.12.2 Cytokine Transgenes

Immunotherapy employing adoptively transferred NK cells is generally accompanied by systemic administration of gamma-cytokines (e.g., IL-2) to promote their in vivo survival and proliferation, as discussed above. However, systemic administration of gamma-cytokines is associated with toxicities and IL-2 mobilizes and activates regulatory T cells, which diminish the anti-tumor efficacy of NK cell adoptive therapy [94]. The transduction of cytokine genes, such as IL-15 or IL-2, into adoptively transferred NK cells could promote their survival, expansion and activation, eliminating the need for systemic gamma-cytokine administration.

Two groups have successfully transduced NK-92 cells with the IL-2 gene using retroviral transduction [191, 192]. These cells proliferated in vitro without exogenous cytokines and produced augmented tumor cytotoxicity. When infused into tumor-bearing mice, IL-2 transduced NK cells exhibited longer survival and elicited greater antitumor responses than non-transduced NK-92 cells stimulated with exogenous IL-2. Ex vivo expanded NK cells have been successfully transduced with a gene for membrane bound IL-15 using retroviral transduction [193]. These cells persisted in vitro for a week without the addition of exogenous cytokines.

9.12.3 NK Cell Activating Receptor Transgenes

The transgene for the high affinity CD16 receptor has been successfully introduced into a (CD16 deficient-) NK cell line using retroviral transduction [144], and into *ex vivo* expanded NK cells using electroporation [194]. In preclinical studies, ADCC of opsonized tumor cells by high affinity CD16-tranduced NK92 cells was significantly greater than that using NK92 cells transduced with the transgene for the low affinity CD16 receptor. Similarly, ADCC of antibody-coated tumor cells by high affinity CD16-tranfected ex vivo expanded NK cells was greater than that achieved by non-transfected ex vivo expanded NK cells possessing the low affinity CD16 receptor (FcγR 158F/F). Adoptive transfer of large numbers of highly active NK cells that have been genetically engineered to express high affinity CD16 receptors could be directed toward any malignancy using tumor-specific monoclonal antibodies.

Another activating receptor that has been successfully introduced into ex vivo expanded NK cells is a chimeric NKG2D receptor (NKG2D-DAP10-CD3ζ). The expression of this chimeric receptor in expanded NK cells increased tumor cytotoxicity compared to mock-transduced expanded NK cells [171]. These cells also mediated effective in vitro cytotoxicity of osteosarcoma, B-cell ALL, T-cell ALL, rhabdomyosarcoma, neuroblastoma, and Ewing sarcoma, and had antitumor activity in a mouse model of osteosarcoma, while the expanded mock-transduced NK cells did not.

9.12.4 *Silencing of NK Cell Inhibitory Receptors by RNA Interference*

Another approach to further enhance the antitumor effect of adoptively transferred cells is to abrogate their sensitivity to inhibitory signals. This can be accomplished through the administration of monoclonal antibodies specific for NK cell inhibitory receptors, as discussed above. A genetic approach to achieve the same goal involves "silencing" NK cell inhibitory receptor genes through the use of short-hairpin RNA (shRNA) technology. shRNA is produced inside the cell from a DNA construct that has been delivered to the nucleus, via viral or other gene therapy vector. The DNA construct encodes a sequence of single stranded RNA and its complement, separated by a "stuffer" fragment. The stuffer fragment allows the RNA molecule to fold back on itself and thus, forms a double-stranded RNA molecule with a hairpin loop. A dicer endonuclease complex generates double-stranded small interfering RNA, which prevents translation of the targeted mRNA and therefore, silences the targeted gene (in this case, an NK inhibitory receptor). This technology has been successfully used to silence the gene for NKG2A using an inducible vector in an NK cell line (NKL) [195] and in IL-2 activated primary NK cells [196]. Silencing the NKG2A gene augmented in vitro cytotoxicity of HLA-E expressing tumor cells [195, 196]. In a xenogeneic mouse model, administering a single dose of NKG2A-silenced NKL cells, along with daily injections of IL-2 to support their survival and proliferation, resulted in slower tumor growth and smaller tumor burden compared to wild type NKL cells or GFP-transduced control NKL cells [195].

9.13 NKT Cells

9.13.1 NKT Cell Biology

NKT cells are a distinct T lymphocyte population possessing features of both innate (NK cells) and adaptive (conventional T cells) immune cells. Like NK cells, they react swiftly to stimuli, modulate immune responses through the production of cytokines and chemokines, and are capable of direct cytotoxicity of target cells. Like conventional T cells, they respond to antigen presentation through a T cell receptor (TCR), though the nature of the TCR and the antigen-presenting molecules are unlike those for conventional T cells. TCRs on NKT cells recognize exogenous and endogenous glycolipids, rather than peptides. In contrast to the highly polymorphic TCRs expressed by αβT cells, the major subset of NKTs express an invariant TCR comprised of a canonical α-chain, Vα24-Jα18, associated with the β chain, Vβ11 (in humans). This subset is called, "invariant" NKT (iNKT) or Type I NKT. The other subset is termed "noninvariant" NKT or Type II NKT, which displays a more heterogeneous αβ usage (preferentially gene segments form Vα1 and Vα3 associated with Vβ8.1/Vβ8.3 in humans) and which responds to distinct glycolipid antigens compared to those of type I NKTs. Both subsets are restricted by the presentation of glycolipid antigens in the context of the MHC class-I-like CD1d molecule. In fact, this feature characterizes NKT cells.

Like many immune cell types, NKT cells appear to have both immune enhancing and immunosuppressive roles. The nature of the NKT cell response is dependent on which subsets are activated, where the iNKT subset is generally immune enhancing and promotes tumor immunity while the noninvariant subset is immunosuppressive. The effector functions employed by iNKT cells include cellular cytotoxicity and cytokine production. Invariant NKT cells can kill target cells directly, through the release of cytotoxic granules and the expression of death receptor ligands (e.g., TRAIL, FasL) that interact with death receptors on the tumor cell surface [167, 197, 198]. Cytokines and chemokines secreted by iNKT cells include IFNγ, IL-2, IL-4, IL-10, IL-13, IL-17, IL-21, IL-22, GM-CSF, TNFα, CCL5, Eotaxin and MIP-1α, and the cytokine/chemokine profile produced depends on which iNKT subsets (e.g. NKT1, NKT2, NKT17, Foxp3+) are responding to antigen. These subsets are programed intrathymically to generate a specific cytokine profile [199, 200]. For tumor immunity, iNKT effector functions enable iNKT cells to directly kill tumor cells and to modulate both the innate and adaptive immune response to cancer.

Invariant NKTs are stimulated to elicit their effector functions through activation by cell-to-cell contact with target cells or antigen presenting cells (APCs). Antigen presenting cells, such as dendritic cells (DCs), B cells, and macrophages, present endogenous glycolipids in the context of the MHC-like molecule, CD1d, to the invariant TCR of iNKT cells. The prototypical glycolipid antigen that potently stimulates iNKT cells is α-galactosylceramide (αGalCer), which is derived from a marine sponge. A number of bacterial, fungal and parasitic glycolipid antigens that stimulate iNKT cells have been discovered, but the identity of tumor specific glycolipid antigens have not yet been determined. It has been shown that the nature of the glycolipid antigen, which determines CD1d-binding kinetics, influences the iNKT response. Non-antigen factors also affect the iNKT response, such as the presence of APC costimulatory molecules, although iNKT cells are less dependent on costimulation compared to conventional naïve T cells. Importantly, since iNKT cells constitutively express surface receptors for pro-inflammatory cytokines, the cytokine milieu in which the interaction between APC and iNKT takes place, greatly influences the iNKT response.

Invariant NKT cells may kill tumor cells either directly or indirectly (Fig. 9.5). Both hematologic malignancies [201–206], and solid tumors [207–210] have been shown to express CD1d on their surface, which may present endogenous glycolipids

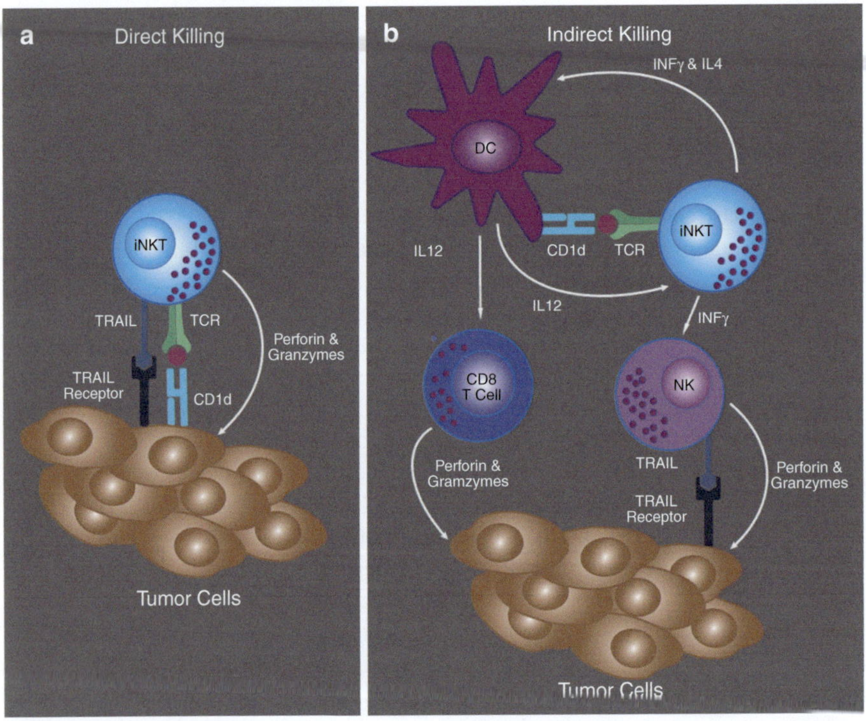

Fig. 9.5 Antitumor activity of iNKT cells. (**a**) iNKT cells directly kill tumor cells through recognition of tumor cell endogenous glycolipids presented by CD1d resulting in the release of cytotoxic granule contents. Tumor cell apoptosis is mediated by iNKT-secreted granzymes and iNKT death receptor ligands (TRAIL, FasL) binding tumor cell death receptors. (**b**) iNKT cells indirectly kill tumor cells by recruiting the cytotoxic function of other immune cells. Tumor cell endogenous glycolipids presented by CD1d on APCs activate iNKT cells, which release cytokines that activate and mature APCs. Bidirectional activation between APCs and iNKT cells results in a cytokine milieu that conscripts innate and adaptive immune antitumor responses

to iNKT cell TCRs and thus, stimulate iNKT cells to directly target the malignancy (Fig. 9.5) [205, 211]. Alternately, iNKT cells may participate in the killing of tumor cells indirectly by recruiting innate and adaptive immune cells, which have cytotoxic effector functions. For instance, DCs may present tumor glycolipid antigen in the context of CD1d to the TCR of iNKT cells, and TCR signaling triggers the rapid release of IFNγ and IL-4. These cytokines, along with CD40/CD40L interactions between DC and iNKT cells promote the maturation and activation of DCs, which can then initiate antigen-specific adaptive lymphocyte responses, including the priming of cytotoxic T lymphocytes. Recruitment of cytolytic cell populations is dependent upon the iNKT-initiation of T_h1 cytokine cascades. In particular, DC production of IL-12 activates NK cells and γδT cells, enlisting an innate immune response. In addition to enhancing innate and adaptive antitumor responses, iNKT cells may also facilitate tumor eradication by killing immunosuppressive tumor associated macrophages or inhibiting their ability to produce pro-angiogenic factors [212, 213].

Observational studies have noted reduced iNKT cell frequency and function in patients with hematologic malignancies [201, 214] and solid tumors [210, 215, 216]. Higher frequency of iNKT cells in peripheral blood of cancer patients, or in tumors, has been correlated with decreased metastases and higher rates of overall and disease-free survival [217–219]. In pediatric patients who received haploidentical HSCT to treat leukemia, reconstitution of iNKT cells in peripheral blood was associated with long-term remissions [133, 220]. However, inferences drawn from such information are challenging since (1) there is large variability in the frequency of iNKT cells between healthy individuals (generally 0.1–0.2% of circulating lymphocytes with a range of undetectable to >1% [134, 221, 222], (2) such changes may be a cause or a consequence of disease, and (3) changes in peripheral cell numbers may reflect recruitment into inflamed tissues, such as tumor sites.

Preclinical studies support a role for iNKT cells in tumor immunosurveillance and control. Tumor growth in a p53 deficient mouse model was greater for animals that were iNKT cell-deficient ($J\alpha18^{-/-}$) compared with wild-type animals [223] and methylcholanthrene (MCA)-induced sarcomas grew in iNKT-deficient mice ($J\alpha281^{-/}$) but not wild type mice [224]. In fact, adoptive transfer of wild type iNKT cells into iNKT-deficient mice dramatically attenuated the growth of MCA-induced sarcomas [224].

Administration of the iNKT glycolipid agonist, αGalCer has been shown in numerous studies to protect against disease progression in tumor-bearing mice [225–231] and this antitumor effect has since been shown to be dependent on IFNγ production and NK cells [232–234]. Moreover, adoptive transfer of αGalCer-pulsed dendritic cells was found to elicit an immune response resulting in rejection of tumor [235], and demonstrated a more potent antitumor effect than αGalCer alone [82]. A number of other compounds show promise for potential translation into clinical studies including αGalCer analogs that contain phenyl group(s) on the lipid tail of αGalCer, which directs iNKT cells toward a

T_h1-skewed response and induces neither NKT cell anergy nor expansion of myeloid derived suppressor cells, despite producing stronger anticancer activity compared with αGalCer [236, 237]. Since preclinical work in mouse tumor models shows a strong correlation between the magnitude of tumor protection afforded by iNKT agonists and the T_h1 cytokine profile (high IFNγ:IL-4 ratio or IFNγ production) [238], there is ongoing research to synthesize iNKT agonists that enhance IFNγ production [236, 239–242].

9.13.2 NKT Cell Immunotherapy

Based on the preclinical data presented above, iNKT cells and iNKT cell agonists have been used for human cancer immunotherapy. Adult patients with solid tumors were treated with soluble αGalCer, which was found to be reasonably safe and well tolerated, [215, 243] but was associated with limited, if any, clinical benefit. Further studies have demonstrated that soluble αGalCer induces iNKT cell anergy [230, 244–246], likely in a PD-1/PD-L1 dependent manner [245]. Another approach used in several small, phase I studies of adult patients with solid tumors was the administration of αGalCer-loaded DCs, which showed expansion of circulating NKT cells and increased serum levels of INFγ and IL12 [244, 247, 248].

Adoptive transfer of in vitro activated iNKT cells into adult patients with non-small cell lung carcinoma resulted in an increased frequency of iNKT cells, NK cell activation and IFNγ release [249]. Yamasaki et al. conducted a phase 2 trial for 10 patients with locally recurrent and operable head and neck squamous cell carcinoma [65]. Patients underwent leukopheresis and then 7 days later received antigen presenting cells (derived from autologous PBMCs that were cultured with GM-CSF and IL-2) by nasal submucosal administration. On day 14, activated Vα24 NKT cells (PBMC cultured for 14 days with IL-2 and αGalCer) were injected intra-arterially via tumor-feeding arteries. Surgical resection of the tumor was performed 2 weeks later. Five patients experienced a PR and 5 had stable disease prior to surgery. Following surgery, tumor tissue was analyzed for Vα24 TCR expression by RT-PCR. This was found to be significantly higher in patients who experienced a PR, compared to those with stable disease or a control group not treated with immunotherapy, suggesting a correlation between NKT tumor infiltration and clinical response.

Another approach to harness the antitumor activity of iNKT cells uses genetic engineering to express a tumor specific CAR. Primary human iNKT cells have been engineered to express a third generation CAR against the GD2 disialoganglioside with CD28 and 4-1BB containing endodomains, which impart in vivo persistence and a striking T_h1-like polarization of NKT cells [250]. In a mouse model of metastatic neuroblastoma, these CAR.GD2 NKT cells localized to tumor sites, had potent antitumor activity and improved long-term survival. A phase I study to treat children with neuroblastoma with CAR.GD2 NKT cells is registered at clinicaltrials.gov (NCT02439788).

References

1. Yu J, Freud AG, Caligiuri MA. Location and cellular stages of natural killer cell development. Trends Immunol. 2013;34:573–82.
2. Campbell JJ, Qin S, Unutmaz D, et al. Unique subpopulations of CD56+ NK and NK-T peripheral blood lymphocytes identified by chemokine receptor expression repertoire. J Immunol. 2001;166:6477–82.
3. Caligiuri MA. Human natural killer cells. Blood. 2008;112:461–9.
4. Strowig T, Brilot F, Munz C. Noncytotoxic functions of NK cells: direct pathogen restriction and assistance to adaptive immunity. J Immunol. 2008;180:7785–91.
5. De Maria A, Bozzano F, Cantoni C, Moretta L. Revisiting human natural killer cell subset function revealed cytolytic CD56(dim)CD16+ NK cells as rapid producers of abundant IFN-gamma on activation. Proc Natl Acad Sci U S A. 2011;108:728–32.
6. Walzer T, Dalod M, Robbins SH, Zitvogel L, Vivier E. Natural-killer cells and dendritic cells: "l'union fait la force". Blood. 2005;106:2252–8.
7. Orange JS. Formation and function of the lytic NK-cell immunological synapse. Nat Rev Immunol. 2008;8:713–25.
8. Chowdhury D, Lieberman J. Death by a thousand cuts: granzyme pathways of programmed cell death. Annu Rev Immunol. 2008;26:389–420.
9. Lieberman J. Mechanisms of granule-mediated cytotoxicity. Curr Opin Immunol. 2003;15:513–5.
10. Chavez-Galan L, Arenas-Del Angel MC, Zenteno E, Chavez R, Lascurain R. Cell death mechanisms induced by cytotoxic lymphocytes. Cell Mol Immunol. 2009;6:15–25.
11. Strasser A, Jost PJ, Nagata S. The many roles of FAS receptor signaling in the immune system. Immunity. 2009;30:180–92.
12. Brandt CS, Baratin M, Yi EC, et al. The B7 family member B7-H6 is a tumor cell ligand for the activating natural killer cell receptor NKp30 in humans. J Exp Med. 2009;206:1495–503.
13. Semeraro M, Rusakiewicz S, Minard-Colin V, et al. Clinical impact of the NKp30/B7-H6 axis in high-risk neuroblastoma patients. Sci Transl Med. 2015;7:283ra255.
14. Glasner A, Ghadially H, Gur C, et al. Recognition and prevention of tumor metastasis by the NK receptor NKp46/NCR1. J Immunol. 2012;188:2509–15.
15. Horton NC, Mathew PA. NKp44 and natural cytotoxicity receptors as damage-associated molecular pattern recognition receptors. Front Immunol. 2015;6:31.
16. Castriconi R, Dondero A, Corrias MV, et al. Natural killer cell-mediated killing of freshly isolated neuroblastoma cells: critical role of DNAX accessory molecule-1-poliovirus receptor interaction. Cancer Res. 2004;64:9180–4.
17. Gilfillan S, Chan CJ, Cella M, et al. DNAM-1 promotes activation of cytotoxic lymphocytes by nonprofessional antigen-presenting cells and tumors. J Exp Med. 2008;205:2965–73.
18. Lakshmikanth T, Burke S, Ali TH, et al. NCRs and DNAM-1 mediate NK cell recognition and lysis of human and mouse melanoma cell lines in vitro and in vivo. J Clin Invest. 2009;119:1251–63.
19. Cooley S, Trachtenberg E, Bergemann TL, et al. Donors with group B KIR haplotypes improve relapse-free survival after unrelated hematopoietic cell transplantation for acute myelogenous leukemia. Blood. 2009;113:726–32.
20. Pende D, Marcenaro S, Falco M, et al. Anti-leukemia activity of alloreactive NK cells in KIR ligand-mismatched haploidentical HSCT for pediatric patients: evaluation of the functional role of activating KIR and redefinition of inhibitory KIR specificity. Blood. 2009;113:3119–29.
21. Venstrom JM, Pittari G, Gooley TA, et al. HLA-C-dependent prevention of leukemia relapse by donor activating KIR2DS1. N Engl J Med. 2012;367:805–16.
22. Chitadze G, Bhat J, Lettau M, Janssen O, Kabelitz D. Generation of soluble NKG2D ligands: proteolytic cleavage, exosome secretion and functional implications. Scand J Immunol. 2013;78:120–9.

23. Kim S, Poursine-Laurent J, Truscott SM, et al. Licensing of natural killer cells by host major histocompatibility complex class I molecules. Nature. 2005;436:709–13.
24. Orr MT, Lanier LL. Natural killer cell education and tolerance. Cell. 2010;142:847–56.
25. Berghuis D, de Hooge AS, Santos SJ, et al. Reduced human leukocyte antigen expression in advanced-stage Ewing sarcoma: implications for immune recognition. J Pathol. 2009;218:222–31.
26. Borowski A, van Valen F, Ulbrecht M, et al. Monomorphic HLA class I-(non-A, non-B) expression on Ewing's tumor cell lines, modulation by TNF-alpha and IFN-gamma. Immunobiology. 1999;200:1–20.
27. Mechtersheimer G, Staudter M, Majdic O, Dorken B, Moldenhauer G, Moller P. Expression of HLA-A,B,C, beta 2-microglobulin (beta 2m), HLA-DR, -DP, -DQ and of HLA-D-associated invariant chain (Ii) in soft-tissue tumors. Int J Cancer. 1990;46:813–23.
28. Peters HL, Yan Y, Solheim JC. APLP2 regulates the expression of MHC class I molecules on irradiated Ewing's sarcoma cells. Oncoimmunology. 2013;2:e26293.
29. Ruggeri L, Capanni M, Urbani E, et al. Effectiveness of donor natural killer cell alloreactivity in mismatched hematopoietic transplants. Science. 2002;295:2097–100.
30. Leung W, Iyengar R, Turner V, et al. Determinants of antileukemia effects of allogeneic NK cells. J Immunol. 2004;172:644–50.
31. Cooley S, Weisdorf DJ, Guethlein LA, et al. Donor killer cell Ig-like receptor B haplotypes, recipient HLA-C1, and HLA-C mismatch enhance the clinical benefit of unrelated transplantation for acute myelogenous leukemia. J Immunol. 2014;192:4592–600.
32. Giebel S, Locatelli F, Lamparelli T, et al. Survival advantage with KIR ligand incompatibility in hematopoietic stem cell transplantation from unrelated donors. Blood. 2003;102:814–9.
33. Hsu KC, Keever-Taylor CA, Wilton A, et al. Improved outcome in HLA-identical sibling hematopoietic stem-cell transplantation for acute myelogenous leukemia predicted by KIR and HLA genotypes. Blood. 2005;105:4878–84.
34. Symons HJ, Leffell MS, Rossiter ND, Zahurak M, Jones RJ, Fuchs EJ. Improved survival with inhibitory killer immunoglobulin receptor (KIR) gene mismatches and KIR haplotype B donors after nonmyeloablative, HLA-haploidentical bone marrow transplantation. Biol Blood Marrow Transplant. 2010;16:533–42.
35. Venstrom JM, Zheng J, Noor N, et al. KIR and HLA genotypes are associated with disease progression and survival following autologous hematopoietic stem cell transplantation for high-risk neuroblastoma. Clin Cancer Res. 2009;15:7330–4.
36. Delgado DC, Hank JA, Kolesar J, et al. Genotypes of NK cell KIR receptors, their ligands, and Fcgamma receptors in the response of neuroblastoma patients to Hu14.18-IL2 immunotherapy. Cancer Res. 2010;70:9554–61.
37. Berg M, Lundqvist A, McCoy P Jr, et al. Clinical-grade ex vivo-expanded human natural killer cells up-regulate activating receptors and death receptor ligands and have enhanced cytolytic activity against tumor cells. Cytotherapy. 2009;11:341–55.
38. Denman CJ, Senyukov VV, Somanchi SS, et al. Membrane-bound IL-21 promotes sustained ex vivo proliferation of human natural killer cells. PLoS One. 2012;7:e30264.
39. Fujisaki H, Kakuda H, Shimasaki N, et al. Expansion of highly cytotoxic human natural killer cells for cancer cell therapy. Cancer Res. 2009;69:4010–7.
40. Iliopoulou EG, Kountourakis P, Karamouzis MV, et al. A phase I trial of adoptive transfer of allogeneic natural killer cells in patients with advanced non-small cell lung cancer. Cancer Immunol Immunother. 2010;59:1781–9.
41. Koehl U, Brehm C, Huenecke S, et al. Clinical grade purification and expansion of NK cell products for an optimized manufacturing protocol. Front Oncol. 2013;3:118.
42. Lim SA, Kim TJ, Lee JE, et al. Ex vivo expansion of highly cytotoxic human NK cells by cocultivation with irradiated tumor cells for adoptive immunotherapy. Cancer Res. 2013;73:2598–607.
43. Somanchi SS, Senyukov VV, Denman CJ, Lee DA. Expansion, purification, and functional assessment of human peripheral blood NK cells. J Vis Exp. 2011;48:2540.
44. Granzin M, Soltenborn S, Muller S, et al. Fully automated expansion and activation of clinical-grade natural killer cells for adoptive immunotherapy. Cytotherapy. 2015;17:621–32.

45. Garg TK, Szmania SM, Khan JA, et al. Highly activated and expanded natural killer cells for multiple myeloma immunotherapy. Haematologica. 2012;97:1348–56.
46. Rujkijyanont P, Chan WK, Eldridge PW, et al. Ex vivo activation of CD56+ immune cells that eradicate neuroblastoma. Cancer Res. 2013;73:2608–18.
47. Zhang H, Cui Y, Voong N, et al. Activating signals dominate inhibitory signals in CD137L/IL-15 activated natural killer cells. J Immunother. 2011;34:187–95.
48. Cho D, Shook DR, Shimasaki N, Chang YH, Fujisaki H, Campana D. Cytotoxicity of activated natural killer cells against pediatric solid tumors. Clin Cancer Res. 2010;16:3901–9.
49. Voskens CJ, Watanabe R, Rollins S, Campana D, Hasumi K, Mann DL. Ex-vivo expanded human NK cells express activating receptors that mediate cytotoxicity of allogeneic and autologous cancer cell lines by direct recognition and antibody directed cellular cytotoxicity. J Exp Clin Cancer Res. 2010;29:134.
50. Spanholtz J, Tordoir M, Eissens D, et al. High log-scale expansion of functional human natural killer cells from umbilical cord blood CD34-positive cells for adoptive cancer immunotherapy. PLoS One. 2010;5:e9221.
51. Grzywacz B, Kataria N, Sikora M, et al. Coordinated acquisition of inhibitory and activating receptors and functional properties by developing human natural killer cells. Blood. 2006;108:3824–33.
52. Woll PS, Grzywacz B, Tian X, et al. Human embryonic stem cells differentiate into a homogeneous population of natural killer cells with potent in vivo antitumor activity. Blood. 2009;113:6094–101.
53. Knorr DA, Ni Z, Hermanson D, et al. Clinical-scale derivation of natural killer cells from human pluripotent stem cells for cancer therapy. Stem Cells Transl Med. 2013;2:274–83.
54. Rezvani K, Rouce RH. The application of natural killer cell immunotherapy for the treatment of cancer. Front Immunol. 2015;6:578.
55. Gong JH, Maki G, Klingemann HG. Characterization of a human cell line (NK-92) with phenotypical and functional characteristics of activated natural killer cells. Leukemia. 1994;8:652–8.
56. Tam YK, Miyagawa B, Ho VC, Klingemann HG. Immunotherapy of malignant melanoma in a SCID mouse model using the highly cytotoxic natural killer cell line NK-92. J Hematother. 1999;8:281–90.
57. Yan Y, Steinherz P, Klingemann HG, et al. Antileukemia activity of a natural killer cell line against human leukemias. Clin Cancer Res. 1998;4:2859–68.
58. Maki G, Klingemann HG, Martinson JA, Tam YK. Factors regulating the cytotoxic activity of the human natural killer cell line, NK-92. J Hematother Stem Cell Res. 2001;10:369–83.
59. Tam YK, Martinson JA, Doligosa K, Klingemann HG. Ex vivo expansion of the highly cytotoxic human natural killer-92 cell-line under current good manufacturing practice conditions for clinical adoptive cellular immunotherapy. Cytotherapy. 2003;5:259–72.
60. Becknell B, Caligiuri MA. Interleukin-2, interleukin-15, and their roles in human natural killer cells. Adv Immunol. 2005;86:209–39.
61. Ferlazzo G, Pack M, Thomas D, et al. Distinct roles of IL-12 and IL-15 in human natural killer cell activation by dendritic cells from secondary lymphoid organs. Proc Natl Acad Sci U S A. 2004;101:16606–11.
62. Konjevic G, Mirjacic Martinovic K, Vuletic A, Babovic N. In-vitro IL-2 or IFN-alpha-induced NKG2D and CD161 NK cell receptor expression indicates novel aspects of NK cell activation in metastatic melanoma patients. Melanoma Res. 2010;20:459–67.
63. Hromadnikova I, Pirkova P, Sedlackova L. Influence of in vitro IL-2 or IL-15 alone or in combination with Hsp-70-derived 14-mer peptide (TKD) on the expression of NK cell activatory and inhibitory receptors. Mediat Inflamm. 2013;2013:405295.
64. Vitale M, Bottino C, Sivori S, et al. NKp44, a novel triggering surface molecule specifically expressed by activated natural killer cells, is involved in non-major histocompatibility complex-restricted tumor cell lysis. J Exp Med. 1998;187:2065–72.
65. Yakes FM, Chinratanalab W, Ritter CA, King W, Seelig S, Arteaga CL. Herceptin-induced inhibition of phosphatidylinositol-3 kinase and Akt Is required for antibody-mediated effects on p 27, cyclin D1, and antitumor action. Cancer Res. 2002;62:4132–41.

66. Skak K, Frederiksen KS, Lundsgaard D. Interleukin-21 activates human natural killer cells and modulates their surface receptor expression. Immunology. 2008;123:575–83.
67. Trotta R, Ciarlariello D, Dal Col J, et al. The PP2A inhibitor SET regulates granzyme B expression in human natural killer cells. Blood. 2011;117:2378–84.
68. Handa K, Suzuki R, Matsui H, Shimizu Y, Kumagai K. Natural killer (NK) cells as a responder to interleukin 2 (IL 2). II. IL 2-induced interferon gamma production. J Immunol. 1983;130:988–92.
69. Hank JA, Kohler PC, Weil-Hillman G, et al. In vivo induction of the lymphokine-activated killer phenomenon: interleukin 2-dependent human non-major histocompatibility complex-restricted cytotoxicity generated in vivo during administration of human recombinant interleukin 2. Cancer Res. 1988;48:1965–71.
70. He XS, Draghi M, Mahmood K, et al. T cell-dependent production of IFN-gamma by NK cells in response to influenza A virus. J Clin Invest. 2004;114:1812–9.
71. Meropol NJ, Porter M, Blumenson LE, et al. Daily subcutaneous injection of low-dose interleukin 2 expands natural killer cells in vivo without significant toxicity. Clin Cancer Res. 1996;2:669–77.
72. Miller JS, Tessmer-Tuck J, Pierson BA, et al. Low dose subcutaneous interleukin-2 after autologous transplantation generates sustained in vivo natural killer cell activity. Biol Blood Marrow Transplant. 1997;3:34–44.
73. Siegel JP, Sharon M, Smith PL, Leonard WJ. The IL-2 receptor beta chain (p 70): role in mediating signals for LAK, NK, and proliferative activities. Science. 1987;238:75–8.
74. Sondel PM, Kohler PC, Hank JA, et al. Clinical and immunological effects of recombinant interleukin 2 given by repetitive weekly cycles to patients with cancer. Cancer Res. 1988;48:2561–7.
75. Trinchieri G, Matsumoto-Kobayashi M, Clark SC, Seehra J, London L, Perussia B. Response of resting human peripheral blood natural killer cells to interleukin 2. J Exp Med. 1984;160:1147–69.
76. Weil-Hillman G, Fisch P, Prieve AF, Sosman JA, Hank JA, Sondel PM. Lymphokine-activated killer activity induced by in vivo interleukin 2 therapy: predominant role for lymphocytes with increased expression of CD2 and leu 19 antigens but negative expression of CD16 antigens. Cancer Res. 1989;49:3680–8.
77. Rosenberg SA, Lotze MT, Muul LM, et al. Observations on the systemic administration of autologous lymphokine-activated killer cells and recombinant interleukin-2 to patients with metastatic cancer. N Engl J Med. 1985;313:1485–92.
78. Bauer M, Reaman GH, Hank JA, et al. A phase II trial of human recombinant interleukin-2 administered as a 4-day continuous infusion for children with refractory neuroblastoma, non-Hodgkin's lymphoma, sarcoma, renal cell carcinoma, and malignant melanoma. A childrens cancer group study. Cancer. 1995;75:2959–65.
79. Lange BJ, Yang RK, Gan J, et al. Soluble interleukin-2 receptor alpha activation in a Children's Oncology Group randomized trial of interleukin-2 therapy for pediatric acute myeloid leukemia. Pediatr Blood Cancer. 2011;57:398–405.
80. Roper M, Smith MA, Sondel PM, et al. A phase I study of interleukin-2 in children with cancer. Am J Pediatr Hematol Oncol. 1992;14:305–11.
81. Ladenstein R, Potschger U, Siabalis D, et al. Dose finding study for the use of subcutaneous recombinant interleukin-2 to augment natural killer cell numbers in an outpatient setting for stage 4 neuroblastoma after megatherapy and autologous stem-cell reinfusion. J Clin Oncol. 2011;29:441–8.
82. Fujii S, Shimizu K, Kronenberg M, Steinman RM. Prolonged IFN-gamma-producing NKT response induced with alpha-galactosylceramide-loaded DCs. Nat Immunol. 2002;3:867–74.
83. Wang J, Sun ZM, Cao LL, Li Q. Biological characteristics of cord blood natural killer cells induced and amplified with IL-2 and IL-15. Zhongguo Shi Yan Xue Ye Xue Za Zhi. 2012;20:731–5.
84. Zamai L, Del Zotto G, Buccella F, et al. Cytotoxic functions and susceptibility to apoptosis of human CD56(bright) NK cells differentiated in vitro from CD34(+) hematopoietic progenitors. Cytometry A. 2012;81:294–302.

85. Rubnitz JE, Inaba H, Ribeiro RC, et al. NKAML: a pilot study to determine the safety and feasibility of haploidentical natural killer cell transplantation in childhood acute myeloid leukemia. J Clin Oncol. 2010;28:955–9.
86. Gamero AM, Ussery D, Reintgen DS, Puleo CA, Djeu JY. Interleukin 15 induction of lymphokine-activated killer cell function against autologous tumor cells in melanoma patient lymphocytes by a CD18-dependent, perforin-related mechanism. Cancer Res. 1995;55:4988–94.
87. Wren L, Parsons MS, Isitman G, et al. Influence of cytokines on HIV-specific antibody-dependent cellular cytotoxicity activation profile of natural killer cells. PLoS One. 2012;7:e38580.
88. Carson WE, Giri JG, Lindemann MJ, et al. Interleukin (IL) 15 is a novel cytokine that activates human natural killer cells via components of the IL-2 receptor. J Exp Med. 1994;180:1395–403.
89. Choi SS, Chhabra VS, Nguyen QH, Ank BJ, Stiehm ER, Roberts RL. Interleukin-15 enhances cytotoxicity, receptor expression, and expansion of neonatal natural killer cells in long-term culture. Clin Diagn Lab Immunol. 2004;11:879–88.
90. Miller JS, Soignier Y, Panoskaltsis-Mortari A, et al. Successful adoptive transfer and in vivo expansion of human haploidentical NK cells in patients with cancer. Blood. 2005;105:3051–7.
91. Moga E, Alvarez E, Canto E, et al. NK cells stimulated with IL-15 or CpG ODN enhance rituximab-dependent cellular cytotoxicity against B-cell lymphoma. Exp Hematol. 2008;36:69–77.
92. Moga E, Canto E, Vidal S, Juarez C, Sierra J, Briones J. Interleukin-15 enhances rituximab-dependent cytotoxicity against chronic lymphocytic leukemia cells and overcomes transforming growth factor beta-mediated immunosuppression. Exp Hematol. 2011;39:1064–71.
93. Roberti MP, Barrio MM, Bravo AI, et al. IL-15 and IL-2 increase Cetuximab-mediated cellular cytotoxicity against triple negative breast cancer cell lines expressing EGFR. Breast Cancer Res Treat. 2011;130:465–75.
94. Bachanova V, Cooley S, Defor TE, et al. Clearance of acute myeloid leukemia by haploidentical natural killer cells is improved using IL-2 diphtheria toxin fusion protein. Blood. 2014;123:3855–63.
95. Conlon KC, Lugli E, Welles HC, et al. Redistribution, hyperproliferation, activation of natural killer cells and CD8 T cells, and cytokine production during first-in-human clinical trial of recombinant human interleukin-15 in patients with cancer. J Clin Oncol. 2015;33:74–82.
96. Schmidt H, Brown J, Mouritzen U, et al. Safety and clinical effect of subcutaneous human interleukin-21 in patients with metastatic melanoma or renal cell carcinoma: a phase I trial. Clin Cancer Res. 2010;16:5312–9.
97. Reddy N, Hernandez-Ilizaliturri FJ, Deeb G, et al. Immunomodulatory drugs stimulate natural killer-cell function, alter cytokine production by dendritic cells, and inhibit angiogenesis enhancing the anti-tumour activity of rituximab in vivo. Br J Haematol. 2008;140:36–45.
98. Wu L, Adams M, Carter T, et al. lenalidomide enhances natural killer cell and monocyte-mediated antibody-dependent cellular cytotoxicity of rituximab-treated CD20+ tumor cells. Clin Cancer Res. 2008;14:4650–7.
99. Berg SL, Cairo MS, Russell H, et al. Safety, pharmacokinetics, and immunomodulatory effects of lenalidomide in children and adolescents with relapsed/refractory solid tumors or myelodysplastic syndrome: a Children's Oncology Group Phase I Consortium report. J Clin Oncol. 2011;29:316–23.
100. Lundqvist A, Abrams SI, Schrump DS, et al. Bortezomib and depsipeptide sensitize tumors to tumor necrosis factor-related apoptosis-inducing ligand: a novel method to potentiate natural killer cell tumor cytotoxicity. Cancer Res. 2006;66:7317–25.
101. Lundqvist A, Berg M, Smith A, Childs RW. Bortezomib treatment to potentiate the antitumor immunity of ex-vivo expanded adoptively infused autologous natural killer cells. J Cancer. 2011;2:383–5.
102. Piperdi B, Ling YH, Liebes L, Muggia F, Perez-Soler R. Bortezomib: understanding the mechanism of action. Mol Cancer Ther. 2011;10:2029–30.

103. Blaney SM, Bernstein M, Neville K, et al. Phase I study of the proteasome inhibitor bortezomib in pediatric patients with refractory solid tumors: a Children's Oncology Group study (ADVL0015). J Clin Oncol. 2004;22:4804–9.
104. Horton TM, Pati D, Plon SE, et al. A phase 1 study of the proteasome inhibitor bortezomib in pediatric patients with refractory leukemia: a Children's Oncology Group study. Clin Cancer Res. 2007;13:1516–22.
105. Messinger Y, Gaynon P, Raetz E, et al. Phase I study of bortezomib combined with chemotherapy in children with relapsed childhood acute lymphoblastic leukemia (ALL): a report from the therapeutic advances in childhood leukemia (TACL) consortium. Pediatr Blood Cancer. 2010;55:254–9.
106. Muscal JA, Thompson PA, Horton TM, et al. A phase I trial of vorinostat and bortezomib in children with refractory or recurrent solid tumors: a Children's Oncology Group phase I consortium study (ADVL0916). Pediatr Blood Cancer. 2013;60:390–5.
107. Horton TM, Drachtman RA, Chen L, et al. A phase 2 study of bortezomib in combination with ifosfamide/vinorelbine in paediatric patients and young adults with refractory/recurrent Hodgkin lymphoma: a Children's Oncology Group study. Br J Haematol. 2015;170:118–22.
108. Armeanu S, Bitzer M, Lauer UM, et al. Natural killer cell-mediated lysis of hepatoma cells via specific induction of NKG2D ligands by the histone deacetylase inhibitor sodium valproate. Cancer Res. 2005;65:6321–9.
109. Skov S, Pedersen MT, Andresen L, Straten PT, Woetmann A, Odum N. Cancer cells become susceptible to natural killer cell killing after exposure to histone deacetylase inhibitors due to glycogen synthase kinase-3-dependent expression of MHC class I-related chain A and B. Cancer Res. 2005;65:11136–45.
110. Son CH, Keum JH, Yang K, et al. Synergistic enhancement of NK cell-mediated cytotoxicity by combination of histone deacetylase inhibitor and ionizing radiation. Radiat Oncol. 2014;9:49.
111. Su JM, Li XN, Thompson P, et al. Phase 1 study of valproic acid in pediatric patients with refractory solid or CNS tumors: a children's oncology group report. Clin Cancer Res. 2011;17:589–97.
112. Fouladi M, Furman WL, et al. Phase I study of depsipeptide in pediatric patients with refractory solid tumors: a Children's Oncology Group report. J Clin Oncol. 2006;24:3678–85.
113. Gupta P, Han SY, Holgado-Madruga M, et al. Development of an EGFRvIII specific recombinant antibody. BMC Biotechnol. 2010;10:72.
114. Baragano Raneros A, Martin-Palanco V, Fernandez AF, et al. Methylation of NKG2D ligands contributes to immune system evasion in acute myeloid leukemia. Genes Immun. 2015;16:71–82.
115. Pfeiffer MM, Burow H, Schleicher S, Handgretinger R, Lang P. Influence of histone deacetylase inhibitors and DNA-methyltransferase inhibitors on the NK cell-mediated lysis of pediatric B-lineage leukemia. Front Oncol. 2013;3:99.
116. Phillips CL, Davies SM, McMasters R, et al. Low dose decitabine in very high risk relapsed or refractory acute myeloid leukaemia in children and young adults. Br J Haematol. 2013;161:406–10.
117. Weng WK, Levy R. Two immunoglobulin G fragment C receptor polymorphisms independently predict response to rituximab in patients with follicular lymphoma. J Clin Oncol. 2003;21:3940–7.
118. Goldman S, Smith L, Galardy P, et al. Rituximab with chemotherapy in children and adolescents with central nervous system and/or bone marrow-positive Burkitt lymphoma/leukaemia: a Children's Oncology Group Report. Br J Haematol. 2014;167:394–401.
119. Yu AL, Gilman AL, Ozkaynak MF, et al. Anti-GD2 antibody with GM-CSF, interleukin-2, and isotretinoin for neuroblastoma. N Engl J Med. 2010;363:1324–34.
120. Cheung NK, Cheung IY, Kushner BH, et al. Murine anti-GD2 monoclonal antibody 3F8 combined with granulocyte-macrophage colony-stimulating factor and 13-cis-retinoic acid in high-risk patients with stage 4 neuroblastoma in first remission. J Clin Oncol. 2012;30:3264–70.

121. Benson DM Jr, Bakan CE, Mishra A, et al. The PD-1/PD-L1 axis modulates the natural killer cell versus multiple myeloma effect: a therapeutic target for CT-011, a novel monoclonal anti-PD-1 antibody. Blood. 2010;116:2286–94.
122. Contardi E, Palmisano GL, Tazzari PL, et al. CTLA-4 is constitutively expressed on tumor cells and can trigger apoptosis upon ligand interaction. Int J Cancer. 2005;117:538–50.
123. Pistillo MP, Tazzari PL, Palmisano GL, et al. CTLA-4 is not restricted to the lymphoid cell lineage and can function as a target molecule for apoptosis induction of leukemic cells. Blood. 2003;101:202–9.
124. Jie HB, Schuler PJ, Lee SC, et al. CTLA-4(+) regulatory T cells increased in cetuximab-treated head and neck cancer patients suppress NK cell cytotoxicity and correlate with poor prognosis. Cancer Res. 2015;75:2200–10.
125. Romano E, Kusio-Kobialka M, Foukas PG, et al. Ipilimumab-dependent cell-mediated cytotoxicity of regulatory T cells ex vivo by nonclassical monocytes in melanoma patients. Proc Natl Acad Sci U S A. 2015;112:6140–5.
126. Simpson TR, Li F, Montalvo-Ortiz W, et al. Fc-dependent depletion of tumor-infiltrating regulatory T cells co-defines the efficacy of anti-CTLA-4 therapy against melanoma. J Exp Med. 2013;210:1695–710.
127. Laurent S, Queirolo P, Boero S, et al. The engagement of CTLA-4 on primary melanoma cell lines induces antibody-dependent cellular cytotoxicity and TNF-alpha production. J Transl Med. 2013;11:108.
128. Merchant MS, Wright M, Baird K, et al. Phase I clinical trial of ipilimumab in pediatric patients with advanced solid tumors. Clin Cancer Res. 2016;22:1364–70.
129. Ferrara C, Grau S, Jager C, et al. Unique carbohydrate-carbohydrate interactions are required for high affinity binding between FcgammaRIII and antibodies lacking core fucose. Proc Natl Acad Sci U S A. 2011;108:12669–74.
130. Forthal DN, Gach JS, Landucci G, et al. Fc-glycosylation influences Fcgamma receptor binding and cell-mediated anti-HIV activity of monoclonal antibody 2G12. J Immunol. 2010;185:6876–82.
131. Ayello J, Berg S, Krailo M, van de Ven C, Ingle A, Lewis D, Harrison L, Blaney S, Adamson P, Cairo M. Lenalidomide significantly enhances circulating serum levels of IL-2 and IL-15 levels, NK expansion and activation and NK and LAK cytotoxicity in children with refractory/recurrent solid tumors: a Children's Oncology Group phase I consoritium report. Blood. 2008;122:3068.
132. Lazar GA, Dang W, Karki S, et al. Engineered antibody Fc variants with enhanced effector function. Proc Natl Acad Sci U S A. 2006;103:4005–10.
133. Loo D, Alderson RF, Chen FZ, et al. Development of an Fc-enhanced anti-B7-H3 monoclonal antibody with potent antitumor activity. Clin Cancer Res. 2012;18:3834–45.
134. Casorati G, de Lalla C, Dellabona P. Invariant natural killer T cells reconstitution and the control of leukemia relapse in pediatric haploidentical hematopoietic stem cell transplantation. Oncoimmunology. 2012;1:355–7.
135. Gumperz JE, Miyake S, Yamamura T, Brenner MB. Functionally distinct subsets of CD1d-restricted natural killer T cells revealed by CD1d tetramer staining. J Exp Med. 2002;195:625–36.
136. Wilcox RA, Tamada K, Strome SE, Chen L. Signaling through NK cell-associated CD137 promotes both helper function for CD8+ cytolytic T cells and responsiveness to IL-2 but not cytolytic activity. J Immunol. 2002;169:4230–6.
137. Melero I, Shuford WW, Newby SA, et al. Monoclonal antibodies against the 4-1BB T-cell activation molecule eradicate established tumors. Nat Med. 1997;3:682–5.
138. Melero I, Johnston JV, Shufford WW, Mittler RS, Chen L. NK1.1 cells express 4-1BB (CDw137) costimulatory molecule and are required for tumor immunity elicited by anti-4-1BB monoclonal antibodies. Cell Immunol. 1998;190:167–72.
139. Kohrt HE, Houot R, Goldstein MJ, et al. CD137 stimulation enhances the antilymphoma activity of anti-CD20 antibodies. Blood. 2011;117:2423–32.
140. Kohrt HE, Houot R, Weiskopf K, et al. Stimulation of natural killer cells with a CD137-specific antibody enhances trastuzumab efficacy in xenotransplant models of breast cancer. J Clin Invest. 2012;122:1066–75.

141. Kohrt HE, Colevas AD, Houot R, et al. Targeting CD137 enhances the efficacy of cetuximab. J Clin Invest. 2014;124:2668–82.
142. Benson DM Jr, Bakan CE, Zhang S, et al. IPH2101, a novel anti-inhibitory KIR antibody, and lenalidomide combine to enhance the natural killer cell versus multiple myeloma effect. Blood. 2011;118:6387–91.
143. Romagne F, Andre P, Spee P, et al. Preclinical characterization of 1-7F9, a novel human anti-KIR receptor therapeutic antibody that augments natural killer-mediated killing of tumor cells. Blood. 2009;114:2667–77.
144. Sola C, Andre P, Lemmers C, et al. Genetic and antibody-mediated reprogramming of natural killer cell missing-self recognition in vivo. Proc Natl Acad Sci U S A. 2009;106:12879–84.
145. Binyamin L, Alpaugh RK, Hughes TL, Lutz CT, Campbell KS, Weiner LM. Blocking NK cell inhibitory self-recognition promotes antibody-dependent cellular cytotoxicity in a model of anti-lymphoma therapy. J Immunol. 2008;180:6392–401.
146. Sola C, Chanuc F, Thielens A, Fuseri N, Morel Y, Blery M, Andre P, Vivier E, Graziano R, Romagne F, Bonnafous C. Anti-tumoral efficacy of therapeutic human anti-KIR antibody (Lirilumab/BMS-986015/IPH2102) in a preclinical xenograft tumor model. J Immunother. Cancer. 2013;1(Suppl 1):P40.
147. Vey N, Bourhis JH, Boissel N, et al. A phase 1 trial of the anti-inhibitory KIR mAb IPH2101 for AML in complete remission. Blood. 2012;120:4317–23.
148. Germain C, Larbouret C, Cesson V, et al. MHC class I-related chain A conjugated to antitumor antibodies can sensitize tumor cells to specific lysis by natural killer cells. Clin Cancer Res. 2005;11:7516–22.
149. von Strandmann EP, Hansen HP, Reiners KS, et al. A novel bispecific protein (ULBP2-BB4) targeting the NKG2D receptor on natural killer (NK) cells and CD138 activates NK cells and has potent antitumor activity against human multiple myeloma in vitro and in vivo. Blood. 2006;107:1955–62.
150. Buhtoiarov IN, Neal ZC, Gan J, et al. Differential internalization of hu14.18-IL2 immunocytokine by NK and tumor cell: impact on conjugation, cytotoxicity, and targeting. J Leukoc Biol. 2011;89:625–38.
151. Lode HN, Xiang R, Dreier T, Varki NM, Gillies SD, Reisfeld RA. Natural killer cell-mediated eradication of neuroblastoma metastases to bone marrow by targeted interleukin-2 therapy. Blood. 1998;91:1706–15.
152. Osenga KL, Hank JA, Albertini MR, et al. A phase I clinical trial of the hu14.18-IL2 (EMD 273063) as a treatment for children with refractory or recurrent neuroblastoma and melanoma: a study of the Children's Oncology Group. Clin Cancer Res. 2006;12:1750–9.
153. Shusterman S, London WB, Gillies SD, et al. Antitumor activity of hu14.18-IL2 in patients with relapsed/refractory neuroblastoma: a Children's Oncology Group (COG) phase II study. J Clin Oncol. 2010;28:4969–75.
154. Shusterman S, London WB, Hank JA, Parisi MT, Shulkin BL, Servases S, Naranjo A, Shimada H, Gan J, Gillies SD, Maris JM, Park JR, Sondel PM. A feasibility and phase II study of the hu14.18-IL2 immunocytokine in combination with GM-CSF and isotretinoin in patients with recurrent or refractory neuroblastoma: a Children's Oncology Group Study. Pediatric Oncol. 2015;33(15):10017.
155. Gleason MK, Verneris MR, Todhunter DA, et al. Bispecific and trispecific killer cell engagers directly activate human NK cells through CD16 signaling and induce cytotoxicity and cytokine production. Mol Cancer Ther. 2012;11:2674–84.
156. Miller JS, Felice M, McElmurry R, McCullar V, Zhou X, Tolar J, Schmohl J, Panoskaltsis-Mortari A, Zhang B, Taras E, Verneris M, Cooley S, Weisdorf D, Blazar B, Vallera D. Trispecific Killer Engagers (TriKEs) that contain IL-15 to make NK cells antigen specific and to sustain their persistence and expansion. Blood. 2015;22:83158.
157. Curti A, Ruggeri L, D'Addio A, et al. Successful transfer of alloreactive haploidentical KIR ligand-mismatched natural killer cells after infusion in elderly high risk acute myeloid leukemia patients. Blood. 2011;118:3273–9.
158. Geller MA, Cooley S, Judson PL, et al. A phase II study of allogeneic natural killer cell therapy to treat patients with recurrent ovarian and breast cancer. Cytotherapy. 2011;13:98–107.

159. Brehm C, Huenecke S, Quaiser A, et al. IL-2 stimulated but not unstimulated NK cells induce selective disappearance of peripheral blood cells: concomitant results to a phase I/II study. PLoS One. 2011;6:e27351.
160. Passweg JR, Tichelli A, Meyer-Monard S, et al. Purified donor NK-lymphocyte infusion to consolidate engraftment after haploidentical stem cell transplantation. Leukemia. 2004;18:1835–8.
161. Rizzieri DA, Dev P, Long GD, et al. Response and toxicity of donor lymphocyte infusions following T-cell depleted non-myeloablative allogeneic hematopoietic SCT from 3-6/6 HLA matched donors. Bone Marrow Transplant. 2009;43:327–33.
162. Shaffer BC, Le Luduec JB, Forlenza C, et al. Phase II study of haploidentical natural killer cell infusion for treatment of relapsed or persistent myeloid malignancies following allogeneic hematopoietic cell transplantation. Biol Blood Marrow Transplant. 2016;22:705–9.
163. Stern M, Passweg JR, Meyer-Monard S, et al. Pre-emptive immunotherapy with purified natural killer cells after haploidentical SCT: a prospective phase II study in two centers. Bone Marrow Transplant. 2013;48:433–8.
164. Yoon SR, Lee YS, Yang SH, et al. Generation of donor natural killer cells from CD34(+) progenitor cells and subsequent infusion after HLA-mismatched allogeneic hematopoietic cell transplantation: a feasibility study. Bone Marrow Transplant. 2010;45:1038–46.
165. Choi I, Yoon SR, Park SY, et al. Donor-derived natural killer cells infused after human leukocyte antigen-haploidentical hematopoietic cell transplantation: a dose-escalation study. Biol Blood Marrow Transplant. 2014;20:696–704.
166. Shah NN, Baird K, Delbrook CP, et al. Acute GVHD in patients receiving IL-15/4-1BBL activated NK cells following T-cell-depleted stem cell transplantation. Blood. 2015;125:784–92.
167. Arai S, Meagher R, Swearingen M, et al. Infusion of the allogeneic cell line NK-92 in patients with advanced renal cell cancer or melanoma: a phase I trial. Cytotherapy. 2008;10:625–32.
168. Altvater B, Landmeier S, Pscherer S, et al. 2B4 (CD244) signaling by recombinant antigen-specific chimeric receptors costimulates natural killer cell activation to leukemia and neuroblastoma cells. Clin Cancer Res. 2009;15:4857–66.
169. Tonn T, Schwabe D, Klingemann HG, et al. Treatment of patients with advanced cancer with the natural killer cell line NK-92. Cytotherapy. 2013;15:1563–158.
170. Alsamah W, Romia Y. Modification of natural killer cells to target tumors. Int J Pharm Clin Res. 2014;6:97–100.
171. Chang YH, Connolly J, Shimasaki N, Mimura K, Kono K, Campana D. A chimeric receptor with NKG2D specificity enhances natural killer cell activation and killing of tumor cells. Cancer Res. 2013;73:1777–86.
172. Chu Y, Ayello J, Lo L, Katz J, Yahr A, et al Expanded natural killer (NK) cells transfected with anti-CD20 chimeric antigen receptor (CAR) mRNA have significant cytotoxicity against poor risk B-Cell (CD20+) leukemia/lymphoma (B-L/L). Blood. 2012;120:abstr. 3007.
173. Imai C, Iwamoto S, Campana D. Genetic modification of primary natural killer cells overcomes inhibitory signals and induces specific killing of leukemic cells. Blood. 2005;106:376–83.
174. Kruschinski A, Moosmann A, Poschke I, et al. Engineering antigen-specific primary human NK cells against HER-2 positive carcinomas. Proc Natl Acad Sci U S A. 2008;105:17481–6.
175. Li L, Liu LN, Feller S, et al. Expression of chimeric antigen receptors in natural killer cells with a regulatory-compliant non-viral method. Cancer Gene Ther. 2010;17:147–54.
176. Ni Z, Knorr DA, Bendzick L, Allred J, Kaufman DS. Expression of chimeric receptor CD4zeta by natural killer cells derived from human pluripotent stem cells improves in vitro activity but does not enhance suppression of HIV infection in vivo. Stem Cells. 2014;32:1021–31.
177. Boissel L, Betancur M, Lu W, et al. Comparison of mRNA and lentiviral based transfection of natural killer cells with chimeric antigen receptors recognizing lymphoid antigens. Leuk Lymphoma. 2012;53:958–65.
178. Boissel L, Betancur M, Wels WS, Tuncer H, Klingemann H. Transfection with mRNA for CD19 specific chimeric antigen receptor restores NK cell mediated killing of CLL cells. Leuk Res. 2009;33:1255–9.
179. Boissel L, Betancur-Boissel M, Lu W, et al. Retargeting NK-92 cells by means of CD19- and CD20-specific chimeric antigen receptors compares favorably with antibody-dependent cellular cytotoxicity. Oncoimmunology. 2013;2:e26527.

180. Chu J, Deng Y, Benson DM, et al. CS1-specific chimeric antigen receptor (CAR)-engineered natural killer cells enhance in vitro and in vivo antitumor activity against human multiple myeloma. Leukemia. 2014;28:917–27.
181. Esser R, Muller T, Stefes D, et al. NK cells engineered to express a GD2 -specific antigen receptor display built-in ADCC-like activity against tumour cells of neuroectodermal origin. J Cell Mol Med. 2012;16:569–81.
182. Jiang H, Zhang W, Shang P, et al. Transfection of chimeric anti-CD138 gene enhances natural killer cell activation and killing of multiple myeloma cells. Mol Oncol. 2014;8:297–310.
183. Liu H, Yang B, Sun T, et al. Specific growth inhibition of ErbB2expressing human breast cancer cells by genetically modified NK92 cells. Oncol Rep. 2015;33:95–102.
184. Muller T, Uherek C, Maki G, et al. Expression of a CD20-specific chimeric antigen receptor enhances cytotoxic activity of NK cells and overcomes NK-resistance of lymphoma and leukemia cells. Cancer Immunol Immunother. 2008;57:411–23.
185. Sahm C, Schonfeld K, Wels WS. Expression of IL-15 in NK cells results in rapid enrichment and selective cytotoxicity of gene-modified effectors that carry a tumor-specific antigen receptor. Cancer Immunol Immunother. 2012;61:1451–61.
186. Schonfeld K, Sahm C, Zhang C, et al. Selective inhibition of tumor growth by clonal NK cells expressing an ErbB2/HER2-specific chimeric antigen receptor. Mol Ther. 2015;23:330–8.
187. Tassev DV, Cheng M, Cheung NK. Retargeting NK92 cells using an HLA-A2-restricted, EBNA3C-specific chimeric antigen receptor. Cancer Gene Ther. 2012;19:84–100.
188. Topfer K, Cartellieri M, Michen S, et al. DAP12-based activating chimeric antigen receptor for NK cell tumor immunotherapy. J Immunol. 2015;194:3201–12.
189. Uherek C, Tonn T, Uherek B, et al. Retargeting of natural killer-cell cytolytic activity to ErbB2-expressing cancer cells results in efficient and selective tumor cell destruction. Blood. 2002;100:1265–73.
190. Zhang G, Liu R, Zhu X, et al. Retargeting NK-92 for anti-melanoma activity by a TCR-like single-domain antibody. Immunol Cell Biol. 2013;91:615–24.
191. Konstantinidis KV, Alici E, Aints A, Christensson B, Ljunggren HG, Dilber MS. Targeting IL-2 to the endoplasmic reticulum confines autocrine growth stimulation to NK-92 cells. Exp Hematol. 2005;33:159–64.
192. Nagashima S, Mailliard R, Kashii Y, et al. Stable transduction of the interleukin-2 gene into human natural killer cell lines and their phenotypic and functional characterization in vitro and in vivo. Blood. 1998;91:3850–61.
193. Imamura M, Shook D, Kamiya T, et al. Autonomous growth and increased cytotoxicity of natural killer cells expressing membrane-bound interleukin-15. Blood. 2014;124:1081–8.
194. Carlsten M, Li L, Su S, Berg M, Reger R, Peshwa M, Childs R. Clinical-grade mRNA electroporation of NK cells: a novel and highly efficient method to genetically reprogram human NK cells for cancer immunotherapy. Blood. 2014;124:2153.
195. Furutani E, Su S, Smith A, Berg M, Childs R (2010). siRNA inactivation of the inhibitory receptor NKG2Azz augments the anti-tumor effects of adoptively transferred NK cells in tumor-bearing hosts. ASH Annual Meeting Abstracts: Orlando.
196. Figueiredo C, Seltsam A, Blasczyk R. Permanent silencing of NKG2A expression for cell-based therapeutics. J Mol Med (Berl). 2009;87:199–210.
197. Kawano T, Nakayama T, Kamada N, et al. Antitumor cytotoxicity mediated by ligand-activated human V alpha24 NKT cells. Cancer Res. 1999;59:5102–5.
198. Nieda M, Nicol A, Koezuka Y, et al. TRAIL expression by activated human CD4(+)V alpha 24NKT cells induces in vitro and in vivo apoptosis of human acute myeloid leukemia cells. Blood. 2001;97:2067–74.
199. Lee YJ, Holzapfel KL, Zhu J, Jameson SC, Hogquist KA. Steady-state production of IL-4 modulates immunity in mouse strains and is determined by lineage diversity of iNKT cells. Nat Immunol. 2013;14:1146–54.
200. Moreira-Teixeira L, Resende M, Devergne O, et al. Rapamycin combined with TGF-beta converts human invariant NKT cells into suppressive Foxp3+ regulatory cells. J Immunol. 2012;188:624–31.

201. Dhodapkar MV, Geller MD, Chang DH, et al. A reversible defect in natural killer T cell function characterizes the progression of premalignant to malignant multiple myeloma. J Exp Med. 2003;197:1667–76.
202. Fais F, Morabito F, Stelitano C, et al. CD1d is expressed on B-chronic lymphocytic leukemia cells and mediates alpha-galactosylceramide presentation to natural killer T lymphocytes. Int J Cancer. 2004;109:402–11.
203. Fais F, Tenca C, Cimino G, et al. CD1d expression on B-precursor acute lymphoblastic leukemia subsets with poor prognosis. Leukemia. 2005;19:551–6.
204. Metelitsa LS, Weinberg KI, Emanuel PD, Seeger RC. Expression of CD1d by myelomonocytic leukemias provides a target for cytotoxic NKT cells. Leukemia. 2003;17:1068–77.
205. Renukaradhya GJ, Khan MA, Vieira M, Du W, Gervay-Hague J, Brutkiewicz RR. Type I NKT cells protect (and type II NKT cells suppress) the host's innate antitumor immune response to a B-cell lymphoma. Blood. 2008;111:5637–45.
206. Xu C, de Vries R, Visser L, et al. Expression of CD1d and presence of invariant NKT cells in classical Hodgkin lymphoma. Am J Hematol. 2010;85:539–41.
207. Chong TW, Goh FY, Sim MY, et al. CD1d expression in renal cell carcinoma is associated with higher relapse rates, poorer cancer-specific and overall survival. J Clin Pathol. 2015;68:200–5.
208. Hix LM, Shi YH, Brutkiewicz RR, Stein PL, Wang CR, Zhang M. CD1d-expressing breast cancer cells modulate NKT cell-mediated antitumor immunity in a murine model of breast cancer metastasis. PLoS One. 2011;6:e20702.
209. Nowak M, Arredouani MS, Tun-Kyi A, et al. Defective NKT cell activation by CD1d+ TRAMP prostate tumor cells is corrected by interleukin-12 with alpha-galactosylceramide. PLoS One. 2010;5:e11311.
210. Tahir SM, Cheng O, Shaulov A, et al. Loss of IFN-gamma production by invariant NK T cells in advanced cancer. J Immunol. 2001;167:4046–50.
211. Fallarini S, Paoletti T, Orsi Battaglini N, Lombardi G. Invariant NKT cells increase drug-induced osteosarcoma cell death. Br J Pharmacol. 2012;167:1533–49.
212. Metelitsa LS. Anti-tumor potential of type-I NKT cells against CD1d-positive and CD1d-negative tumors in humans. Clin Immunol. 2011;140:119–29.
213. Song L, Asgharzadeh S, Salo J, et al. Valpha24-invariant NKT cells mediate antitumor activity via killing of tumor-associated macrophages. J Clin Invest. 2009;119:1524–36.
214. Chen YH, Chiu NM, Mandal M, Wang N, Wang CR. Impaired NK1+ T cell development and early IL-4 production in CD1-deficient mice. Immunity. 1997;6:459–67.
215. Giaccone G, Punt CJ, Ando Y, et al. A phase I study of the natural killer T-cell ligand alpha-galactosylceramide (KRN7000) in patients with solid tumors. Clin Cancer Res. 2002;8:3702–9.
216. Molling JW, Kolgen W, van der Vliet HJ, et al. Peripheral blood IFN-gamma-secreting Valpha24+Vbeta11+ NKT cell numbers are decreased in cancer patients independent of tumor type or tumor load. Int J Cancer. 2005;116:87–93.
217. Molling JW, Langius JA, Langendijk JA, et al. Low levels of circulating invariant natural killer T cells predict poor clinical outcome in patients with head and neck squamous cell carcinoma. J Clin Oncol. 2007;25:862–8.
218. Najera Chuc AE, Cervantes LA, Retiguin FP, Ojeda JV, Maldonado ER. Low number of invariant NKT cells is associated with poor survival in acute myeloid leukemia. J Cancer Res Clin Oncol. 2012;138:1427–32.
219. Tachibana T, Onodera H, Tsuruyama T, et al. Increased intratumor Valpha24-positive natural killer T cells: a prognostic factor for primary colorectal carcinomas. Clin Cancer Res. 2005;11:7322–7.
220. de Lalla C, Rinaldi A, Montagna D, et al. Invariant NKT cell reconstitution in pediatric leukemia patients given HLA-haploidentical stem cell transplantation defines distinct CD4+ and CD4- subset dynamics and correlates with remission state. J Immunol. 2011;186:4490–9.
221. Lee PT, Benlagha K, Teyton L, Bendelac A. Distinct functional lineages of human V(alpha)24 natural killer T cells. J Exp Med. 2002;195:637–41.

222. Montoya CJ, Pollard D, Martinson J, et al. Characterization of human invariant natural killer T subsets in health and disease using a novel invariant natural killer T cell-clonotypic monoclonal antibody, 6B11. Immunology. 2007;122:1–14.
223. Swann JB, Uldrich AP, van Dommelen S, et al. Type I natural killer T cells suppress tumors caused by p53 loss in mice. Blood. 2009;113:6382–5.
224. Crowe NY, Smyth MJ, Godfrey DI. A critical role for natural killer T cells in immunosurveillance of methylcholanthrene-induced sarcomas. J Exp Med. 2002;196:119–27.
225. Ambrosino E, Terabe M, Halder RC, et al. Cross-regulation between type I and type II NKT cells in regulating tumor immunity: a new immunoregulatory axis. J Immunol. 2007;179:5126–36.
226. Hayakawa Y, Rovero S, Forni G, Smyth MJ. Alpha-galactosylceramide (KRN7000) suppression of chemical- and oncogene-dependent carcinogenesis. Proc Natl Acad Sci U S A. 2003;100:9464–9.
227. Kawano T, Cui J, Koezuka Y, et al. Natural killer-like nonspecific tumor cell lysis mediated by specific ligand-activated Valpha14 NKT cells. Proc Natl Acad Sci U S A. 1998;95:5690–3.
228. Kobayashi E, Motoki K, Uchida T, Fukushima H, Koezuka Y. KRN7000, a novel immunomodulator, and its antitumor activities. Oncol Res. 1995;7:529–34.
229. Morita M, Motoki K, Akimoto K, et al. Structure-activity relationship of alpha-galactosylceramides against B16-bearing mice. J Med Chem. 1995;38:2176–87.
230. Parekh VV, Wilson MT, Olivares-Villagomez D, et al. Glycolipid antigen induces long-term natural killer T cell anergy in mice. J Clin Invest. 2005;115:2572–83.
231. Swann JB, Coquet JM, Smyth MJ, Godfrey DI. CD1-restricted T cells and tumor immunity. Curr Top Microbiol Immunol. 2007;314:293–323.
232. Hayakawa Y, Takeda K, Yagita H, et al. Critical contribution of IFN-gamma and NK cells, but not perforin-mediated cytotoxicity, to anti-metastatic effect of alpha-galactosylceramide. Eur J Immunol. 2001;31:1720–7.
233. Nakagawa R, Nagafune I, Tazunoki Y, et al. Mechanisms of the antimetastatic effect in the liver and of the hepatocyte injury induced by alpha-galactosylceramide in mice. J Immunol. 2001;166:6578–84.
234. Smyth MJ, Crowe NY, Pellicci DG, et al. Sequential production of interferon-gamma by NK1.1(+) T cells and natural killer cells is essential for the antimetastatic effect of alpha-galactosylceramide. Blood. 2002;99:1259–66.
235. Shimizu K, Goto A, Fukui M, Taniguchi M, Fujii S. Tumor cells loaded with alpha-galactosylceramide induce innate NKT and NK cell-dependent resistance to tumor implantation in mice. J Immunol. 2007;178:2853–61.
236. Chang YJ, Huang JR, Tsai YC, et al. Potent immune-modulating and anticancer effects of NKT cell stimulatory glycolipids. Proc Natl Acad Sci U S A. 2007;104:10299–304.
237. Huang JR, Tsai YC, Chang YJ, et al. alpha-Galactosylceramide but not phenyl-glycolipids induced NKT cell anergy and IL-33-mediated myeloid-derived suppressor cell accumulation via upregulation of egr2/3. J Immunol. 2014;192:1972–81.
238. O'Konek JJ, Illarionov P, Khursigara DS, et al. Mouse and human iNKT cell agonist beta-mannosylceramide reveals a distinct mechanism of tumor immunity. J Clin Invest. 2011;121:683–94.
239. Aspeslagh S, Li Y, Yu ED, et al. Galactose-modified iNKT cell agonists stabilized by an induced fit of CD1d prevent tumour metastasis. EMBO J. 2011;30:2294–305.
240. Carreno LJ, Saavedra-Avila NA, Porcelli SA. Synthetic glycolipid activators of natural killer T cells as immunotherapeutic agents. Clin Transl Immunology. 2016;5:e69.
241. Schmieg J, Yang G, Franck RW, Tsuji M. Superior protection against malaria and melanoma metastases by a C-glycoside analogue of the natural killer T cell ligand alpha-Galactosylceramide. J Exp Med. 2003;198:1631–41.
242. Wu TN, Lin KH, Chang YJ, et al. Avidity of CD1d-ligand-receptor ternary complex contributes to T-helper 1 (Th1) polarization and anticancer efficacy. Proc Natl Acad Sci U S A. 2011;108:17275–80.

243. Schneiders FL, Scheper RJ, von Blomberg BM, et al. Clinical experience with alpha-galactosylceramide (KRN7000) in patients with advanced cancer and chronic hepatitis B/C infection. Clin Immunol. 2011;140:130–41.
244. Ishikawa A, Motohashi S, Ishikawa E, et al. A phase I study of alpha-galactosylceramide (KRN7000)-pulsed dendritic cells in patients with advanced and recurrent non-small cell lung cancer. Clin Cancer Res. 2005;11:1910–7.
245. Parekh VV, Lalani S, Kim S, et al. PD-1/PD-L blockade prevents anergy induction and enhances the anti-tumor activities of glycolipid-activated invariant NKT cells. J Immunol. 2009;182:2816–26.
246. Uldrich AP, Crowe NY, Kyparissoudis K, et al. NKT cell stimulation with glycolipid antigen in vivo: costimulation-dependent expansion, Bim-dependent contraction, and hyporesponsiveness to further antigenic challenge. J Immunol. 2005;175:3092–101.
247. Chang DH, Osman K, Connolly J, et al. Sustained expansion of NKT cells and antigen-specific T cells after injection of alpha-galactosyl-ceramide loaded mature dendritic cells in cancer patients. J Exp Med. 2005;201:1503–17.
248. Nieda M, Okai M, Tazbirkova A, et al. Therapeutic activation of Valpha24+Vbeta11+ NKT cells in human subjects results in highly coordinated secondary activation of acquired and innate immunity. Blood. 2004;103:383–9.
249. Motohashi S, Ishikawa A, Ishikawa E, et al. A phase I study of in vitro expanded natural killer T cells in patients with advanced and recurrent non-small cell lung cancer. Clin Cancer Res. 2006;12:6079–86.
250. Heczey A, Liu D, Tian G, et al. Invariant NKT cells with chimeric antigen receptor provide a novel platform for safe and effective cancer immunotherapy. Blood. 2014;124:2824–33.

Chapter 10
Cancer Vaccines in Pediatrics

Miho Nakajima and Shakeel Modak

Abstract Cancer vaccines are antigen-specific biological agents that stimulate the immune system's ability to fight malignancy. In children, cancer vaccines have the potential for far-reaching benefits while avoiding short and long-term toxicities associated with chemotherapy and radiotherapy. However, obstacles to their use in pediatrics include a paucity of tumor-specific antigens, severe chemotherapy-related immunosuppression, and relatively little interest in the pharmaceutical industry to devote major resources to develop immunotherapies for rare malignancies. Cancer vaccines seek to recruit a sustained cellular immune response against tumor antigens. This requires activation of CD4+ and CD8+ T-cells; in addition NK cell involvement is probably significant. In children with neuroblastoma the early success of a humoral vaccine suggests that B-cell responses are also important. In this chapter we focus on the current status of pediatric cancer vaccines with an emphasis on current and completed clinical trials, and on approaches that might inform future directions in their use.

Keywords Cancer vaccines • Pediatrics • Neuroblastoma • Active immunity

10.1 Introduction

Cancer vaccines are antigen-specific biological agents that stimulate the immune system's ability to fight malignancy. As opposed to passive immunotherapy that is mediated by antibodies or infused immune cells, cancer vaccines are a form of active immunotherapy. Vaccines against infectious agents such as human papillomavirus [1] and hepatitis B [2], when administered to children or young adults, have been proven to prevent adult-onset infection-associated cervical and liver carcinomas respectively. However, in the therapeutic setting, cancer vaccines have yet to achieve their full potential as illustrated by the fact that thus far, only one vaccine [3] has been approved by the Food and Drug Administration (FDA) of the United States for cancer therapy compared to several dozen anti-cancer antibodies. In children, effective

M. Nakajima, M.D. • S. Modak, M.D., M.R.C.P. (✉)
Department of Pediatrics, Memorial Sloan Kettering Cancer Center, 1275 York Avenue,
New York, NY 10065, USA
e-mail: modaks@mskcc.org

J.C. Gray, A. Marabelle (eds.), *Immunotherapy for Pediatric Malignancies*,
https://doi.org/10.1007/978-3-319-43486-5_10

anti-cancer immunotherapy in general, and cancer vaccines in particular, has the potential for far-reaching benefits while avoiding the short and long-term toxicities associated with chemotherapy, radiotherapy, or even toxicities related to other immunotherapies such as graft versus host disease (GVHD) following allogeneic bone marrow transplant. Most cancer vaccines seek to recruit a sustained cellular immune response against tumor antigens. This cellular immune response requires activation of CD4+ and CD8+ T-cells; in addition NK cell involvement is likely to be important. In children with neuroblastoma the early success of a humoral vaccine against neuroblastoma [4] suggests that B-cell responses are at least as important.

Obstacles to the use of cancer vaccines in children are even more significant than in adults: few tumor-specific antigens have been identified in pediatric malignancies; children with high-risk malignancies receive aggressive chemotherapy rendering them severely immunosuppressed and unable to exploit cancer vaccines; and there is relatively little interest in the pharmaceutical industry to devote major resources to develop specific immunotherapies for rare malignancies such as those occurring in children. Recent events in the drug development arena provide some hope for expanding the role of immunotherapy in pediatric oncology: the first FDA approval of a monoclonal antibody specifically targeted against a pediatric tumor (dinutuximab for neuroblastoma) [5] and the contemporaneous introduction of the anti-CD19 immunotherapeutic agents blinatumomab [6] and chimeric antigen receptor transduced T-cells in the treatment of both adults and children [7] with leukemia. In this chapter we will focus on the current status of cancer vaccines in children with an emphasis on current and completed clinical trials (Tables 10.1 and 10.2), and on approaches that might inform future directions in their use.

10.1.1 Tumor Antigens for Cancer Vaccines

Unlike viral antigens, tumor-associated antigens are usually non-mutated self antigens for which T-cell tolerization has resulted in a lack of high affinity T-cells, resulting in suboptimal immunological responses. In adults, the discovery of mutation-associated neoantigens has vastly expanded the pool of antigens that can potentially be used for immunotherapy [8]. Most pediatric malignancies have far fewer genetic mutations thus restricting a strategy aimed at neoantigens [9]. Cancer-testis antigens such as MAGE and NY-ESO-1 [10] and oncofetal antigens such as alpha-fetoprotein (AFP) constitute another category of antigens for cancer vaccines in children. However, these might have low immunogenicity [11]. Immune responses have been difficult to elicit against oncogenic proteins resulting from the chromosomal translocations commonly observed in pediatric sarcomas [12]. None of the current paediatric tumor targets meet the NCI criteria for an "ideal" tumor antigen [13]. In pediatric oncology, the most commonly targeted tumor antigens for immunotherapy are non-mutated antigens, e.g. GD2 for solid tumors [4]. Whole tumor cell vaccines might overcome the limited availability of antigens; however they are fraught with difficulties in standardization.

Table 10.1 Pediatric cancer vaccines using whole tumor cells, peptides, glycolipids and anti-idiotypes: completed and ongoing clinical trials

Antigen	Adjuvant	Disease/s	Clinicaltrials.gov identifier (if available)	Status	Results (if published)
Whole cell vaccines					
Autologous whole cells					
Transfected NB	IL-2	NB	NCT00048386	Completed	[22]
Transfected NB	IL-2 and lymphotactin	NB	NCT00062855	Completed	[24]
Leukemia+ transfected fibroblasts	IL2 and CD40 ligand	Acute leukemia	NCT00058799	Completed	[28]
Transfected sarcoma	GM-CSF	Sarcoma	NCT00258687	Completed	[30]
Transfected sarcoma	GM-CSF and RNAibi-shRNA^{furin}	Sarcoma	NCT01061840	Completed	[31]
Allogeneic whole cells					
Transfected NB cell line	IL-2	NB	NCT00186862	Completed	[37]
Transfected NB cell line	IL-2 and lymphotactin	NB	NCT00703222	Completed	[38]
Transfected NB cell lines	IL-2 and lymphotactin (+ cyclophosphamide)	NB	NCT01192555	Completed	–
Allogeneic tumor lysate	Imiquimod	GBM	NCT01400672	Completed	–
Peptides					
L-MTP-PE	None	OS	NCT00631631	Completed	[51]
EphA2, IL-13Rα2 + survivin	Montanide and poly-ICLC	Glioma	NCT01130077 NCT02358187	Recruiting	[53, 54]
EphA2, IL-13Rα2 + survivin	Imiquimod	Glioma	NCT01795313	Recruiting	–
WT1	Post-allo transplant	Leukemia, lymphoma	NCT00923910	Completed	–
Telomerase	GM-CSF	Sarcoma, brain tumors	NCT00069940	Completed	–

(continued)

Table 10.1 (continued)

Antigen	Adjuvant	Disease/s	Clinicaltrials.gov identifier (if available)	Status	Results (if published)
Patient-specific peptides	HSP gp96	Glioma	NCT02722512	Recruiting	–
Glycolipids					
GD2 and GM3	KLH, OPT-821 and BG	NB	NCT00911560	Recruiting	[97]
Anti-idiotypes					
GD2-mimic A1G4		GD2+ solid tumors	NCT00003023	Completed	–
GD2-mimic 1A7		NB	–	Completed	[103]
GM3-mimic racotumomab		Solid tumors	NCT01598454	Completed	[106]

Abbreviations: *BG* β-D-Glucan, *Bi-shRNA* bifunctional short hairpin RNA, *CD40* cluster of differentiation 40, *EphA2* ephrin type-A receptor 2, *GBM* Glioblastoma multiforme, *GM-CSF* granulocyte macrophage colony-stimulating factor, *HSP Gp96* heat shock protein glucose—regulated protein 96, *IFN* interferon, *IL2* interleukin-2, *IL13Ra2* interleukin-13 receptor subunit alpha-2, *KLH* keyhole limpet hemocyanin, *L-MTP-PE* liposome-encapsulated muramyl tripeptide phosphadylethanolamine, *NB* neuroblastoma, *OS* osteosarcoma, *Poly-ICLC* polyinosinic-polycytidylic acid stabilized with poly-L-lysine and carboxymethylcellulose, *WT1* Wilms' tumor suppressor gene

Table 10.2 DC Vaccines in pediatric oncology: completed and ongoing clinical trials

Antigen/tumor type	Adjuvant	Clinicaltrials.gov identifier if available	Status	Results (if published)
Autologous tumor lysate				
Brain tumors	None	None	Completed	[111]
Glioblastoma	None	NCT00576537	Completed	–
Brain tumors	Imiquimod	NCT01902771	Recruiting	–
Glioblastoma and Brain stem glioma	None	NCT00576641	Completed	–
Glioma	None	NCT00107185	Completed	[111]
Brain tumors and Sarcoma	None	NCT02496520	Recruiting	–
Brain tumors	Imiquimod	NCT01808820	Recruiting	–
Sarcoma	Gemcitabine	NCT01803152	Recruiting	–
Osteosarcoma	KLH	–	Completed	[118]
Non Hodgkins lymphoma	None	NCT00006434	Completed	–
Neuroblastoma	Autotransplant	NCT02745756	Recruiting	–
Solid tumors	Autotransplant	NCT00405327	Completed	[116]
Solid tumors	None	NCT02533895	Completed	–
Solid tumors	Autotransplant+IL7	NCT00923351	Completed	[115]
Solid tumors	KLH, LPS, IFN	–	Completed	[121]
Solid tumors	KLH	–	Completed	[120]
Tumor stem cells				
Brain tumors	None	NCT01171469	Completed	[114]
Peptide				
Cancer testis Antigens				
Neuroblastoma and Sarcoma	Decitabine	NCT01241162	Completed	[10]
Brain tumor	Decitabine	NCT02332889	Terminated	–
Fusion peptides				
Ewing and ARMS	Autotransplant +IL2	NCT00001566	Completed	[12]
Total tumor RNA				
Medulloblastoma	Autotransplant and expanded T cells	NCT01326104	Recruiting	–
Neuroblastoma	Autotransplant	–	Completed	[119]
Brain tumor	None	–	Completed	[113]

Abbreviations: *DC* Dendritic cells, *IFN* Interferon, IL2: Interleukin-2, *IL-7* Interleukin-7, *KLH* Keyhole limpet hemocyanin, *LPS* Lipopolysaccharides

10.1.2 Adjuvants for Cancer Vaccines

Potent adjuvants are critical to the success of tumor vaccines both by enhancing activation of T-helper cells and antigen enhancing cells, and by modulating the immunosuppressive effect of the tumor microenvironment. Some adjuvants serve as or induce damage-associated molecular patterns and/or pathogen-associated molecular patterns that are recognized by receptors on innate immune cells. These pattern recognition receptors (PRR), when activated elicit the activation of a cascade of immune responses that can be directed against the adjuvant-associated tumor antigens. Other adjuvants, by being opsonized or phagocytosed, serve as delivery agents to direct tumor antigens into antigen-presenting cells [14]. Some cancer vaccination approaches incorporate adjuvants within the vaccine, e.g. viral vectors contain numerous PRR ligands [15], and DNA vaccines contain inbuilt PRRs [16]. However, most vaccines require adjuvants for optimal activation of antigen presenting cells. Immunostimulant adjuvants used in pediatric oncology include beta glucan, imiquimod, keyhole limpet hemocyanin (KLH), montanide, the QS-21 analog OPT-21 and cytokines.

10.1.3 Cancer Vaccines in Pediatric Oncology: Other Clinical Considerations

Besides selection of antigen and adjuvants, several other factors can influence the effectiveness of tumor vaccines. Optimal antigen delivery to maximize concentration in antigen presenting cells is critical [17], as is the immunological fitness of the patient. Young children have an immature immune system as a whole having had a relatively short time to build an immune memory response to most antigens. In addition most children with high-risk cancer receive highly immunosuppressive cytotoxic therapies further limiting their ability to utilize vaccines. Many pediatric tumors have low or absent HLA expression thus limiting T-cell recognition and responses. Moreover, vaccines are likely to be effective only in the adjuvant setting and not as monotherapy. Therefore the timing of anti-cancer vaccination is a fundamental consideration; vaccines are likely to elicit responses only after immune reconstitution has taken place after recovery from the effects of conventional lymphosuppressive therapies. Finally, the rarity of pediatric malignancies poses unique obstacles to the conduct of clinical trials, especially since vaccines are unlikely to be effective in the setting of measurable disease. The development of validated biomarkers to measure efficacy in the setting of "minimal disease" is critical to the successful evaluation of vaccines in children. All of the above challenges have yet to be overcome in pediatric oncology and indeed in oncology in general. Nevertheless, recent developments in the use of early phase clinical trials of cancer vaccines in children offer encouragement for considering their wider use.

10.2 Types of Cancer Vaccines

Tumor antigens can be presented by several methods and cancer vaccines can be classified based on the types of platforms that present antigens to the immune system (Tables 10.1 and 10.2).

10.2.1 Whole Tumor Cell Vaccines

By presenting several tumor antigens, vaccines derived from whole tumor cells can potentially overcome issues related to tumor heterogeneity and stimulate a polyclonal T cell response. This property is particularly attractive for pediatric tumors which have a unique antigen repertoire compared to adult malignancies. The first tumor cell vaccines used irradiated tumor cells admixed with non-specific immunostimulants such as Mycobacterium bovis and BCG for recurrent melanoma [18]. Current approaches use autologous or allogeneic tumor cells administered along with adjuvants.

10.2.1.1 Autologous Tumor Cell Vaccines

Autologous tumor cell vaccines, individualized formulations prepared using irradiated autologous tumor cells obtained from the patient, have distinct advantages as therapeutic agents: (a) they could reflect the actual antigen repertoire within the patient's tumors, thus obviating the need to identify tumor antigens, (b) they can present a wide range of tumor antigens in the context of self-major histocompatibility antigens. Disadvantages include: (a) their autologous nature reduces immunogenicity (b) their production is time-consuming and requires large amounts of tumor tissues, and (c) due to the presence of normal self antigens, the development of autoimmunity is a potential concern. In adults, autologous tumor cell derived vaccines, when gene-modified with cytokines such as IL2, IFN-gamma or GM-CSF, or co-stimulatory molecules such as B7-1, elicit a range of immunostimulatory responses in patients including recruitment and maturation of dendritic cells and priming of T-cells [19–21].

Autologous tumor cell vaccines have been tested in several clinical trials in children and young adults. IL2-adenovector-transduced un-irradiated autologous tumor cell vaccines were used to treat ten children with relapsed neuroblastoma in a phase I study in which each patient received up to 10^8 autologous tumor cells which were obtained from disrupted tumor biopsy or bone marrow samples and isolated using immunocytology. A local inflammatory response as well as a systemic immune response was observed with a rise in circulating activated T-cells, a smaller increase in circulating NK cells, development of IgG antitumor antibody and increased cytotoxic T-cell activity specifically against autologous tumor cells. One patient each had complete and partial response. There was a suggestion of correlation of anti-tumor activity with co-existing anti-tumor T-cells [22]. In an attempt to improve responses, based on preclinical data favoring the combination of chemokine and cytokines in T-cell activation [23], the investigators used the adenovirus platform to transfect autologous neuroblastoma cells with IL-2 and lymphotactin, a chemokine that encourages lymphocyte chemotaxis, and performed a phase I study [24]. Adverse events were mild and a local inflammatory response was again observed. Favorable immune responses were observed as measured by ELISPOT assays. However, no clinical anti-tumor responses were noted.

Leukemia cells generally lack costimulatory surface molecules which are crucial for T-cell activation. This T-cell unresponsiveness could be overcome by direct stimulation via the CD40/CD40 ligand (CD40 L) pathway. CD40 is expressed on B-cells and B-cell blasts and its ligand on activated T-cells and antigen presenting cells. CD40/CD40L interactions lead to T-cell-dependent B cell activation, T-cell priming and expression of co-stimulatory molecules by leukemia cells [25–27]. Irradiated autologous leukemia blasts were admixed with separate populations of autologous skin fibroblasts genetically modified to secrete IL2 and CD40L. These were administered subcutaneously to patients (including seven children) with acute lymphoblastic or acute myeloid leukemia in cytological remission. Patients were noted to have increased numbers of circulating CD4+, CD8+ and activated CD3+DR+ lymphocytes. A 10-890 fold increase in leukemia-reactive cytotoxic CD4+ and CD8+ T-cells was also seen. Two patients made antibodies against recipient derived leukemic blasts. Clinical efficacy could not be determined since patients were in remission prior to study entry [28].

GM-CSF-transfected autologous tumor cells have been used to treat adults with various malignancies since the late 1990s [29]. However, only one study has reported on their use in children. In a phase I trial, autologous tumor cells engineered by adenoviral-mediated gene transfer to secrete GM-CSF were used to treat patients, including three children, with metastatic alveolar soft-part and clear cell sarcoma. Although tumor regressions were not seen, vaccination induced dendritic cell infiltration, and stimulated T-cell and antibody responses. Interestingly, tumor biopsies showed PD-1 positive CD8+ T-cells in association with PD-L1-expressing sarcoma cells suggesting that PD-1 blockade might improve the efficacy of vaccine [30].

More complex genetic engineering yielded a vaccine with triple functionality: autologous tumor cells (to present patient-specific tumor antigens), transfected with GM-CSF (for dendritic cell recruitment and activation) and RNAibi-shRNA^{furin} (to block endogenous TGFβ and reverse immune tolerance). This vaccine was used to treat 12 patients (including eight <20 years of age) with Ewing sarcoma. No significant adverse events were noted; tumor-specific responses were observed on ELISPOT and one partial response was noted [31].

10.2.1.2 Allogeneic Tumor Cell Vaccines

Allogeneic tumor cell vaccines use irradiated cancer cell lines known to express specific tumor antigens and have several advantages over autologous tumor cell vaccines: (a) they can be mass produced and standardized using Good Manufacturing Practice processes at a relatively low production cost [32], and (b) protocols to modify and optimize such vaccines can be easily implemented and the product can be used in multiple treating centers. Using antigenically well defined cell lines helps their clinical outcome to be more comparable and analyzable. Disadvantages include: (a) recognition of allo-antigens by the patient could lead to destruction of the injected allogeneic tumor cells or interference with the recognition of vaccine antigens [33], and (b) tumor antigens expressed on allogeneic vaccines might not reflect the antigen repertoire of the patient's tumor [34]. Irradiation can enhance tumor antigen recognition by antigen presenting cells [35], but can also release intracellular immunosuppressive molecules [36].

Patients with high-risk relapsed neuroblastoma were treated with 10^4–10^7 IL2-gene-modified allogeneic cells. An HLA-A1,2 positive cell line derived from a patient with disseminated neuroblastoma transfected with a retroviral vector coding for huIL-2 was used [37]. Although therapy was safe and local inflammatory responses were noted, systemic immune responses were far inferior to those observed with IL-2-transfected autologous neuroblastoma vaccine [22] and no tumor regressions were observed. The investigators concluded that the paucity of systemic immune responses was possibly related to the use of an allogeneic product with different antigen expression from autologous tumor. In contrast, when a composite vaccine consisting of the above IL-2 transfected cell line along with the same cell line transfected (via electroporation) with lymphotactin was administered to children with advanced neuroblastoma, improved systemic immune responses were noted, (i.e. expansion of T-cell, NK cells, eosinophils and increase in serum cytokine levels). 15/21 patients treated made specific IgG antibodies and three patients had objective tumor responses [38]. The chemokine lymphotactin might have contributed to this response; however the two groups of patients were not matched for disease status or prior immunosuppressive therapies. In an effort to increase antigen diversity, the IL-2 and lymphotactin secreting neuroblastoma cell line was combined with a second unmodified neuroblastoma cell line and a phase I/II trial initiated in 2010. Patients with advanced neuroblastoma also received metronomic cyclophosphamide with the objective of suppressing regulatory T-cells (clinicaltrials.gov identifier NCT01192555), but results have not yet been published.

10.2.1.3 Allogeneic Tumor Cell Lysates

For immunotherapy, tumor cell lysates are usually used to pulse antigen-presenting cells ex vivo, however, clinical investigators have used direct injection of tumor lysates [39], though their poor immunogenicity requires combination with immune adjuvants. Such an approach has not been applied in pediatric oncology, however, a clinical trial combining a tumor lysate derived from a glioblastoma cell line in combination with the adjuvant imiquimod is being considered for children with glioma (clinicaltrials.gov identifier NCT01400672).

Overall autologous or allogeneic whole tumor cell vaccines have not been associated with significant toxicities in adults, but clinical benefit has not been proven in phase III studies thus far. Small early phase studies have been performed in pediatric oncology but patients with minimal residual disease who are most likely to benefit have not been studied at all.

10.2.2 Peptide Based Vaccines

Peptide based vaccines are among the most common strategies for to elicit therapeutic immune responses in adults and children. Their use is based on the rationale that neoplastic cells express tumor-associated antigens and peptides derived from these antigens can be immunogenic. Peptide vaccines are almost always administered in conjunction with immune adjuvants in order to elicit an immune response. Short peptides do not require processing by antigen-presenting cells and bind directly to HLA class I molecules to be presented to T-cells. Their activity is therefore MHC class restricted. Furthermore, class I HLA molecules of non-professional APCs might also be bound in the absence of co-stimulatory molecules leading to tolerization [17]. Synthetic long peptides (25–35 amino acids in length) on the other hand require processing in APCs prior to MHC binding allowing a more physiologically appropriate antigen presentation. Longer peptides often harbor both CD4+ and CD8+ epitopes, thus eliciting a more balanced T-helper/suppressor response. Moreover, the use of synthetic long peptides avoids the need for MHC selection [40].

In pediatric oncology, liposomal muramyl-tripeptide-phosphatidylethanolamine (L-MTP-PE; mifamurtide) is the peptide that has undergone the most extensive clinical testing. MTP-PE, a synthetic peptide derived from muramyl dipeptide, a glycan found in bacterial cell walls, activates and enhances function of monocytes and macrophages [41, 42]. MTP-PE was formulated into liposomes leading to improved immune activation and pharmacokinetics [43, 44]. L-MTP-PE was noted to have anti-tumor activity against osteosarcoma in *in vitro* and *in vivo* studies and in dogs developing spontaneous osteosarcoma [45–47]. Early phase studies established the toxicity profile and recommended phase II dose. Adverse events included nausea, chills, myalgia, and malaise and were common, though serious events such as hemorrhagic pericarditis were rare [48, 49]. L-MTP-PE was found to induce fibrosis in osteosarcoma lung metastases in patients [50]. A seminal randomized clinical trial investigated if the addition of ifosfamide and/or L-MTP-PE to standard chemotherapy could improve event-free survival in patients with newly diagnosed non-metastatic osteosarcoma. 662 patients were treated, 348 receiving L-MTP-PE in an adjuvant setting. Patients receiving both ifosfamide and L-MTP-PE had the best outcome with a 3 year-EFS of 78%, but a definitive conclusion of the efficacy of each agent could not be drawn since an interaction was observed between ifosfamide and L-MTP-PE [51]. A follow-up analysis of the study cohorts demonstrated improved 6-year overall survival in patients receiving L-MTP-PE ($p = 0.03$) with a trend towards improved event-free survival ($p = 0.08$) [52]. A possible benefit for patients with metastatic osteosarcoma treated on an open access protocol was also suggested [53]. Currently L-MTP-PE is approved for the treatment of osteosarcoma by the European Medicines Agency, but remains an investigational agent in the United States [54].

Other peptide strategies directed at pediatric malignancies have thus far only been tested in early phase or pilot studies. The peptide epitopes for the glioma-associated antigens EphA2, interleukin-13 receptor alpha2 (IL-13Rα2) and survivin were administered along with two adjuvants, montanide-ISA-151 and polyinosinic-polycytidilic acid stabilized by lysine and carboxymethylcellulose (poly-ICLC), to children with malignant high-grade and low grade gliomas. No major toxicities were encountered. IFN-γ-ELISPOT responses to one or more antigens were observed in most patients, and pseudoprogression followed by partial regressions in a minority of patients [55, 56]. Children with WT1 expressing malignancies including leukemia were treated with a modified WT1 peptide restricted to HLA-A*24:02. Montanide ISA51 was used as an adjuvant [57]. A similar approach was used to immunize children with acute leukemia following allogeneic stem cell transplantation [58]. However, clinical and immune responses were inconsistent.

In general, vaccination with peptides is often associated with immune responses: both humoral and cellular; however, clinical responses are rarely observed and no peptide vaccine has been approved as an anti-cancer treatment [59]. The reasons for poor anticancer activity are multifactorial. Immunoediting by tumor cells results in limited expression of tumor antigens and immunostimulatory signals, the tumor microenvironment is often immunosuppressive, and targeting of single as opposed to multiple epitopes might be ineffective. Malignancies arising in adults are often caused by multiple mutations that result in the emergence of neoantigens which can be presented in the context of HLA molecules. T-cells reactive to neoantigens are unlikely to be subject to immune tolerization and are likely to express high affinity receptors potentially leading to enhanced tumor cell cytotoxicity. HLA-restricted neoantigen-derived peptides ("neoepitopes") are now being tested in adults with advanced cancers [60]. Such an approach has limitations in children due to the paucity of somatic mutations in pediatric malignancies [61].

10.2.3 Viral and Bacterial Vector-Based Vaccines

Viruses and bacteria can serve as vaccines when used as vectors for the delivery of tumor antigens to immune cells. In addition oncolytic viruses have the potential to release tumor antigens that can elicit immune responses. A genetically engineered oncolytic herpes virus engineered to secrete GM-CSF recently received FDA approval for the treatment of melanoma [62]. Bacteria and viruses used as vaccines, albeit attenuated, have complex arrays of antigens that can trigger immunity via multiple pathways. Viral infection often results in expression of MHC-restricted peptides that can enhance the immune response. However, these vectors are strongly immunogenic and can elicit neutralizing antibodies that could preclude boosting. Clinical trials in adults have utilized attenuated organisms with low intrinsic immunogenicity. Viruses tested include pox [63], vaccinia [64], adenovirus [65], and herpes simplex viruses. Bacteria include Listeria monocytogenes [66] and Salmonella typhi [67]. In general, some early phase trials of viral-based vaccines appear to show clinical and immune responses, though pivotal phase III studies have yet to demonstrate a clear benefit. Oncolytic viruses [68] including Pexa-vec [69], a vaccinia virus engineered to secrete GM-CSF have been tested in early phase studies in children with cancer, but viral or bacterial vector-based vaccines have not been yet been tested. Preclinical studies in pediatric cancer models showing promise include using orally administered Salmonella typhimurium as a vector to deliver tumor antigens such as survivin [70] and MYCN [71] against neuroblastoma.

10.2.4 DNA and RNA Vaccines

Once injected, antigen-coding genes inserted into a bacterial plasmid are taken up by host cells, processed and presented as antigen. DNA vaccines can induce both MHC class I and II restricted cellular and humoral immune responses [72]. In addition, plasmids themselves can stimulate innate immune responses via interaction with toll-like receptors and other DNA sensors, thus acting as immune adjuvants [73, 74]. RNA vaccines are processed similarly but the injected mRNA does not require entry into the nucleus, since translation to antigen occurs within the cytoplasm itself [75]. Recent advances in recombinant technology have allowed plasmid genes to be manipulated to produce vaccines for multiple antigens to account for tumor heterogeneity [76], and to enhance their adjuvant effect [77]. Other advantages include ease and economy of production and convenience of administration (intradermal, intramuscular or via gene gun or electroporation) of single or multiple doses [16]. The safety of nucleic acid vaccines has been established in clinical trials in adults with cancer, but their efficacy has been sub-optimal specifically due to low immunogenicity [78, 79]. Anti-tumor DNA and RNA vaccines have not yet been tested in children. Preclinical studies have tested DNA vaccines coding for MYCN [71], tyrosine hydroxylase [80] and survivin [70] for neuroblastoma, and targeted acute lymphoblastic lymphoma with a BCR-ABL DNA vaccine [81]. In addition, DNA vaccines encoding for peptides mimicking GD2, the most common tumor antigen expressed on neuroblastoma, have been tested in mouse models [82].

10.2.5 Glycolipid Vaccines

Multiple types of cancer cells express glycolipids on the cell surface. The ganglioside GD2 has been the main tumor antigen targeted for therapy in high-risk neuroblastoma. GD2 is highly expressed on neuroblastoma cell surface on almost all tumors at diagnosis and relapse and is not immunomodulated off cell surface. In addition GD2 is expressed on a broad range of other solid tumors including osteosarcoma, melanoma and small cell lung cancer. Expression on normal tissues is restricted to nerve cells [83, 84]. GD3 is also expressed on neuroblastoma and other pediatric tumors, though in general at a lower density on cell surface [85, 86]. Other glycolipids such as GM2, GM3, Globo H, Lewis antigens and mucins have been targeted as tumor antigens for cancer immunotherapy in adults [87]. However, glycolipids when used alone have major disadvantages as tumor antigens for use as cancer vaccines. They are not recognized by T cells and yield short-lived, T-independent type II, low-affinity IgM responses which are rarely converted to IgG production. These responses can lead to immune tolerance [88]. To overcome these drawbacks, carbohydrate vaccines must be used in combination with a protein carrier and strong adjuvants. Such an approach can switch immune response to T-dependence and has been successful in developing vaccines against bacterial carbohydrate antigens, initially for Haemophilus influenza type b and subsequently for Streptococcus pneumoniae and Neisseria meningococcus [89]. For gangliosides, conjugation with the carrier molecule KLH was associated with the most robust immune response in mouse models [90].

In the only glycolipid cancer vaccine tested in children, a bivalent anti-GD2 and GD3 vaccine was prepared by conjugating the gangliosides with KLH. Two other immune adjuvants were administered in conjunction: OPT-821 and yeast-derived adjuvant (1 → 3),(1 → 6)-β-D-Glucan (BG). The former is a saponin-derived mixture of two glycosides related to the previously clinically tested adjuvant QS-21 [91, 92]. The latter has been evaluated in large studies in adults with cancer and found to be safe and effective in eliciting immune responses [93]. β-glucans are naturally occurring glucose polymers that have multiple immune stimulant effects. In preclinical studies, β-glucans were shown to potentiate NK cell cytotoxicity, activate macrophages and cytotoxic T cells, enhance antibody responses, induce cytokines and activate complement pathway [94]. In mouse models, both yeast and barley-derived β-glucans synergized with complement-activating antibodies including 3F8 and rituximab for anti-tumor effect [95, 96]. In a phase I clinical trial the anti-tumor activity of barley-derived (1 → 3),(1 → 4)-β-D-Glucan (BG) in combination with 3F8 was demonstrated to be safe and was associated with significant immune responses. Objective tumor responses were observed in 13/22 patients with refractory or relapsed advanced neuroblastoma including BM CR in 33% [97]. The adjuvants OPT-821 and BG were combined with the KLH-conjugated gangliosides GD2 and GD3 and tested in patients with resistant neuroblastoma in a phase I study in which the dose of OPT-821 was escalated. Gangliosides and OPT-821 were injected subcutaneously while BG was administered orally. Treatment was well tolerated with grade 1 local reactions being typical. One patient had transient grade 3 elevation of hepatic enzymes. Neuropathic pain characteristic of anti-GD2 monoclonal antibody therapy was not observed. 12/15 patients developed anti-GD2 and/or anti-GD3 titers. All 15 treated patients received the vaccine in second remission after experiencing relapse: an ultra-high risk population which historically would be expected to have another relapse within 12–24 months. Intriguingly 12/15 patients remain in continued remission with a median follow up of >5 years after completing therapy (Fig. 10.1), although seroconversion did not correlate with survival. Based on these encouraging data, a phase II trial is currently open; eligibility criteria include high-risk neuroblastoma patients in second remission as well as first remission patients who have completed anti-GD2 monoclonal antibody therapy (clinicaltrials.gov identifier NCT00911560) [4].

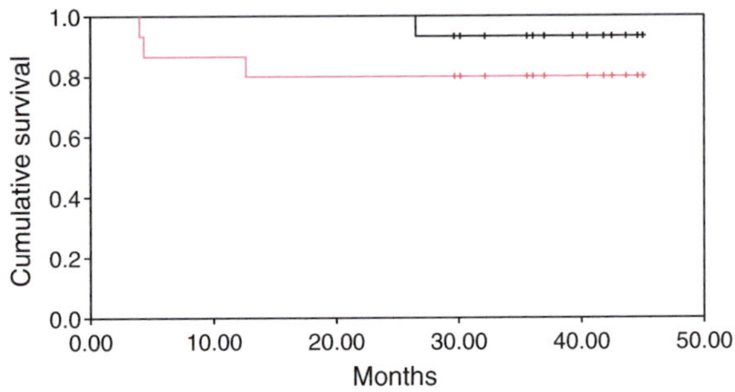

Fig. 10.1 Relapse-free survival (*red*) and overall survival (*black*) in patients receiving bivalent gangliosides vaccine

10.2.6 Anti-idiotype Vaccines

Harnessing the anti-idiotype system has the potential to break the immunotolerance associated with tumor antigen-based vaccines [98, 99]. Patients receiving treatment with monoclonal antibodies can mount an immune response to the latter. A subset of this response is constituted of anti-idiotypic antibodies which can mimic the three dimensional structure of the original antigen and induce the production of anti-anti idiotypic Abs. Such an approach was first shown to be effective in adults with lymphoma treated with individualized anti-idiotypic antibody [100]. In children with neuroblastoma treated with the murine anti-GD2 antibody 3F8, the development of human anti-mouse (HAMA) and anti-anti idiotypic antibodies was associated with a significantly improved progression-free and overall survival while non-idiotypic antibody responses (anti-mouse IgG3 or anti-tumor nuclear HUD antigen) had no impact on survival [101]. The prognostic value of elevated HAMA titers (used as surrogate for anti-anti-idiotype antibodies) was confirmed in a larger study of neuroblastoma patients treated with 3F8 plus GM-CSF in remission [102]. Based on this observation, the rat monoclonal antibody A1G4 raised against 3F8 as a GD2 mimic was used to treat patients with GD2-positive tumors (clinicaltrials.gov NCT00003023). Twenty-four patients were treated on a phase I study. No significant toxicities were observed and several patients remain alive several years after immunization. MAb1A7, a second anti-idiotypic rat antibody mimicking GD2 but derived against the anti-GD2 antibody ch14G2a has also undergone clinical investigation in neuroblastoma. Thirty one patients were treated, all generated anti-1A7 titers, and serum from some exhibited complement-mediated cytotoxicity [103]. A chimeric GD2 mimic ganglidiximab [104] has been characterized pre-clinically. The first report of an anti-idiotype antibody in pediatric oncology was on the GM3 mimic racotumomab. In this phase I study in children, racotumomab was demonstrated to be safe and to elicit IgG and IgM responses in children with solid tumors [105]. Racotumomab improved survival in adults with non-small cell lung cancer [106].

10.2.7 Antigen Presenting Cell Vaccines

Another promising approach is vaccination using antigen-loaded antigen presenting cells such as monocytes, activated B cells and dendritic cells (DCs). DCs are considered to be a nexus of immunity due to their ability to present captured antigen to T cells, capacity to stimulate naïve and memory CD8+ T cells, NK cells, B cells and CD4 helper-T cells efficiently, and their localization at the site of antigen exposure such as skin, lymph nodes and intestinal mucosa. Immature DCs are known to be able to present self or tumor antigen to T cells leading to immune tolerance [107]. DC vaccines can be generated from autologous or allogeneic sources using peripheral blood mononuclear cells, hematopoietic progenitor cells or monocytes. DCs are typically loaded with tumor antigens ex-vivo using whole tumor lysates, peptides or tumor mRNA before injection. Strategies to enhance DC function include *in vitro* maturation using cytokine cocktails and co-administration of adjuvants. Routes of administration include intravenous, intradermal, subcutaneous and intratumoral [108]. Numerous clinical trials of DCs have been carried out for malignancies in adults. Sipuleucel-T, a patient-specific DC vaccine produced by exposing the autologous peripheral blood mononuclear cells to a fusion protein consisting of prostatic acid phosphatase and GM-CSF [109], was approved by the FDA for the treatment of prostate cancer in 2010, and remains the only anti-cancer vaccine with FDA-approval. However, subsequent DC vaccine studies have been disappointing in general [110].

In pediatrics, several high-risk malignancies have been targeted by DC vaccines in small, early phase trials. Children with high-grade gliomas and other brain tumors were treated with DCs pulsed with autologous tumor lysate [111, 112] or autologous whole tumor RNA [113]. These studies demonstrated the feasibility of producing DC vaccines in children and treatment was not associated with major adverse events. No significant clinical or immunological responses were observed. Another novel approach was to pulse autologous DCs with apoptotic bodies derived from an allogeneic brain tumor cell line (GBM6-AD). Apoptotic bodies have been shown to display multiple tumor antigens. Treatment was safe and there was a suggestion of immune response with increased intracellular IL-17a detected in some patients [114].

In the largest published study of DC vaccines in pediatric sarcomas, 29 patients with metastatic or relapsed disease (age range: 6-38 years) received combination immunotherapy consisting of autologous lymphocytes, DCs pulsed with autologous tumor lysate and KLH, and recombinant huIL17 after standard treatment for their malignancy. IFNγ production in response to tumor lysate was noted even prior to immunotherapy, though its frequency increased after immunotherapy, and clinical outcome was superior in patients exhibiting such a response. Delayed hypersensitivity was not observed against tumor lysate. Patient survival appeared to be higher than that in historical controls [115]. A monocyte plus DC vaccine derived from peripheral blood mononuclear cells pulsed with peptides derived from breakpoint regions of fusion proteins was administered to 16 patients with rhabdomyosarcoma and Ewing sarcoma. No significant clinical or immune responses were observed [116]. Marginal clinical and immunological responses were also reported in studies of an autologous tumor lysate and KLH-pulsed DC vaccine in children with relapsed solid tumors [117, 118], and in studies of patients with neuroblastoma [119] and other solid tumors [120] immunized with autologous tumor RNA pulsed DCs administered after autologous bone marrow transplant. In another study, a combination of mature and semi-mature DCs were pulsed with autologous tumor lysates, KLH, lipopolysaccharide and interferon gamma. Children with extracranial tumors receiving this product uniformly mounted a T-cell response to KLH but only a minority responded to the tumor antigen [121]. In an effort to upregulate tumor antigens on cancer cells, children with relapsed/refractory solid tumors were treated with decitabine, a demethylating agent that has been shown to upregulate cancer germline genes, prior to administration of DCs pulsed with overlapping peptides derived from the cancer testis antigens MAGE-A1, MAGE-A3 and NY-ESO-1. Therapy was well tolerated apart from decitabine-related myelosuppression. Six of nine evaluable patients showed T-cell responses to the cancer-testis antigens and one patient had an objective clinical response [10].

WT1 peptide pulsed DCs have shown clinical benefit in adults with AML treated in minimal residual disease state with responses correlating with T-cell and NK cell responses [122]. In an anecdotal report, a 15-year old boy with AML received WT1 peptide pulsed allogeneic DCs generated from a sibling donor. No GVHD was seen, WT1-specific immune responses were detected and the patient maintained a prolonged remission [123].

Efforts to enhance the anti-tumor effect of DC vaccines include manipulating the immunosuppressive tumor microenvironment, identifying more potent DC subsets [124], combination with implantable scaffolds [125] and DC-derived exosomes [126]. Several of these strategies are being tested in adults. The optimal use for DCs, as for all cancer vaccines, is likely to be in the setting of minimal residual disease and/or in combination with other anti-cancer agents.

10.3 Future Directions in Development of Pediatric Cancer Vaccines

Cancer vaccines, more than other forms of immunotherapy, have proven safety both in adults and children. If the potential for efficacy can be realized, children with high-risk cancers can derive profound benefits from a vaccination approach since adverse events related to cytotoxic therapies can be severe and lifelong. Pediatric patients have been enrolled and treated on clinical trials involving most types of cancer vaccines, however, unique challenges to their wider use have yet to be overcome. These include identification of appropriate tumor antigens, a better understanding and targeting of the tumor microenvironment, timing and integration into effective multimodality chemotherapy regimens, and optimization of immune monitoring.

10.3.1 Identification of Tumor Targets for Cancer Vaccines

Unlike in adult cancers, the low frequency of somatic mutations and downregulation of MHC class I in most pediatric malignancies have hampered respectively, the identification of neoantigens and the targeting of internal proteins with cancer vaccines. However, newer genomic technologies have yielded interesting candidates for solid tumors in children which will require validation [127]. Immune checkpoint molecules are obvious targets for inhibition but have not been well characterized on pediatric tumors. Early phase studies of the checkpoint blockade inhibiting antibodies nivolumab, pembrolizumab and atezolizumab are under way in children, and once safety is established, they could be combined rationally with cancer vaccines.

10.3.2 Manipulating the Tumor Microenvironment

The tumor microenvironment contains a range of immunosuppressive cells including Tregs and myeloid-derived suppressor cells. These secrete several cytokines and chemokines that can negatively impact DC and T cell function. Furthermore deprivation of nutrients and hypoxia in the tumor microenvironment can lead to further immune suppression. Lymphocytes also require additional co-stimulatory signals to maintain activation and avoid anergy. Improvements in vaccine design such as optimizing the choice of adjuvant and combination with other therapies such as checkpoint inhibitors and Treg suppressive chemotherapy such as cyclophosphamide [128] or temozolomide [129] have the potential to reverse the immunosuppressive effect of the tumor microenvironment and enhance the effect of cancer vaccines [130].

10.3.3 Monitoring Effectiveness of Vaccines

Optimizing strategies for vaccination against cancer is critical to their success. Unfortunately animal experiments have not accurately predicted outcomes in humans. Early phase trials in patients with bulky disease are not likely to demonstrate efficacy and might lead to discarding a possibly effective treatment for minimal residual disease. Furthermore, these clinical results might not be relevant to the goal of eradicating minimal disease. Defining predictive immunological and patient-specific biomarkers can improve the judicious use of cancer vaccines. Several international consortia have recently proposed guidelines for the optimization of vaccine monitoring in adult cancer patients, but they have not considered the specific needs and challenges of children with cancer [131, 132].

10.3.4 Integrating Vaccines into Multimodality Therapy for Pediatric Malignancies

Children with high-risk malignancies are often treated with multimodality therapies that significantly affect immune function. On the one hand, chemotherapy and radiotherapy, by inducing cell death, can release tumor antigens which could be taken by endogenous antigen presenting cells and enhance immune response against cancer. The abscopal effect occasionally seen after radiotherapy is likely to be mediated by immune mechanisms [133]. Specific chemotherapeutic agents, by depleting the tumor microenvironment of Tregs and tumor macrophages, might enhance the effect of vaccines. However, in general, the high doses of chemotherapy administered to children with cancer are highly myelosuppressive and immune recovery is necessary for cancer vaccines to be effective. Cancer vaccines could be combined with immune checkpoint inhibitors as discussed above. Another approach could be to administer cancer vaccines after anti-idiotype antibodies have had the opportunity to develop in patients following antibody therapy. This is being investigated at Memorial Sloan Kettering Cancer Center (Fig. 10.2). Patients with high-risk neuroblastoma initially undergo high-dose chemotherapy and surgery to achieve complete remission. They then receive passive immunotherapy with anti-GD2 antibodies

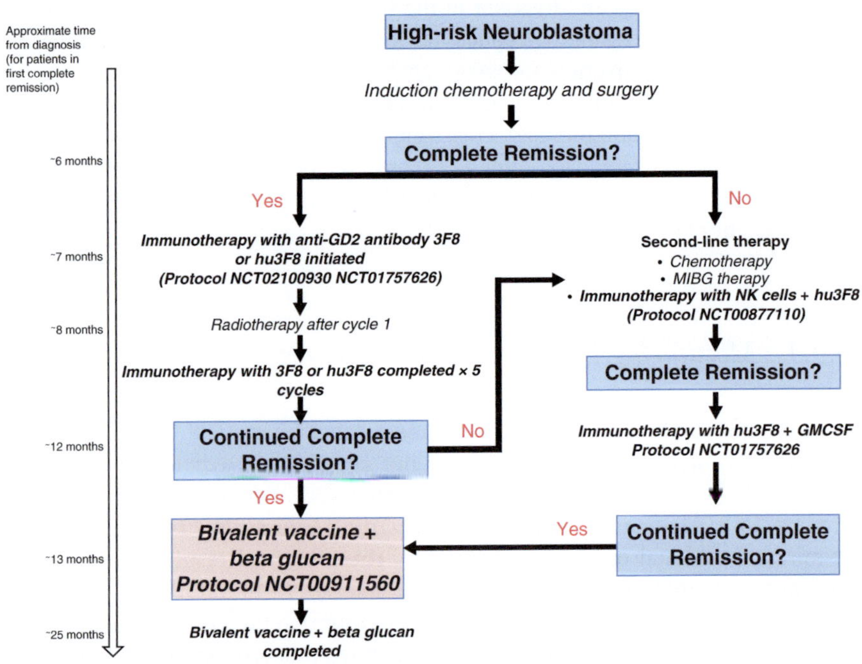

Fig. 10.2 Integration of passive and active immunotherapy into conventional multimodality therapy for high-risk neuroblastoma: the Memorial Sloan Kettering Cancer Center approach. Abbreviations: *CR* complete remission, *VGPR* very good partial remission

during a phase when T-cell recovery has not occurred. This is followed by anti-GD2 vaccination (>6 months after high-dose chemotherapy is complete) at a point when T-cell recovery is expected. The hypothesis is that passive immunotherapy elicits an anti-idiotype response which can then be boosted by anti-GD2 vaccination. In addition to immune recovery, disease status is also relevant for the timing of cancer vaccines. Vaccines are most likely to be efficacious in the setting of minimal residual disease (MRD). Early detection and treatment of MRD has been effective in the management of childhood leukemia. Assays have now been developed for MRD of blood or bone marrow metastases in solid tumors such as neuroblastoma [134, 135]. These could be utilized to measure the efficacy of immunotherapies such as vaccines that are ideally introduced when disease cannot be detected by conventional modalities.

10.4 Conclusions

The judicious and effective use of cancer vaccines in children will require several obstacles to be overcome, many of them common to those faced in adult oncology. These include choosing the right antigens and types of vaccines, developing an understanding of immune recovery after cytotoxic therapy to optimize timing and integration of vaccines into multimodality therapy, and developing strategies to combine vaccines with other modalities of immunotherapy. Although most vaccines have a good safety record in adults, the unique physiology of young children will require careful monitoring for unintended toxicities. In addition, the rarity of pediatric cancer poses unique challenges of trial design and regulatory approval. However, the recent introduction of state-of-the-art immunotherapies into the field of pediatric oncology provides hope that more children can be treated with cancer vaccines.

Acknowledgements We thank Dr. Nai-Kong V. Cheung for reviewing the manuscript and Joe Olechnowicz for editorial assistance.

References

1. Herrero R, Gonzalez P, Markowitz LE. Present status of human papillomavirus vaccine development and implementation. Lancet Oncol. 2015;16:e206–16.
2. Zanetti AR, Van Damme P, Shouval D. The global impact of vaccination against hepatitis B: a historical overview. Vaccine. 2008;26:6266–73.
3. Kantoff PW, Higano CS, Shore ND, et al. Sipuleucel-T immunotherapy for castration-resistant prostate cancer. N Engl J Med. 2010;363:411–22.
4. Kushner BH, Cheung IY, Modak S, et al. Phase I trial of a bivalent gangliosides vaccine in combination with beta-glucan for high-risk neuroblastoma in second or later remission. Clin Cancer Res. 2014;20:1375–82.

5. Yu AL, Gilman AL, Ozkaynak MF, et al. Anti-GD2 antibody with GM-CSF, interleukin-2, and isotretinoin for neuroblastoma. N Engl J Med. 2010;363:1324–34.
6. Hoffman LM, Gore L. Blinatumomab, a bi-specific anti-CD19/CD3 BiTE((R)) antibody for the treatment of acute lymphoblastic leukemia: perspectives and current pediatric applications. Front Oncol. 2014;4:63.
7. Maude SL, Frey N, Shaw PA, et al. Chimeric antigen receptor T cells for sustained remissions in leukemia. N Engl J Med. 2014;371:1507–17.
8. Schumacher TN, Schreiber RD. Neoantigens in cancer immunotherapy. Science. 2015;348:69–74.
9. Vogelstein B, Papadopoulos N, Velculescu VE, et al. Cancer genome landscapes. Science. 2013;339:1546–58.
10. Krishnadas DK, Shusterman S, Bai F, et al. A phase I trial combining decitabine/dendritic cell vaccine targeting MAGE-A1, MAGE-A3 and NY-ESO-1 for children with relapsed or therapy-refractory neuroblastoma and sarcoma. Cancer Immunol Immunother. 2015;64:1251–60.
11. Butterfield LH. Cancer vaccines. BMJ. 2015;350:h988.
12. Mackall CL, Rhee EH, Read EJ, et al. A pilot study of consolidative immunotherapy in patients with high-risk pediatric sarcomas. Clin Cancer Res. 2008;14:4850–8.
13. Cheever MA, Allison JP, Ferris AS, et al. The prioritization of cancer antigens: a national cancer institute pilot project for the acceleration of translational research. Clin Cancer Res. 2009;15:5323–37.
14. Temizoz B, Kuroda E, Ishii KJ. Vaccine adjuvants as potential cancer immunotherapeutics. Int Immunol. 2016;28:329–38.
15. Larocca C, Schlom J. Viral vector-based therapeutic cancer vaccines. Cancer J. 2011;17:359–71.
16. Yang B, Jeang J, Yang A, et al. DNA vaccine for cancer immunotherapy. Hum Vaccin Immunother. 2014;10:3153–64.
17. Bijker MS, van den Eeden SJ, Franken KL, et al. CD8+ CTL priming by exact peptide epitopes in incomplete Freund's adjuvant induces a vanishing CTL response, whereas long peptides induce sustained CTL reactivity. J Immunol. 2007;179:5033–40.
18. Seigler HF, Shingleton WW, Pickrell KL. Intralesional BCG, intravenous immune lymphocytes, and immunization with neuraminidase-treated tumor cells to manage melanoma: A clinical assessment. Plast Reconstr Surg. 1975;55:294–8.
19. Abdel-Wahab Z, Weltz C, Hester D, et al. A Phase I clinical trial of immunotherapy with interferon-gamma gene-modified autologous melanoma cells: monitoring the humoral immune response. Cancer. 1997;80:401–12.
20. Soiffer R, Hodi FS, Haluska F, et al. Vaccination with irradiated, autologous melanoma cells engineered to secrete granulocyte-macrophage colony-stimulating factor by adenoviral-mediated gene transfer augments antitumor immunity in patients with metastatic melanoma. J Clin Oncol. 2003;21:3343–50.
21. Fishman M, Hunter TB, Soliman H, et al. Phase II trial of B7-1 (CD-86) transduced, cultured autologous tumor cell vaccine plus subcutaneous interleukin-2 for treatment of stage IV renal cell carcinoma. J Immunother. 2008;31:72–80.
22. Bowman L, Grossmann M, Rill D, et al. IL-2 adenovector-transduced autologous tumor cells induce antitumor immune responses in patients with neuroblastoma. Blood. 1998;92:1941–9.
23. Dilloo D, Bacon K, Holden W, et al. Combined chemokine and cytokine gene transfer enhances antitumor immunity. Nat Med. 1996;2:1090–5.
24. Russell HV, Strother D, Mei Z, et al. Phase I trial of vaccination with autologous neuroblastoma tumor cells genetically modified to secrete IL-2 and lymphotactin. J Immunother. 2007;30:227–33.
25. Faassen AE, Dalke DP, Berton MT, et al. CD40-CD40 ligand interactions stimulate B cell antigen processing. Eur J Immunol. 1995;25:3249–55.

26. Grewal IS, Xu J, Flavell RA. Impairment of antigen-specific T-cell priming in mice lacking CD40 ligand. Nature. 1995;378:617–20.
27. Schoenberger SP, Toes RE, van der Voort EI, et al. T-cell help for cytotoxic T lymphocytes is mediated by CD40-CD40L interactions. Nature. 1998;393:480–3.
28. Rousseau RF, Biagi E, Dutour A, et al. Immunotherapy of high-risk acute leukemia with a recipient (autologous) vaccine expressing transgenic human CD40L and IL-2 after chemotherapy and allogeneic stem cell transplantation. Blood. 2006;107:1332–41.
29. Dranoff G, Soiffer R, Lynch T, et al. A phase I study of vaccination with autologous, irradiated melanoma cells engineered to secrete human granulocyte-macrophage colony stimulating factor. Hum Gene Ther. 1997;8:111–23.
30. Goldberg JM, Fisher DE, Demetri GD, et al. Biologic activity of autologous, granulocyte-macrophage colony-stimulating factor secreting alveolar soft-part sarcoma and clear cell sarcoma vaccines. Clin Cancer Res. 2015;21:3178–86.
31. Ghisoli M, Barve M, Mennel R, et al. Three year follow up of GMCSF/bi-shRNAfurin DNA transfected autologous tumor immunotherapy (Vigil) in metastatic advanced Ewing's sarcoma. Mol Ther. 2016;24(8):1478–83.
32. Parmiani G, Pilla L, Maccalli C, et al. Autologous versus allogeneic cell-based vaccines? Cancer J. 2011;17:331–6.
33. Ehlken H, Schadendorf D, Eichmuller S. Humoral immune response against melanoma antigens induced by vaccination with cytokine gene-modified autologous tumor cells. Int J Cancer. 2004;108:307–13.
34. Ueda R, Shiku H, Pfreundschuh M, et al. Cell surface antigens of human renal cancer defined by autologous typing. J Exp Med. 1979;150:564–79.
35. Sharma A, Bode B, Wenger RH, et al. Gamma-radiation promotes immunological recognition of cancer cells through increased expression of cancer-testis antigens in vitro and in vivo. PLoS One. 2011;6:e28217.
36. Klopp AH, Spaeth EL, Dembinski JL, et al. Tumor irradiation increases the recruitment of circulating mesenchymal stem cells into the tumor microenvironment. Cancer Res. 2007;67:11687–95.
37. Bowman L, Grossmann M, Rill D, et al. Interleukin-2 gene-modified allogeneic tumor cells for treatment of relapsed neuroblastoma. Hum Gene Ther. 1998;9:1303–11.
38. Rousseau RF, Haight AE, Hirschmann-Jax C, et al. Local and systemic effects of an allogeneic tumor cell vaccine combining transgenic human lymphotactin with interleukin-2 in patients with advanced or refractory neuroblastoma. Blood. 2003;101:1718–26.
39. Sondak VK, Sosman JA. Results of clinical trials with an allogenic melanoma tumor cell lysate vaccine: Melacine. Semin Cancer Biol. 2003;13:409–15.
40. Melief CJ, van Hall T, Arens R, et al. Therapeutic cancer vaccines. J Clin Invest. 2015;125:3401–12.
41. Key ME, Talmadge JE, Fogler WE, et al. Isolation of tumoricidal macrophages from lung melanoma metastases of mice treated systemically with liposomes containing a lipophilic derivative of muramyl dipeptide. J Natl Cancer Inst. 1982;69:1189–98.
42. Koff WC, Fidler IJ, Showalter SD, et al. Human monocytes activated by immunomodulators in liposomes lyse herpesvirus-infected but not normal cells. Science. 1984;224:1007–9.
43. Schroit AJ, Fidler IJ. Effects of liposome structure and lipid composition on the activation of the tumoricidal properties of macrophages by liposomes containing muramyl dipeptide. Cancer Res. 1982;42:161–7.
44. Dieter P, Ambs P, Fitzke E, et al. Comparative studies of cytotoxicity and the release of TNF-alpha, nitric oxide, and eicosanoids of liver macrophages treated with lipopolysaccharide and liposome-encapsulated MTP-PE. J Immunol. 1995;155:2595–604.
45. Kleinerman ES, Snyder JS, Jaffe N. Influence of chemotherapy administration on monocyte activation by liposomal muramyl tripeptide phosphatidylethanolamine in children with osteosarcoma. J Clin Oncol. 1991;9:259–67.

46. MacEwen EG, Kurzman ID, Rosenthal RC, et al. Therapy for osteosarcoma in dogs with intravenous injection of liposome-encapsulated muramyl tripeptide. J Natl Cancer Inst. 1989;81:935–8.
47. Fidler IJ, Fogler WE, Brownbill AF, et al. Systemic activation of tumoricidal properties in mouse macrophages and inhibition of melanoma metastases by the oral administration of MTP-PE, a lipophilic muramyl dipeptide. J Immunol. 1987;138:4509–14.
48. Urba WJ, Hartmann LC, Longo DL, et al. Phase I and immunomodulatory study of a muramyl peptide, muramyl tripeptide phosphatidylethanolamine. Cancer Res. 1990;50:2979–86.
49. Anderson P. Liposomal muramyl tripeptide phosphatidyl ethanolamine: ifosfamide-containing chemotherapy in osteosarcoma. Future Oncol. 2006;2:333–43.
50. Kleinerman ES, Gano JB, Johnston DA, et al. Efficacy of liposomal muramyl tripeptide (CGP 19835A) in the treatment of relapsed osteosarcoma. Am J Clin Oncol. 1995;18:93–9.
51. Meyers PA, Schwartz CL, Krailo M, et al. Osteosarcoma: a randomized, prospective trial of the addition of ifosfamide and/or muramyl tripeptide to cisplatin, doxorubicin, and high-dose methotrexate. J Clin Oncol. 2005;23:2004–11.
52. Meyers PA, Schwartz CL, Krailo MD, et al. Osteosarcoma: the addition of muramyl tripeptide to chemotherapy improves overall survival—a report from the Children's Oncology Group. J Clin Oncol. 2008;26:633–8.
53. Anderson PM, Meyers P, Kleinerman E, et al. Mifamurtide in metastatic and recurrent osteosarcoma: a patient access study with pharmacokinetic, pharmacodynamic, and safety assessments. Pediatr Blood Cancer. 2014;61:238–44.
54. Meyers PA, Chou AJ. Muramyl tripeptide-phosphatidyl ethanolamine encapsulated in liposomes (L-MTP-PE) in the treatment of osteosarcoma. Adv Exp Med Biol. 2014;804:307–21.
55. Pollack IF, Jakacki RI, Butterfield LH, et al. Immune responses and outcome after vaccination with glioma-associated antigen peptides and poly-ICLC in a pilot study for pediatric recurrent low-grade gliomas. Neuro Oncol. 2016;18:1157–68.
56. Pollack IF, Jakacki RI, Butterfield LH, et al. Antigen-specific immune responses and clinical outcome after vaccination with glioma-associated antigen peptides and polyinosinic-polycytidylic acid stabilized by lysine and carboxymethylcellulose in children with newly diagnosed malignant brainstem and nonbrainstem gliomas. J Clin Oncol. 2014;32:2050–8.
57. Sawada A, Inoue M, Kondo O, et al. Feasibility of cancer immunotherapy with WT1 peptide vaccination for solid and hematological malignancies in children. Pediatr Blood Cancer. 2016;63:234–41.
58. Hashii Y, Sato-Miyashita E, Matsumura R, et al. WT1 peptide vaccination following allogeneic stem cell transplantation in pediatric leukemic patients with high risk for relapse: successful maintenance of durable remission. Leukemia. 2012;26:530–2.
59. Pol J, Bloy N, Buque A, et al. Trial watch: peptide-based anticancer vaccines. Oncoimmunology. 2015;4:e974411.
60. Hirayama M, Nishimura Y. The present status and future prospects of peptide-based cancer vaccines. Int Immunol. 2016;28:319–28.
61. Lawrence MS, Stojanov P, Polak P, et al. Mutational heterogeneity in cancer and the search for new cancer-associated genes. Nature. 2013;499:214–8.
62. Andtbacka RH, Kaufman HL, Collichio F, et al. Talimogene laherparepvec improves durable response rate in patients with advanced melanoma. J Clin Oncol. 2015;33:2780–8.
63. DiPaola RS, Chen YH, Bubley GJ, et al. A national multicenter phase 2 study of prostate-specific antigen (PSA) pox virus vaccine with sequential androgen ablation therapy in patients with PSA progression: ECOG 9802. Eur Urol. 2015;68:365–71.
64. Quoix E, Lena H, Losonczy G, et al. TG4010 immunotherapy and first-line chemotherapy for advanced non-small-cell lung cancer (TIME): results from the phase 2b part of a randomised, double-blind, placebo-controlled, phase 2b/3 trial. Lancet Oncol. 2016;17:212–23.
65. Alvarez RD, Barnes MN, Gomez-Navarro J, et al. A cancer gene therapy approach utilizing an anti-erbB-2 single-chain antibody-encoding adenovirus (AD21): a phase I trial. Clin Cancer Res. 2000;6:3081–7.

66. Le DT, Wang-Gillam A, Picozzi V, et al. Safety and survival with GVAX pancreas prime and Listeria Monocytogenes-expressing mesothelin (CRS-207) boost vaccines for metastatic pancreatic cancer. J Clin Oncol. 2015;33:1325–33.
67. Niethammer AG, Lubenau H, Mikus G, et al. Double-blind, placebo-controlled first in human study to investigate an oral vaccine aimed to elicit an immune reaction against the VEGF-receptor 2 in patients with stage IV and locally advanced pancreatic cancer. BMC Cancer. 2012;12:361.
68. Burke MJ, Ahern C, Weigel BJ, et al. Phase I trial of Seneca Valley Virus (NTX-010) in children with relapsed/refractory solid tumors: a report of the Children's Oncology Group. Pediatr Blood Cancer. 2015;62:743–50.
69. Cripe TP, Ngo MC, Geller JI, et al. Phase 1 study of intratumoral Pexa-Vec (JX-594), an oncolytic and immunotherapeutic vaccinia virus, in pediatric cancer patients. Mol Ther. 2015;23:602–8.
70. Fest S, Huebener N, Bleeke M, et al. Survivin minigene DNA vaccination is effective against neuroblastoma. Int J Cancer. 2009;125:104–14.
71. Stermann A, Huebener N, Seidel D, et al. Targeting of MYCN by means of DNA vaccination is effective against neuroblastoma in mice. Cancer Immunol Immunother. 2015;64:1215–27.
72. Rice J, Ottensmeier CH, Stevenson FK. DNA vaccines: precision tools for activating effective immunity against cancer. Nat Rev Cancer. 2008;8:108–20.
73. Kobiyama K, Jounai N, Aoshi T, et al. Innate immune signaling by, and genetic adjuvants for DNA vaccination. Vaccines (Basel). 2013;1:278–92.
74. Ishii KJ, Kawagoe T, Koyama S, et al. TANK-binding kinase-1 delineates innate and adaptive immune responses to DNA vaccines. Nature. 2008;451:725–9.
75. McNamara MA, Nair SK, Holl EK. RNA-based vaccines in cancer immunotherapy. J Immunol Res. 2015;2015:794528.
76. Fioretti D, Iurescia S, Fazio VM, et al. DNA vaccines: developing new strategies against cancer. J Biomed Biotechnol. 2010;2010:174378.
77. Zhu D, Stevenson FK. DNA gene fusion vaccines against cancer. Curr Opin Mol Ther. 2002;4:41–8.
78. Staff C, Mozaffari F, Haller BK, et al. A phase I safety study of plasmid DNA immunization targeting carcinoembryonic antigen in colorectal cancer patients. Vaccine. 2011;29:6817–22.
79. Ribas A, Weber JS, Chmielowski B, et al. Intra-lymph node prime-boost vaccination against Melan A and tyrosinase for the treatment of metastatic melanoma: results of a phase 1 clinical trial. Clin Cancer Res. 2011;17:2987–96.
80. Huebener N, Fest S, Hilt K, et al. Xenogeneic immunization with human tyrosine hydroxylase DNA vaccines suppresses growth of established neuroblastoma. Mol Cancer Ther. 2009;8:2392–401.
81. Kochling J, Rott Y, Arndt S, et al. Prevention and synergistic control of Ph(+) ALL by a DNA vaccine and 6-mercaptopurine. Vaccine. 2012;30:5949–55.
82. Bolesta E, Kowalczyk A, Wierzbicki A, et al. DNA vaccine expressing the mimotope of GD2 ganglioside induces protective GD2 cross-reactive antibody responses. Cancer Res. 2005;65:3410–8.
83. Suzuki M, Cheung NK. Disialoganglioside GD2 as a therapeutic target for human diseases. Expert Opin Ther Targets. 2015;19:349–62.
84. Modak S, Cheung NK. Disialoganglioside directed immunotherapy of neuroblastoma. Cancer Invest. 2007;25:67–77.
85. Zhang S, Cordon-Cardo C, Zhang HS, et al. Selection of tumor antigens as targets for immune attack using immunohistochemistry 1. Focus on gangliosides. Int J Cancer. 1997;73:42–9.
86. Dobrenkov K, Ostrovnaya I, Gu J, et al. Oncotargets GD2 and GD3 are highly expressed in sarcomas of children, adolescents, and young adults. Pediatr Blood Cancer. 2016;63:1780–5.
87. Heimburg-Molinaro J, Lum M, Vijay G, et al. Cancer vaccines and carbohydrate epitopes. Vaccine. 2011;29:8802–26.

88. Durrant LG, Noble P, Spendlove I. Immunology in the clinic review series; focus on cancer: glycolipids as targets for tumour immunotherapy. Clin Exp Immunol. 2012;167:206–15.
89. Makela PH. Vaccines, coming of age after 200 years. FEMS Microbiol Rev. 2000;24:9–20.
90. Helling F, Shang A, Calves M, et al. GD3 vaccines for melanoma: superior immunogenicity of keyhole limpet hemocyanin conjugate vaccines. Cancer Res. 1994;54:197–203.
91. Kim SK, Ragupathi G, Cappello S, et al. Effect of immunological adjuvant combinations on the antibody and T-cell response to vaccination with MUC1-KLH and GD3-KLH conjugates. Vaccine. 2000;19:530–7.
92. Ragupathi G, Gardner JR, Livingston PO, et al. Natural and synthetic saponin adjuvant QS-21 for vaccines against cancer. Expert Rev Vaccines. 2011;10:463–70.
93. Eggermont AM, Suciu S, Rutkowski P, et al. Adjuvant ganglioside GM2-KLH/QS-21 vaccination versus observation after resection of primary tumor > 1.5 mm in patients with stage II melanoma: results of the EORTC 18961 randomized phase III trial. J Clin Oncol. 2013;31:3831–7.
94. Vannucci L, Krizan J, Sima P, et al. Immunostimulatory properties and antitumor activities of glucans: review. Int J Oncol. 2013;43:357–64.
95. Cheung NK, Modak S. Oral (13),(14)-beta-D-glucan synergizes with antiganglioside GD2 monoclonal antibody 3F8 in the therapy of neuroblastoma. Clin Cancer Res. 2002;8:1217–23.
96. Modak S, Koehne G, Vickers A, et al. Rituximab therapy of lymphoma is enhanced by orally administered (13),(14)-D-beta-glucan. Leuk Res. 2005;29:679–83.
97. Modak S, Kushner BH, Kramer K, et al. Anti-GD2 antibody 3F8 and barley-derived (13),(14)-beta--glucan: A Phase I study in patients with chemoresistant neuroblastoma. Oncoimmunology. 2013;2:e23402.
98. McCarthy H, Ottensmeier CH, Hamblin TJ, et al. Anti-idiotype vaccines. Br J Haematol. 2003;123:770–81.
99. Ladjemi MZ. Anti-idiotypic antibodies as cancer vaccines: achievements and future improvements. Front Oncol. 2012;2:158.
100. Meeker TC, Lowder J, Maloney DG, et al. A clinical trial of anti-idiotype therapy for B cell malignancy. Blood. 1985;65:1349–63.
101. Cheung NK, Guo HF, Cheung IY. Correlation of anti-idiotype network with survival following anti-G(D2) monoclonal antibody 3F8 therapy of stage 4 neuroblastoma. Med Pediatr Oncol. 2000;35:635–7.
102. Cheung NK, Cheung IY, Kushner BH, et al. Murine anti-GD2 monoclonal antibody 3F8 combined with granulocyte-macrophage colony-stimulating factor and 13-Cis-retinoic acid in high-risk patients with stage 4 neuroblastoma in first remission. J Clin Oncol. 2012;30:3264–70.
103. Batova A, Yu A, Strother D, et al. Promising results of a pilot trial of a GD2 directed anti-idiotypic antibody as a vaccine for high-risk neuroblastoma. Proc ASCO. 2004;22:8511.
104. Eger C, Siebert N, Seidel D, et al. Generation and characterization of a human/mouse chimeric GD2-mimicking anti-idiotype antibody ganglidiximab for active immunotherapy against neuroblastoma. PLoS One. 2016;11:e0150479.
105. Cacciavillano W, Sampor C, Venier C, et al. A phase I study of the anti-idiotype vaccine racotumomab in neuroblastoma and other pediatric refractory malignancies. Pediatr Blood Cancer. 2015;62:2120–4.
106. Alfonso S, Valdes-Zayas A, Santiesteban ER, et al. A randomized, multicenter, placebo-controlled clinical trial of racotumomab-alum vaccine as switch maintenance therapy in advanced non-small cell lung cancer patients. Clin Cancer Res. 2014;20:3660–71.
107. Goyvaerts C, Breckpot K. Pros and cons of antigen-presenting cell targeted tumor vaccines. J Immunol Res. 2015;2015:785634.
108. Constantino J, Gomes C, Falcao A, et al. Antitumor dendritic cell-based vaccines: lessons from 20 years of clinical trials and future perspectives. Transl Res. 2016;168:74–95.
109. Patel PH, Kockler DR. Sipuleucel-T: a vaccine for metastatic, asymptomatic, androgen-independent prostate cancer. Ann Pharmacother. 2008;42:91–8.

110. Bloy N, Pol J, Aranda F, et al. Trial watch: dendritic cell-based anticancer therapy. Oncoimmunology. 2014;3:e963424.
111. Lasky JL 3rd, Panosyan EH, Plant A, et al. Autologous tumor lysate-pulsed dendritic cell immunotherapy for pediatric patients with newly diagnosed or recurrent high-grade gliomas. Anticancer Res. 2013;33:2047–56.
112. Ardon H, De Vleeschouwer S, Van Calenbergh F, et al. Adjuvant dendritic cell-based tumour vaccination for children with malignant brain tumours. Pediatr Blood Cancer. 2010;54:519–25.
113. Caruso DA, Orme LM, Neale AM, et al. Results of a phase 1 study utilizing monocyte-derived dendritic cells pulsed with tumor RNA in children and young adults with brain cancer. Neuro Oncol. 2004;6:236–46.
114. Olin MR, Low W, McKenna DH, et al. Vaccination with dendritic cells loaded with allogeneic brain tumor cells for recurrent malignant brain tumors induces a CD4(+)IL17(+) response. J Immunother Cancer. 2014;2:4.
115. Merchant MS, Bernstein D, Amoako M, et al. Adjuvant immunotherapy to improve outcome in high-risk pediatric sarcomas. Clin Cancer Res. 2016;22:3182–91.
116. Dagher R, Long LM, Read EJ, et al. Pilot trial of tumor-specific peptide vaccination and continuous infusion interleukin-2 in patients with recurrent Ewing sarcoma and alveolar rhabdomyosarcoma: an inter-institute NIH study. Med Pediatr Oncol. 2002;38:158–64.
117. Geiger JD, Hutchinson RJ, Hohenkirk LF, et al. Vaccination of pediatric solid tumor patients with tumor lysate-pulsed dendritic cells can expand specific T cells and mediate tumor regression. Cancer Res. 2001;61:8513–9.
118. Himoudi N, Wallace R, Parsley KL, et al. Lack of T-cell responses following autologous tumour lysate pulsed dendritic cell vaccination, in patients with relapsed osteosarcoma. Clin Transl Oncol. 2012;14:271–9.
119. Caruso DA, Orme LM, Amor GM, et al. Results of a phase I study utilizing monocyte-derived dendritic cells pulsed with tumor RNA in children with stage 4 neuroblastoma. Cancer. 2005;103:1280–91.
120. Suminoe A, Matsuzaki A, Hattori H, et al. Immunotherapy with autologous dendritic cells and tumor antigens for children with refractory malignant solid tumors. Pediatr Transplant. 2009;13:746–53.
121. Dohnal AM, Witt V, Hugel H, et al. Phase I study of tumor Ag-loaded IL-12 secreting semi-mature DC for the treatment of pediatric cancer. Cytotherapy. 2007;9:755–70.
122. Van Tendeloo VF, Van de Velde A, Van Driessche A, et al. Induction of complete and molecular remissions in acute myeloid leukemia by Wilms' tumor 1 antigen-targeted dendritic cell vaccination. Proc Natl Acad Sci U S A. 2010;107:13824–9.
123. Saito S, Yanagisawa R, Yoshikawa K, et al. Safety and tolerability of allogeneic dendritic cell vaccination with induction of Wilms tumor 1-specific T cells in a pediatric donor and pediatric patient with relapsed leukemia: a case report and review of the literature. Cytotherapy. 2015;17:330–5.
124. Haniffa M, Shin A, Bigley V, et al. Human tissues contain CD141hi cross-presenting dendritic cells with functional homology to mouse CD103+ nonlymphoid dendritic cells. Immunity. 2012;37:60–73.
125. Liu Y, Xiao L, Joo KI, et al. In situ modulation of dendritic cells by injectable thermosensitive hydrogels for cancer vaccines in mice. Biomacromolecules. 2014;15:3836–45.
126. Romagnoli GG, Zelante BB, Toniolo PA, et al. Dendritic cell-derived exosomes may be a tool for cancer immunotherapy by converting tumor cells into immunogenic targets. Front Immunol. 2014;5:692.
127. Orentas RJ, Yang JJ, Wen X, et al. Identification of cell surface proteins as potential immunotherapy targets in 12 pediatric cancers. Front Oncol. 2012;2:194.
128. Heylmann D, Bauer M, Becker H, et al. Human CD4+CD25+ regulatory T cells are sensitive to low dose cyclophosphamide: implications for the immune response. PLoS One. 2013;8:e83384.

129. Iversen TZ, Brimnes MK, Nikolajsen K, et al. Depletion of T lymphocytes is correlated with response to temozolomide in melanoma patients. Oncoimmunology. 2013;2:e23288.
130. van der Burg SH, Arens R, Ossendorp F, et al. Vaccines for established cancer: overcoming the challenges posed by immune evasion. Nat Rev Cancer. 2016;16:219–33.
131. Butterfield LH, Palucka AK, Britten CM, et al. Recommendations from the iSBTc-SITC/FDA/NCI Workshop on Immunotherapy Biomarkers. Clin Cancer Res. 2011;17:3064–76.
132. Romero P, Banchereau J, Bhardwaj N, et al. The human vaccines project: a roadmap for cancer vaccine development. Sci Transl Med. 2016;8:334ps9.
133. Deloch L, Derer A, Hartmann J, et al. Modern radiotherapy concepts and the impact of radiation on immune activation. Front Oncol. 2016;6:141.
134. Cheung NK, Ostrovnaya I, Kuk D, et al. Bone marrow minimal residual disease was an early response marker and a consistent independent predictor of survival after anti-GD2 immunotherapy. J Clin Oncol. 2015;33:755–63.
135. Chicard M, Boyault S, Colmet Daage L, et al. Genomic copy number profiling using circulating free tumor DNA highlights heterogeneity in neuroblastoma. Clin Cancer Res. 2016;22:5564–73.

Chapter 11
Immune Adjuvants and Cytokine Therapies

Vito Pistoia, Ignazia Prigione, and Lizzia Raffaghello

Abstract The term "adjuvant" derives from the Latin verb "adiuvare" that means to provide aid. An immune adjuvant (IA) is a chemical substance of heterogeneous nature that is administered together with a vaccine to potentiate the immune response to the relevant antigen. IA were originally developed to sustain immunity to bacterial and viral antigens in the context of preventive vaccinations against pathogens. More recently, the progress of cancer immunotherapy has fostered the search for IA, in various formulations, able to stimulate the immune response of cancer patients to tumor antigens.

Cytokines are molecules released by different cell types in the extracellular milieu that play essential roles in intercellular communication. Cytokines represent a category of IA, and will be discussed here in detail, as they have already achieved widespread use in pediatric oncology.

Keywords Pediatric tumors • Immune response • Immunotherapy • Immune adjuvants • Cytokines

11.1 Cytokines in Pediatric Oncology

The primary aim of using cytokines in tumor-bearing patients is to achieve the activation of the host immune system, in order to promote elimination of cancer cells. Different strategies have been developed to achieve this aim, including:

1. *Direct administration of recombinant cytokines.*
2. *In vitro activation of immune effector cells by incubation with cytokines*; activated cells that include lymphokine activated killer (LAK) cells, cytotoxic

V. Pistoia, M.D. (✉)
Immunology Area, Bambino Gesù Pediatric Hospital, Viale San Paolo 15, Rome 00146, Italy
e-mail: vito.pistoia@opbg.net

I. Prigione, Ph.D. • L. Raffaghello, Ph.D.
Laboratory of Oncology, Translational Research and Laboratory Medicine, Istituto Giannina Gaslini, Via Gaslini, 5, Genoa 16147, Italy
e-mail: ignaziaprigione@gaslini.org; lizziaraffaghello@gaslini.org

J.C. Gray, A. Marabelle (eds.), *Immunotherapy for Pediatric Malignancies*,
https://doi.org/10.1007/978-3-319-43486-5_11

T lymphocytes (CTL) [1], natural killer (NK) cells [2], cytokine induced killer (CIK) cells [3] and chimeric antigen receptor (CAR) T lymphocytes [4] are subsequently re-infused in the patient.
3. *Administration of cytokines in the form of cytokine gene therapy*; whereby tumor cells are transfected with cytokine encoding genes and infused (sometimes in combination with other IA) [5].
4. *Administration of cytokines as fusion proteins*: in which a cytokine is fused to an antibody moiety allowing targeting of the former directly to tumor cells or to the tumor microenvironment [6].

The experience gathered from the clinical use of cytokines in pediatric oncology has translated into further refinements. For instance, subcutaneous (s.c.) administration of recombinant interleukin-2 (rIL2) has proved to be better tolerated than intravenous administration of the same cytokine. Cytokines such as rIL-2 and recombinant granulocyte-macrophage colony stimulating factor (rGM-CSF) have been administered with tumor specific monoclonal antibodies with the aim of increasing the efficiency of cancer cell killing by NK cells and macrophages, respectively, through antibody-dependent cell cytotoxicity (ADCC). Vaccination with cytokine-transfected cancer cells, although promising, requires cumbersome and costly procedures [7]. Although cytokine-antibody fusion proteins still hold promise, the results obtained so far in the clinical setting have been inferior to the expectations, and novel strategies are needed to re-evaluate such molecules.

Cytokines may also be used in pediatric oncology to support haematopoiesis, an indication that is independent of their IA effect [8, 9]. Granulocyte-colony stimulating factor (G-CSF), which promotes differentiation of myeloid progenitors along the granulocytic lineage, and at a lesser extent, GM-CSF, which stimulates generation of mature granulocytes and monocytes/macrophages from myeloid progenitors, are both used for this purpose [10]. Erythropoietin (EPO), and thrombopoietin (TPO) or related molecules, that induce the differentiation of erythroid progenitors or megakaryocytes to mature red blood cells or platelets, respectively, have not been widely used in pediatric patients receiving chemotherapy.

G-CSF has different mechanisms of action that are context-dependent, (a) it accelerates the recovery of neutrophils after high dose chemotherapy and hematopoietic stem cell (HSC) transplantation; (b) it mobilizes $CD34^+$ HSC from the bone marrow to the circulating compartment, thus allowing their collection for transplantation [11]. Plerixafor, an antagonist of CXCR4, the main receptor (R) for the chemokine CXCL12, also mobilizes $CD34^+$ HSC from the bone marrow and is used in the clinic [12]; (c) it activates neutrophils, that play a central role in the defense from fungal and bacterial infections, and has been shown to protect from mucositis; (d) finally, G-CSF has been administered to patients with acute myeloid leukemia (AML) to sensitize tumor cells, that express G-CSFR, to cycle-specific chemotherapeutic drugs. This latter indication for G-CSF use that extends also to GM-CSF has also been associated with risk of stimulating proliferation and invasiveness of the AML cells [10].

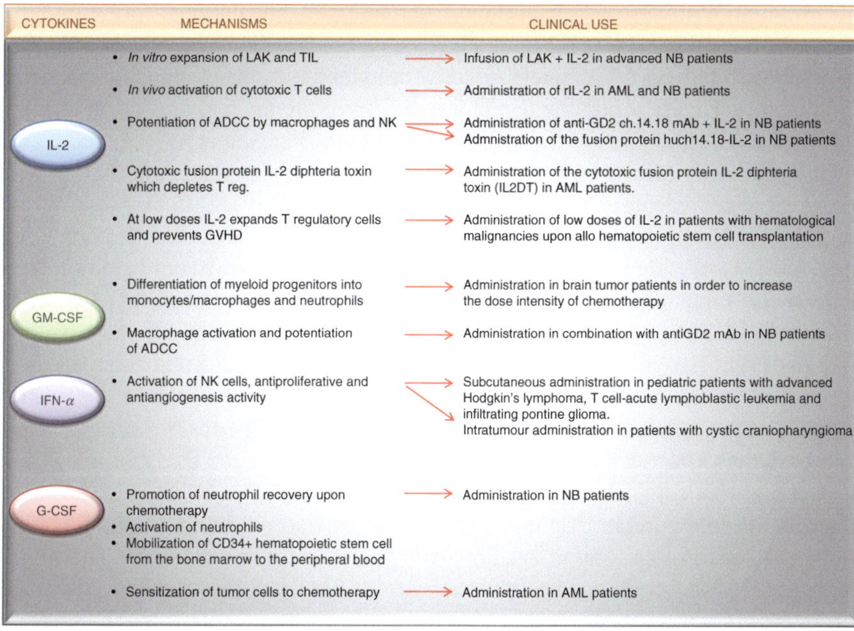

Fig. 11.1 Mechanisms and clinical use of cytokines in pediatric oncology. The Figure summarizes the mechanisms underlying the clinical use of cytokines in pediatric oncology. Details and references are reported in the main text. Abbreviations: *LAK* Lymphokine Activated Killer cells, *TIL* Tumor Infiltrating Lymphocytes, *NB* Neuroblastoma, *AML* Acute Myeloid Leukemia, *ADCC* Antibody-dependent Cell-mediated Cytotoxicity, *NK* Natural Killer cells, *GD2* Disialoganglioside 2

A similar note of caution must be raised about the use of G-CSF to accelerate granulocyte recovery in neuroblastoma patients. Although the cytokine accelerates neutrophil recovery after autologous HSC transplant in these patients [13] it has been recently reported that G-CSF acts as survival and growth factor for neuroblastoma cancer stem cells [14]. There is therefore theoretical risk of the favorable hematopoietic effects of G-CSF being outweighed by tumor promoting activity.

The principal cytokines that have been administered to pediatric oncology patients are IL-2, GM-CSF and interferon (IFN)-alpha. Their applications will be discussed in detail (Fig. 11.1).

11.1.1 Interleukin-2

IL-2 is produced mostly by activated T lymphocytes and acts a growth factor for the same cells upon binding to a heterotrimeric receptor composed of three chains; the α chain (CD25), the β chain (CD122) and the γ chain (CD132). These three chains are differentially expressed in different immune cell populations, forming complexes with varying affinity for IL-2. The α chain binds to IL-2 with low affinity, the βγ complex binds IL-2 with intermediate affinity and transduces signal in NK cells and memory T cells, while the receptor made up of the three chains displays high affinity for IL-2 and operates in activated T cells and T regulatory (Treg) cells. The γ chain of the IL-2R is also referred to as common γ chain since it is shared with other cytokines receptors, namely those for IL-4, IL-7, IL-9, IL-15 and IL-21 [15]. IL-2 and the IL-2R related transcription factor STAT-5 are indispensable in order to induce the expression of the transcription factor Foxp3 and differentiation of Treg cells in the thymus [16]. Quite recently it has been demonstrated that signaling through the IL-2R plays an essential role not only in the maintenance of mature Treg cells, but also in their suppressor function, and that STAT5 deficiency in Treg cells results in loss of suppressor function [17]. These results point to a key role of IL-2R-STAT5 signaling in linking the differentiation and the maintenance of Treg cells and their functional activities.

The first clinical studies with IL-2 in pediatric oncology date back to the early nineties, when a number of phase I trials were carried out in children with solid malignancies. The first approach involved the in vitro expansion of autologus peripheral blood lymphocytes, cultured with IL-2 in order to generate LAK cells, a mixture of activated NK cells and a lower proportion of activated T lymphocytes expressing predominantly, although not exclusively, CD8. LAK cells displayed a potent cytolytic activity *in vitro* against a broad spectrum of hematopoietic and non hematopoietic tumor cell lines and caused tumor regression in pre-clinical models of human cancer [17]. On the basis of this pre-clinical evidence, a number of different clinical trials were conducted in adult cancer patients, who received high concentrations of LAK cells together with high dose IL-2 in order to maintain the activation state of the LAK cells and allow their *in vivo* expansion [17]. A small number of similar studies were carried out in pediatric cancer patients. In one of these, that is discussed as an example, fifteen children with advanced metastatic neuroblastoma were enrolled in a phase II trial using IL-2 and LAK cells. Twelve of them had relapsed after intensive chemotherapy and autologous HSC transplantation and three had primary refractory disease following conventional chemotherapy. IL-2 was administered as continuous infusion at the dose of 18×10^6 international units (UI)/m^2 for 5 days, followed by a 6 day break and a second cycle of IL-2. Leukapheresis was performed to harvest lymphocytes during the rest period. LAK cells were expanded in culture containing IL-2 for 4 days and injected together with IL-2 in the second cycle. Two patients died due to treatment-related toxicities, one for cardiotoxicity, and the other from respiratory distress. No significant clinical response was detected and immune monitoring did not reveal significant changes of the immunological profile during treatment [18].

Altogether, clinical trials conducted with IL-2 and LAK cells failed to produce benefits and were toxic; in addition, the procedures to expand LAK cells *in vitro* were cumbersome and costly. A development in the methodology was next elaborated in which IL-2 was used to drive *in vitro* expansion of autologous tumor-infiltrating lymphocytes (TILs) rather than peripheral blood lymphocytes, followed by infusion in the patients together with IL-2. TILs were predominantly $CD8^+$ cytotoxic T lymphocytes enriched for cells capable of killing *in vitro* autologous tumor cells in a HLA-restricted manner. This therapeutic approach produced some appreciable results in the two most immunogenic adult tumors, i.e. malignant melanoma and renal carcinoma, but was not developed in pediatric oncology [1]. In subsequent studies, rIL-2 was administered alone without LAK or TIL cells, based upon the assumption that IL-2 could activate *in vivo* cytotoxic T cells with anti-tumor activity. A few clinical trials were carried out in pediatric patients affected with neuroblastoma or AML. Different schedules were used ranging from continuous infusion to i.v. bolus administration, with various doses of IL-2. Toxicities were dose-dependent and similar to those reported in adult cancer patients treated with similar schedules, including fever, vascular leak, hypotension, tachycardia, rash, thrombocytopenia, elevated transaminase, electrolyte disturbance and hyperglicemia [19–23]. In a study performed in neuroblastoma patients, rIL2 alone (administered first as i.v. bolus and then s.c) was shown to prolong disease-free survival in neuroblastoma patients [24]. A dose-finding study conducted by the European Network SIOPEN showed that 6×10^6 IU/m^2 IL-2 administered in six 5-day cycles every 2 weeks had relatively low toxicity and induced a sustained increase of circulating NK cells, suggesting that this regimen could be delivered in an outpatient setting [25].

A further step in the use of IL-2 in oncology has been the combination of this cytokine with an antibody specific for a tumor-associated antigen or the engineering of IL-2 with the single chain variable fragment (scFv) of tumor specific antibody to generate a fusion protein. In pediatric oncology, both of these approaches have been clinically tested in neuroblastoma.

GD2 is a ganglioside expressed at high density and with good selectivity by human neuroblastoma cells. GD2 represents therefore a suitable TAA for antibody targeting, and anti-GD2 mAbs have been administered to neuroblastoma patients in different studies [26, 27]. The major mechanism whereby the chimeric ch14.18 mAbs kills neuroblastoma cells is thought to be antibody-dependent cell cytotoxicity (ADCC). In ADCC, IgG1 and IgG3 mAbs bind target cells through the Fragment antigen binding F(ab)2 and effector cells, represented by NK cells, macrophages and neutrophils, bind antibody-coated targets through the Fragment crystallizable (Fc) portion of the latter molecules. GM-CSF and IL-2 potentiate ADCC by activating macrophages and NK cells, respectively. Based upon these premises, a phase III clinical trial was designed in the U.S. in which the ch.14.18 mAb was administered to NB patients in association with GM-CSF, IL-2 and isotretinoin [28], a retinoid previously investigated in neuroblastoma patients after myeloablative therapy and hematopoietic stem cell rescue [29]. The combination of the antibody with these cytokines was found to be feasible, with significant but manageable toxicity. Second, the efficacy of immunotherapy with ch.14.18, GM-CSF, IL-2 and isotretinoin was compared to standard therapy (isotretinoin alone) in a cohort of neuroblastoma patients who had responded to induction therapy and HSC transplantation. Combination immunotherapy improved significantly patient outcome with regard to event-free survival and overall survival [28].

An interesting fusion protein has been produced by fusing an IL-2 moiety with the scFv fragment of a humanized version of the anti-GD2 ch14.18 mAb (hu14.18-IL2) [30]. This fusion protein bridges GD2$^+$ neuroblastoma cells with activated NK cells and kills tumor cells through ADCC and, at a lesser extent, complement activation. Pre-clinical experiments showed that hu14.18-IL2 displayed higher anti-tumor activity against neuroblastoma cells than the combination of ch14.18 mAb and IL-2. A phase I clinical trials was performed in pediatric patients with neuroblastoma or melanoma, another malignancy of neuroectodermal origin sharing GD2 expression [31]. This study demonstrated that the fusion protein was biologically active and well tolerated. More recently, a phase II study conducted in patients with neuroblastoma has demonstrated that hu14.18-IL2 induced some objective responses in patients with non-bulky disease [32]. Altogether, the results obtained with the fusion protein have been inferior to the expectations and further studies are needed to find the right place for this molecule in neuroblastoma treatment. In this respect, pre-clinical studies have demonstrated good therapeutic activity of the fusion protein following intratumoral injection.

IL-2 diphteria toxin (IL2DT) is a recombinant cytotoxic fusion protein composed of the amino acid sequences for diphteria toxin followed by truncated amino acid sequences for IL-2. IL2DT selectively depletes CD25 expressing T cells, including Treg cells. In a clinical trial that enrolled 57 refractory AML patients including a proportion of pediatric patients, all of them were treated with lymphodepleting cyclophosphamide and fludarabine followed by haploidentical NK cell infusion and IL-2 administration. Fifteen patients received host Treg depletion with IL2DT. Depletion of Treg cells with the fusion protein improved the efficacy of haploidentical NK cell therapy [33].

The already mentioned activity of IL-2 on Treg cells may represent a double edge sword when the cytokine is administered to tumor-bearing patients. On one hand the cytokine activates anti-cancer cytotoxic effector cells, but on the other hand it expands Treg cells that dampen immune responses to tumor cells [34]. In principle, this problem can be solved switching to other IL-2 related cytokines such as IL-7 or IL-15, that activate immune effector mechanism without expanding Treg cells [35].

However, IL-2 activity on Treg cells has been exploited for prophylaxis of graft versus host disease (GVHD), that has been associated with low levels of circulating CD4$^+$, CD25$^+$, FoxP3$^+$ Treg cells. The latter cells express high levels of IL-2R and therefore can selectively expand *in vivo* in response to low IL-2 doses that are insufficient to activate effector T cells; under these conditions, GVHD may be prevented. Indeed, ultra low doses of IL-2, i.e. $1–2 \times 10^5$ IU/m^2/dose s.c. three times per week for 6 weeks, followed by additional 6 weeks if the previous treatment was tolerated, accelerated recovery of Treg cells in pediatric patients receiving allo SCT compared to a control group that did not receive IL-2. All patients had hematologic malignancies (AML, acute lymphoblastic leukemia or non-Hodgkin lymphoma). No IL-2 related toxicities were observed and the IL-2 group showed a lower incidence of viral infections and GVHD [36].

11.1.2 Granulocyte-Macrophage Colony Stimulating Factor

GM-CSF is a hematopoietic growth factor that stimulates the differentiation of myeloid progenitors into the monocytic/macrophagic and neutrophilic lineages. GM-CSF binds to a heterodimeric receptor composed of the α and β subunits, the latter participating also in the formation of the IL-3 and IL-5 receptors. It is a potent macrophage activator and can therefore potentiate ADCC.

The first pediatric trial in which GM-CSF was administered had the aim of increasing the dose intensity of cyclophosphamide in children with malignant brain tumors, glioma and PNET. GM-CSF was used by virtue of its hematopoietic stimulating activity. The regimen was demonstrated to allow double the dose of cyclophosphamide to be administered, and neutrophil recovery was accelerated [37].

Three GM-CSF based studies have been conducted in neuroblastoma patients. In the first two, GM-CSF was administered in combination with the murine anti-GD2 mAb 3F8 or the chimeric anti-GD2 mAb ch14.18. The former study was a phase II trial in which patients resistant to intensive therapy, either shortly after diagnosis or at relapse, were enrolled. The combination of 3F8 mAb and GM-CSF was found to be well tolerated and complete bone marrow remission was reported in 12/15 patients treated for resistance to induction therapy and 5/10 patients resistant to treatment at relapse [38].

The design of the second study was different since the neuroblastoma patients enrolled had recently received autologous HSC transplant. A total of 79 courses of GM-CSF plus ch14.18 mAb were administered, the main toxicities being severe neuropathic pain, fever, nausea or vomiting, grade 3 recurrent urticaria, and grade 4 vomiting. All of these toxicities were manageable. The maximum tolerated dose of ch14.18 mAbs was 40 $mg/m^2/d$ for 4 days when administered in association with GM-CSF [39].

In a recent phase II trial, 79 patients without prior progressive disease were treated for persistent osteomedullary neuroblastoma with the 3F8 mAb and GM-CSF. This latter combination was found to be highly active against chemoresistant neuroblastoma and the toxicities were manageable [40].

11.1.3 Interferon Alpha (IFN-α)

IFN-α is an immunomodulatory cytokine produced by leucocytes that activates NK cells and also has antiproliferative and antiangiogenic activities. IFN-α has been tested in numerous clinical trials enrolling adult cancer patients and is still being used in malignant melanoma, hairy cell leukemia and AIDS-related Kaposi's sarcoma. Few pediatric studies have been conducted. In one of them, 15 patients younger than 18 years with newly diagnosed stage III melanoma were treated with adjuvant biotherapy consisting of an induction therapy whereby IFN-α was administered at very high dose i.v. followed by a maintenance therapy in which the cytokine was administered at low dose s.c. Such treatment that was prolonged until 48 weeks was feasible and associated with tolerable toxicity [41].

Additional pediatric clinical trials were carried out in (a) patients with advanced Hodgkin's lymphoma who had recovered hematologically after high dose chemotherapy and autologous HSC transplant [42]; (b) patients with chemotherapy resistant T cell-acute lymphoblastic leukemia (T-ALL) [43], and (c) infiltrating pontine glioma [44]. In these studies, IFN-α was administered predominantly s.c., treatment was tolerated although some severe side effects were reported, and evidence for therapeutic activity was limited or absent.

IFN-α has also been administered intratumorally (3 M units/dose for a total of 36 M per cycle) to nine pediatric patients suffering from cystic craniopharyngioma using intratumoral catheters inserted by a subfrontal approach. Craniopharingioma can be radically removed by surgery but severe neurological or endocrine sequelae may occur. In this study, the lesions disappeared completely in seven cases and a partial reduction of the tumor size was observed in the two remaining cases. These effects persisted for at least 1 year and 8 months. Minor side effects were observed [45].

Recently, pegylated IFN-alpha2b has been tested as maintenance therapy in patients with osteosarcoma showing good histologic response to induction chemotherapy in the frame of the EURAMOS-1 study. Patients younger than 40 and older than 5 received two cycles of preoperative MAP (methotrexate, doxorubicin, and cisplatin), and underwent macroscopically complete surgery of primary tumor. If histological response was good and there was no evidence of disease progression, patients were randomized to receive four additional MAP cycles with or without IFN-alpha2b (0.5–1.0 μg/kg weekly after chemotherapy until 2 years after registration). MAP and MAP plus IFN-alpha 2b regimens had superimposable activity [46].

In conclusion, current evidence indicates that cytokines may serve as IA to stimulate patient immune response against pediatric cancer cells in selected situations (Fig. 11.1). Further investigation is needed to exploit the full potential of this group of IA. Numerous ongoing clinical trials aim at evaluating the feasibility and/or efficacy of various approaches of immunotherapy for pediatric tumors. Some of these studies involve the use of cytokines as IA, for example the NCT00258687 trial is based on an autologus vaccine composed of cancer cells expressing GM-CSF (GVAX), while the NCT00923351 trial makes use of tumor lysate pulsed autologous dendritic cells with autologous lymphocytes with or without rIL-7, and the NCT01192555 employs IL-2 or lymphotactin gene modified allogeneic neuroblastoma cells as vaccine [47].

11.2 Immune Adjuvants Other Than Cytokines

Beside cytokines, there are additional IAs that have been classified recently in two main categories, immunopotentiators and delivery systems. An immunopotentiator boosts the innate immune response by activating pattern recognition receptors, and

Table 11.1 Main adjuvant class with representative examples and clinical application in pediatric oncology

Class	Examples	Clinical use
Immunopotentiators/ bacterial products	1. Muramyl dipeptide (MDP) 2. Monophosphoryl lipid A (MPL) 3. Saponins 4. Oligonucleotides 5. Chemokines 6. Cytokines 7. Bacterial products (LPS) and their synthetic derivatives targeting mostly TLR including: • Gram-bacteria lipopolysaccharide (LPS) and derivatives (e.g. lipid A and MPL) • Polyriboinosinic-polycytidylic acid (poly I:C) • Imiquimod and resiquimod • CpG oligonucleotides	Subcutaneous administration of 852A, a systemic TLR-7 agonist in patients with advanced hematologic malignancies. Autologous dendritic cells plus imiquimod and decitabine in sarcoma and glioma and NB patients.
Delivery systems	1. Alum adjuvant 2. Calcium phosphate 3. Liposomes 4. Emulsions (oil/water, water/oil emulsions and free fatty acid such as Montanide)	Intradermal administration of Montanide ISA-51 in children with relapsed or refractory solid and hematological malignancies. Subcutaneous administration of glioma associated antigens (GAAs emulsified with Montanide + poly-ICLC) in diffuse brainstem gliomas and other low and high-grade gliomas
Polymeric microspheres	Biodegradable and biocompatible microspheres incorporating antigens of various types	
Carbohydrate based adjuvants	Complex carbohydrates of natural origin (gamma-inulin, glucans, xylans)	

Abbreviations: *TLR* Toll like receptors, *NB* neuroblastoma

specifically toll-like receptors (TLRs). If the adjuvant stimulates antigen uptake by antigen presenting cells (APCs) it is defined a delivery system. Additional categories of IAs are polymeric microsphere adjuvants, carbohydrate based adjuvants and bacterial products (Table 11.1) [47–53].

Before reviewing IA in detail, two historical compounds that have been administered to patients as immune stimulants in the early age of tumor immunotherapy deserve mention. The first is the Bacillus of Calmette and Guerin (BCG), an attenuated strain of Mycobacterium bovis closely related to Mycobacteriun tuberculosis. BCG has been administered to adult patients with different cancers, especially bladder cancer, in order to stimulate innate immune responses against cancer cells. Now this compound is virtually abandoned due to the strong granulomatous reactions induced and the related toxicity. Interestingly, BCG activates host immune cells not only through TLR2 and TLR4 [54], but also through TLR9 possibly by virtue of its immunostimlatory CpG motifs [55].

The second compound of historical interest is OK-432, a lyophilized biological preparation of different Streptococcus Pyogenes substrains treated with Benzylpenicillin, which is known as Picibanil. Picibanil has sclerosing activities and has been clinically tested in children with cystic hygroma [56] or lymphangiomas [57] with favorable results.

The vast majority of traditional vaccines contain aluminum based compounds as adjuvant, that stimulate weak T helper (Th)2 responses with production of antibodies and fail to induce Th1 or CTL responses. This latter feature is not ideal for cancer vaccines that need to stimulate immune responses dominated by IFN-γ production in order to overcome tumor-mediate immune suppression. In principle, cancer vaccine IAs must be endowed with two major properties; the ability to stimulate immune effector cells and the ability to generate memory immune responses. These latter requisites are not easily found in a single IA. Thus, for example, IL-12 and IFN-α are potent inducers of T cell differentiation towards effector cells, whereas ligands of tumor necrosis factor (TNF) receptors such as OX-40, 4–1BB and CD27 favor preferential differentiation of T cells along the memory pathway. On this basis, it is not unusual that two different adjuvants are combined to potentiate the immune response to cancer vaccines.

Among the various IAs, only a few encompassing TLR-3, −4, 7/8 and 9-agonists represent promising cancer immunotherapeutic agents and have been included in the ranked National Cancer Institute's list of immune drugs with high potential to treat cancer [53].

Most TLR agonists induce IL-12 or IFN-α production and thereby promote generation of T effector cells. TLR agonists that have been widely investigated include (a) Gram- bacteria lipopolysaccharide (LPS) and derivatives (e.g. lipid A and MPL), (b) polyriboinosinic-polycytidylic acid (Poly I:C), a synthetic analog of viral dsRNA that stimulates endosomal TLR-3, (c) the synthetic low-molecular weight imidazoquinolines imiquimod and resiquimod that induce cytokine production, costimulatory molecule and HLA I/II expression in APC by triggering TLR7 and, in the case of resiquimod only, TLR8, and (d) CpG oligonucleotides that bind TLR9 and activate innate immunity, cytokine production and Th1 differentiation [52].

Another IA family that has been used in cancer vaccinology is that of adjuvant emulsions, that include oil/water (O/W) and water/oil (WO) emulsions as free fatty acid, Montanide, and others. The best characterized IAs of this group are Montanides, that are based on purified squalene and squalene emulsified with highly purified mannide mono-oleate. There are different types of Montanide, including ISA 50 V, 51 and 720, that are W/O emulsions, and ISA 206, that is a W/O-in-water emulsion [53].

A further group of IA is liposome adjuvants that are particles composed of non viral lipids utilized to deliver antigens and adjuvants. Liposomes enhance humoral and cellular immunity to protein and polysaccharide antigens and help extend the half-life of antigens in blood, thus allowing higher antigen exposure to APCs after vaccination.

Table 11.1 summarizes the main categories of IA and their mechanisms of action.

IAs have been widely used to increase the immunogenicity of cancer vaccines in adult patients, whereas few studies incorporating IAs other than cytokines have been published in pediatric oncology. The first clinical trial, that included both pediatric and adult patients, investigated the prolonged subcutaneous administration of 852A, a systemic TLR7 agonist, to activate innate immune responses in patients with advanced hematologic malignancies. 825A activates APCs, leading to production of cytokines (IFN-α, TNF), upregulation of CCR7 driving migration of DCs to lymph nodes, and expression on APCs of co-stimulatory molecules necessary for T cell activation. Patients received 825A s.c. at the initial dose of 0.6 mg/m^2 twice weekly and escalated by 0.2 mg/m^2 after every two doses as tolerated to the targeted dose of 1.2 mg/m^2. The drug was safely administered at the latter dose, with evidence of good tolerability and clinical activity in hematologic malignancies [58].

Another study was a phase I/II trial of Wilms tumor 1 (WT1) peptide vaccination for children with relapsed or refractory solid and hematological malignancies. The WT1 gene maintains the oncogenic functions of tumor cells and is expressed in different types of malignancies. WT1 peptide was thawed, emulsified with Montanide ISA-51 at a 1:1 weight ratio and injected intradermally in various body regions at different concentrations (0.5–3 mg) depending on the weight of the patient. WT1 peptide vaccination was performed every week 12 times. Vaccination proved to be safe and to induce WT1-specific T cell responses. Of the two groups of patients studied; those patients who received vaccination after allogeneic HSC transplant displayed the highest rate of complete remission, likely due to the more favorable immune environment [59]. The results of this study are consistent with those from two previous pediatric clinical trials, the first performed in children and young adults with various malignancies, the second in leukemic patients at high risk of relapse who had received allogeneic HSC transplantation [60, 61].

Diffuse brainstem gliomas and other high-grade gliomas of childhood are poor prognosis malignancies for which different glioma associated antigens (GAAs) have been identified; these include EphrinA2, IL-13Rα2 and survivin. In a recent study, GAA-specific immune responses and clinical outcome were evaluated in 26 glioma patients treated with irradiation or irradiation and concurrent chemotherapy and subjected to vaccination with HLA-A2 restricted peptides from the above mentioned GAAs. The latter were emulsified in Montanide ISA-51 and injected s.c. Patients received concurrent intramuscular injections of the TLR3 ligand poly-ICLC (30 μg/kg) every 3 weeks for a total of 8 vaccines. Poly-ICLC is the already mentioned poly-IC stabilized with lysine and carboxymethylcellulose. Thus, in this trial, two IAs were associated, i.e. Montanide ISA-51, a vaccine delivery vehicle shown to promote in pre-clinical models sustained generation of antigen-specific CTLs, and Poly-ICLC, that was shown to increase the efficacy of GAA-directed vaccinations both in pre-clinical models and in adult glioma patients. Toxicities were predominantly local reactions at the injection site and flu-like symptoms that waned in a couple days and were easily manageable. In a half of patients specific immune responses to GAA-associated peptides were detected. Five children showed symptomatic pseudo progression that was controlled with dexamethasone and was associated with prolonged survival. Two children had partial responses and two had prolonged disease-free status after surgery [62].

More recently, the same group has published a pilot study in which 14 low-grade glioma patients were enrolled and vaccinated following exactly the same schedule. The results obtained confirm those of the previous study, showing that vaccination was generally well tolerated and providing preliminary evidence for immunological and clinical activity of the vaccine plus adjuvant [63].

A number of clinical trials based upon immunotherapy of pediatric tumors are ongoing. Although the approaches are heterogenous (e.g. vaccination with TAA peptides, tumor lysate pulsed autologous dendritic cells) the IAs most commonly administered are Montanide ISA-51, poly-IC and imiquimod [47].

In conclusion, clinical trials in which cytokines and/or other immune adjuvants have been administered to enhance the immune response of pediatric patients against autologous tumor cells are so far limited in number, but these approaches appear feasible and promising (Table 11.1). The landscape of cancer immunotherapy is evolving quickly and new scenarios are emerging which will soon impact on the reprogramming of anti-tumor immunity in pediatric oncology. Examples of new players in this field are the concept of immunogenic cell death whereby some chemotherapeutic drugs concur to enhance tumor immunogenicity, targeting of immune checkpoints such as PD-1 or CTLA-4 and their ligands which reinstate dampened anti-tumor immune responses, and the development of CAR T cells, whose dramatic efficacy in hematologic malignancies has been already established.

References

1. Rosenberg SA, et al. Cancer immunotherapy: moving beyond current vaccines. Nat Med. 2004;10:909–91.
2. Dahlberg CI, et al. Natural killer cell-based therapies targeting cancer: possible strategies to gain and sustain anti-tumor activity. Front Immunol. 2016;6:605.
3. Chung MJ, et al. Phase II clinical trial of ex vivo-expanded cytokine-induced killer cells therapy in advanced pancreatic cancer. Cancer Immunol Immunother. 2014;63:939–46.
4. Sadelain M. CAR therapy: the CD19 paradigm. J Clin Invest. 2016;125:3392–400.
5. Brenner MK. Gene-modified cells for stem cell transplantation and cancer therapy. Hum Gene Ther. 2014;25(7):563–9.
6. Young PA, et al. Antibody-cytokine fusion proteins for treatment of cancer: engineering cytokines for improved efficacy and safety. Semin Oncol. 2016;41:623–36.
7. Bowman IL, et al. IL-2 adenovector-transduced autologous tumor cells induce antitumor immune responses in patients with neuroblastoma. Blood. 1998;92:1941–9.
8. Welte K, et al. A randomized phase-III study of the efficacy of granulocyte colony-stimulating factor in children with high-risk acute lymphoblastic leukemia. Berlin-Frankfurt-Munster Study Group. Blood. 1996;87:3143–50.
9. Lehrnbecher T, Creutzig U. Myeloid growth factors as anti-infective measures in children with leukemia and lymphoma. Expert Rev Hematol. 2009;2:159–72.
10. Smith TJ, et al. Recommendations for the use of WBC growth factors: American society of clinical oncology clinical practice guideline update. J Clin Oncol. 2015;33:3199–212.

11. Kanakry CG, et al. Modern approaches to HLA-haploidentical blood or marrow transplantation. Nat Rev Clin Oncol. 2016;13(1):10–24.
12. Keating GM. Plerixafor: a review of its use in stem-cell mobilization in patients with lymphoma or multiple myeloma. Drugs. 2011;71:1623–47.
13. Ladenstein R, et al. Randomized trial of prophylactic granulocyte colony stimulating factor during rapid COJEC induction in pediatric patients with high-risk neuroblastoma. J Clin Oncol. 2010;28:3516–24.
14. Agarwal S, et al. G-CSF promotes neuroblastomatumorigenicity and metastasis via STAT3-dependent cancer stem cell activation. Cancer Res. 2015;75:2566–79.
15. Arenas-Ramirez N, et al. Interleukin-2: biology design and application. Trends Immunol. 2015;36:763–77.
16. Furtado GC, et al. Interleukin 2 signaling is required for $CD4^+$ regulatory T cell function. J Exp Med. 2002;196:851–7.
17. Rosenberg SA, et al. NIH conference. New approaches to the immunotherapy of cancer using interleukin-2. Ann Intern Med. 1988;108:853–64.
18. Negrier S, et al. Interleukin-2 and lymphokine-activated killer cells in 15 children with advanced metastatic neuroblastoma. J Clin Oncol. 1991;9:1363–70.
19. Pais RC, et al. Phase I study of recombinant human interleukin-2 for pediatric malignancies: feasibility of outpatient therapy. A pediatric oncology group study. J Immunother. 1992;12:138–46.
20. Truitt RL, et al. Immunological evaluation of pediatric cancer patients receiving recombinant interleukin-2 in a phase I trial. J Immunother. 1991;11:274–85.
21. Valteau-Couanet D, et al. Phase I-II study of interleukin-2 after high-dose chemotherapy and autologous bone marrow transplantation in poorly responding neuroblastoma. Bone Marrow Transplant. 1995;16:515–20.
22. Bauer M, et al. A phase II trial of human recombinant interleukin-2 administered as a 4-day continuous infusion for children with refractory neuroblastoma, non-Hodgkin's lymphoma, sarcoma, renal cell carcinoma, and malignant melanoma. A children cancer group study. Cancer. 1995;75:2959–65.
23. Sievers EL, et al. Feasibility, toxicity, and biologic response of interleukin-2 after consolidation chemotherapy for acute mylogenous leukemia: a report from the Children's cancer group. J Clin Oncol. 1998;16:914–9.
24. Pession A, et al. Immunotherapy with low dose recombinant interleukin-2 after high dose chemotherapy and autologous stem cell transplantation in neuroblastoma. Br J Cancer. 1998;78:528–33.
25. Ladenstein R, et al. Dose finding study for the use of subcutaneous recombinant interleukin-2 to augment natural killer cell numbers in an outpatient setting for stage 4neuroblastoma after megatherapy and autologous stem-cell reinfusion. J Clin Oncol. 2011;29:441–8.
26. Yu AL, et al. Phase I trial of a human-mouse chimeric anti-disialoganglioside monoclonal antibody ch14.18 in patients with refractory neuroblastoma and osteosarcoma. J Clin Oncol. 1998;19:4189–94.
27. Simon T, et al. Consolidation treatment with chimeric anti-GD2-antibody ch14.18 in children older than 1 year with metastatic neuroblastoma. J Clin Oncol. 2004;22(17):3549–57.
28. Yu AL, et al. Anti-GD2 antibody with GM-CSF, interleukin-2, and isotretinoin for neuroblastoma. N Engl J Med. 2010;363:1324–34.
29. Villablanca JG, et al. Phase I trial of 13-cis-retinoic acid in children with neuroblastoma following bone marrow transplantation. J Clin Oncol. 1995;13(4):894–901.
30. Yamane BH, et al. The development of antibody-IL2 based immunotherapy with hu14.18-IL2 (EMD-273063) in melanoma and neuroblastoma. Expert Opin Investig Drugs. 2009;18:991–1000.
31. Osenga KL, et al. A phase I clinical trial of the hu14.18-IL2 (EMD 273063) as a treatment for children with refractory of recurrent neuroblastoma and melanoma. Clin Cancer Res. 2006;12:1750–9.

32. Shusterman S, et al. Antitumor activity of huch14.18-IL2 in patients with relapsed/refractory neuroblastoma: a Children's oncology group (COG) phase II study. J Clin Oncol. 2010;28:4969–75.
33. Bachanova V, et al. Clearance of acute myeloid leukemia by haploidentical natural killer cells is improved using IL-2 diphteria toxin fusion protein. Blood. 2014;123:3855–63.
34. Zhang H, et al. Lymphopenia and interleukin-2 therapy alter homeostasis of $CD4^{-}CD25^{+}$ regulatory T cells. Nat Med. 2005;11:1238–43.
35. Shah NN, et al. Acute GVHD in patients receiving IL-15/4-1 BBL activated NK cells following T-cell-depleted stem cell transplantation. Blood. 2015;125:784–92.
36. Kennedy-Nasser AA, et al. Ultra low-dose IL-2 for GVHD prophylaxis after allogeneic hematopoietic stem cell transplantation mediates expansion of regulatory T cells without diminishing antiviral and antileukemic activity. Clin Cancer Res. 2014;20:2215–25.
37. Abrahamsen TG, et al. A phase I and II trial of dise-intensified cyclophosphamide and GM-CSF in pediatric malignant brain tumors. J Pediatr Hematol Oncol. 1995;17:134–9.
38. Kushner BH, et al. Phase II trial of the anti-G(D2) monoclonal antibody 3F8 and granulocyte-macrophage colony-stimulating factor for neuroblastoma. J Clin Oncol. 2001;19:4189–94.
39. Ozkaynak MF, et al. Phase I study of chimeric human/murine anti-ganglioside G(D2) monoclonal antibody (ch14.18) with granulocyte-macrophage colony-stimulating factor in children with neuroblastoma immediately after hematopoietic stem-cell transplantation: a Children's cancer group study. J Clin Oncol. 2000;18:4077–85.
40. NKV C, et al. Key role for myeloid cells: phase II results of anti-G_{D2} antibody 3F8 plus granlocyte-macrophage colony stimulating factor for chemoresistant osteomedullary neuroblastoma. Int J Cancer. 2014;135:2199–205.
41. Navid F, et al. The feasibility of adjuvant interferon α-2b in children with high-risk melanoma. Cancer. 2005;103:780–7.
42. Petropoulos D, et al. Interferon-a after autologous stem cell transplantation in pediatric patients with advanced Hodgkin's lymphoma. Bone Marrow Transplant. 2006;38:345–9.
43. Lauer SJ, et al. Recombinant alpha-2B interferon treatment for childhood T-lymphoblastic leukemia disease in relapse. A pediatric oncology group phase II study. Cancer. 1994;74:197–202.
44. Warren K, et al. A phase 2 study of pegylated interferon α-2b (PEG-intron) in children with diffuse intrinsic pontine glioma. Cancer. 2012;118:3607–13.
45. Cavalheiro S, et al. Use of interferon alpha in intratumoral chemotherapy for cystic craniopharyngioma. Childs Nerv Syst. 2005;21:719–24.
46. Bielack SS, et al. Methotrexate, doxorubicin, and Cisplatin (MAP) plus maintenance pegylated interferon Alfa-2b versus MAP alone in patients with resectable high-grade osteosarcoma and good histologicresponse to preoperative MAP: first results of the EURAMOS-1 good response randomized controlled trial. J Clin Oncol. 2015;33:2279–87.
47. Mackall CL, et al. Immune-based therapies for childhood cancer. Nat Rev Clin Oncol. 2014;11:693–703.
48. Cicchelero L, et al. Various ways to improve whole cancer cell vaccine. Exper Rev Vaccines. 2014;13:721–35.
49. Berzofsky JA, et al. Strategies to use immune modulators in therapeutic vaccine against cancer. Semin Oncol. 2012;29:348–57.
50. Banday AH, et al. Cancer vaccine adjuvants-recent clinical progress and future perspectives. Immunopharmacol Immunotoxicol. 2015;37:1–11.
51. Capitini CM, et al. Immune-based therapeutics for pediatric cancer. Expert Opin Biol Ther. 2010;10:161–78.
52. Steinhagen F, et al. TLR-based immune adjuvants. Vaccine. 2011;29:3341–55.
53. Tefit NJ, Serra V. Outlining novel cellular adjuvant products for therapeutic vaccines against cancer. Expert Rev Vaccines. 2011;10:1207–20.
54. Heldwein KA, et al. TLR2 and TLR4 serve distinct roles in the host immune response against Mycobacterium Bovis BCG. J Leuk Biol. 2003;74:277–86.

55. Von Meyenn F, et al. Toll-like receptor 9 contributes to recognition of Mycobacterium Bovis bacillus Calmette-Guerin by Flt3-ligand generated dendritic cells. Immunobiology. 2006;211:557–65.
56. Ogita S, et al. Intracystic injection of OK-432: anew sclerosing therapy for cystic hygroma in children. Br J Surg. 1987;74:690–1.
57. Laranne J, et al. OK-432 (Picibanil) therapy for lymphangiomas in children. Eur Arch Otorhinolaryngol. 2002;259:274–8.
58. Weigel B, et al. Prolonged subcutaneous administration of 825A, a novel systemic toll-like receptor 7 agonist, to activate innate immune responses in patients with advanced hematologic malignancies. Am J Hematol. 2012;87:953–6.
59. Sawada A, et al. Feasibility of cancer immunotherapy with WT1 peptide vaccination for solid and hematological malignancies in children. Pediatr Blood Cancer. 2016;63:234–41.
60. Hashii Y, et al. WT1 peptide immunotherapy for cancer in children and young adults. Pediatr Blood Cancer. 2010;55:352–5.
61. Hashii Y, et al. WT1Peptide vaccination following allogeneic stem cell transplantation in pediatric leukemic patients with high risk for relapse. Successful maintenance of durable remission. Leukemia. 2012;26:530–2.
62. Pollack IF, et al. Antigen-specific immune responses and clinical outcome after vaccination with glioma-associated antigen peptides and polyinosinic-polycytidylic acid stabilized by lysine and carboxymethyl cellulose in children with newly diagnosed malignant brainstem and non brainstem gliomas. J Clin Oncol. 2014;32:2050–8.
63. Pollack IF, et al. Immune responses and outcome after vaccination with glioma-associated antigen peptides and poly-ICLC in a pilot study for pediatric recurrent low-grade gliomas. Neuro-Oncology. 2016;18(8):1157–68. doi:10.1093/neuonc/now026.

Chapter 12
Immune Biomarkers in Paediatric Malignancies

Michaela Semeraro, Claudia Pasqualini, and Nathalie Chaput

Abstract During the last decade, biomarkers have played an increasingly important role in the development of novel targeted cancer therapies. Since such treatments are rarely effective in all patients, predictive biomarkers to identify those most likely to benefit from a specific therapy are useful. Identification of biomarkers may also improve our understanding of how treatments work, as well as resistance mechanisms, and thus be used not only to anticipate clinical benefit but also the toxicity of a candidate drug. This applies similarly to the identification of immunological biomarkers associated with immunotherapies. The objective of such immunomonitoring is to identify prognostic but also predictive immune biomarkers in patients. Today, reliable identification of biomarkers is a necessary step to personalized treatment for cancer patients. An evaluation of the immune profile and/or the molecular profile of the tumor is expected to optimize the treatment for a better chance of therapeutic benefit. This can also apply to pediatric tumors. Here we will describe the main immunological biomarkers that have been described in patients with pediatric tumor.

M. Semeraro (✉)
Unité de Recherche Clinique et Centre d'Investigation Clinique 1419, Paris Descartes-Université Sorbonne Paris Cité, Hôpital Universitaire Necker Enfants malades Assistance Publique-Hôpitaux de Paris, 149 Rue de Sèvres, 75015 Paris, France

Unité INSERM 1015 Gustave Roussy Cancer Campus, Villejuif, France
e-mail: michaela.semeraro@aphp.fr

C. Pasqualini
Laboratoire d'immunomonitoring en Oncologie UMS 3655 CNRS / US 23 INSERM, Gustave Roussy Cancer Campus, Villejuif, France

Département de, Cancérologie de l'Enfant et de l'Adolescent, Gustave Roussy Cancer Campus, Villejuif, France

N. Chaput
Laboratoire de Thérapie Cellulaire, Gustave Roussy Cancer Campus, Villejuif, France

Laboratoire d'immunomonitoring en Oncologie UMS 3655 CNRS / US 23 INSERM, Gustave Roussy Cancer Campus, Villejuif, France

Département de, Cancérologie de l'Enfant et de l'Adolescent, Gustave Roussy Cancer Campus, Villejuif, France

J.C. Gray, A. Marabelle (eds.), *Immunotherapy for Pediatric Malignancies*,
https://doi.org/10.1007/978-3-319-43486-5_12

Keywords Paediatric malignancies • Immune biomarkers • Tumour-associated macrophages • T lymphocytes • Natural killer (NK) cells • Cytokines • Chemokines • Glycoproteins • Immune checkpoint

12.1 Introduction

The need for significant molecular biomarkers of survival, response and/or toxicity in cancer treatment is particularly strong in the era of personalized medicine [1]. The increasing development of immunotherapy strategies requires immunologic biomarkers to improve the clinical efficacy of immunotherapies and our ability to stratify patients rationally for therapeutic intervention [2]. Accurate biomarkers are critical for earlier diagnosis, improved precision of administration of expensive and potentially toxic therapies in selected patients, and for monitoring therapeutic effects and disease progression. Recent technical improvements in evaluations of immune cells *in situ* and immune monitoring of children with cancer [3–5] have provided data confirming that immune cells play a key role in paediatric cancer development and progression. A number of potentially promising immune biomarkers have emerged [6, 7], but most remain to be validated.

In order to obtain a long-term immune response, researchers focus on discovering immune targets specifics for the different types of children cancers but also understanding the mechanism underlying immune response or immune escape [8, 9].

Subsequently, two major tasks are important for paediatric oncologists working on immunotherapies:

- Identify predictive biomarkers for stratifying and sub grouping patients in order to ascertain the most responsive patient subgroup
- Perform longitudinal immune monitoring to test the effects of the immunotherapies in patients and, as ultimate goal, defining the surrogate immune function parameters which correlate with disease response and/or toxicities related to these immunotherapies. These studies will help (1) to define the best combinatorial strategies and (2) to better anticipate and treat immune-related toxicities.

Nevertheless, understanding a young children's immune status can be challenging for clinicians and investigators due to the limited availability of biosamples (especially for repeated blood samples). It is therefore vital that technologies that yield the most of information from the least material possible are identified.

Immune monitoring is essential to providing translational research during cancer immunotherapy. It consists of monitoring and characterizing quantitatively and/or qualitatively an immune response (Fig. 12.1). There are to date very few valid tests for routine clinical use; moreover, currently most biomarkers in adult or paediatric cancers are retrospectively validated, then a prospective evaluation and a robust development of a technique are needed in order to validate the predictive role of a

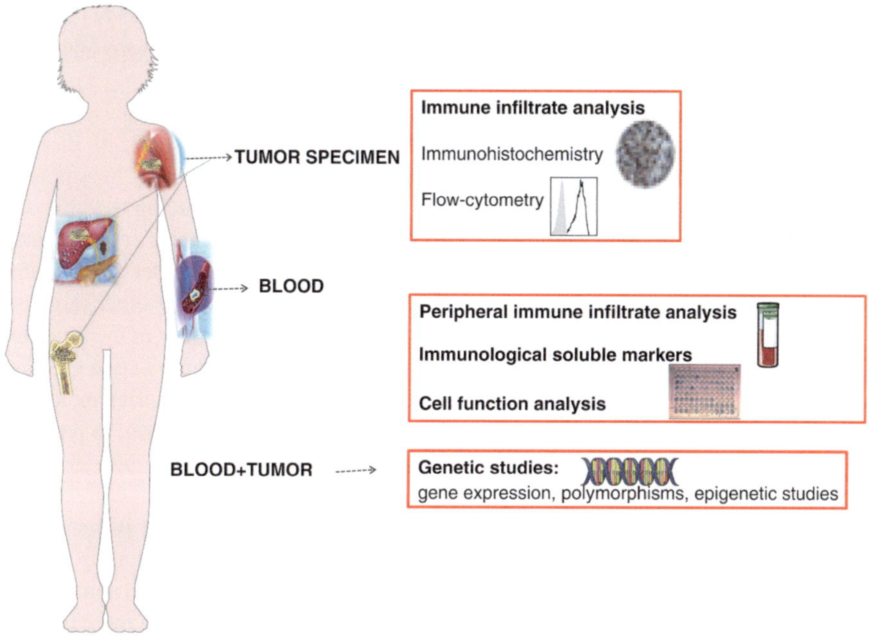

Fig. 12.1 The immunomonitoring tools in paediatric oncology: the tumor specimen and the peripheral blood can be informative to determine the tumor and the host immune profile

biomarkers [10]. Particularly in paediatric oncology, harmonization of the immune monitoring methods is fundamental, but challenging.

Different compartments can be analysed to establish an immune profile in paediatric cancer patients (Fig. 12.1):

- The tumour specimen: if the tumour sample is available (after surgery or biopsy), the analysis of the immune infiltrate can potentially be evaluated by immunohistochemistry or flow-cytometry. In the latter case, disaggregation of the tumour is needed. In the case of paediatric cancers that have metastasizes to the bone marrow then, bone marrow aspirations also potentially represent a tool for the immune monitoring [11–13].
- Blood sample: in paediatric patients the volume and frequency with which blood that can be taken, is limited. Nevertheless three blood compartments are available for immune monitoring: the mononuclear cells (T, B, NK lymphocytes, monocytes, dendritic cells), the serum where several immunological soluble markers could be analyzed (cytokines, chemokines, soluble receptors, soluble ligands) and the whole blood where an exhaustive immune phenotype and cellular quantification can be done, including analysis of the neutrophil population.

Successful immune-monitoring technology requires standardizion and validation of immune assays to ensure reliability of both cellular and soluble biomarkers (e.g. immunohistochemistry, flow-cytometry, ELISA). Standardized assays [14, 15] are now available to analyze secreted cytokines, cell subsets and functions and gene expression.

Conventional therapies often establish a state of minimal residual disease in paediatric cancer patients, but in which there remains a significant risk of disease relapse. This may offer a window where some form of immunotherapy may potentially be effective in eradicating remaining tumour cells, and reducing the chances of relapse [16]. Although significant progress has been made in in recent years, further efforts are needed in the field of paediatric oncology in order to combine immune therapies with each other or with conventional therapies or other targeted therapies, to fully utilize the natural complexity and interactive nature of the immune system. To achieve this goal major efforts are needed to identify predictive cellular and soluble biomarkers specific for each disease. As with adult malignancies,, a biomarker requires some specific characteristics for clinical application, in particular it has to be accurately measured, feasible to measure and it has to be validated. A biomarker may be useful at several time points: predicting the possible risk of disease, improving the detection of cancer and support the probability of benefit or toxicity from an immunotherapy approach. A better knowledge of naturally occurring immune effector mechanisms in paediatric oncology has led to novel approaches such as unconjugated and conjugated monoclonal antibodies (mAbs), and chimeric antigen receptors (CARs) which have proved their effectiveness in phase I-II and III trials [17, 18]. Nevertheless, compared to adult cancer patients, there are no validated immune biomarkers in clinical practice. The majority of studies on the interaction between the immune system and cancer cells have been performed in adult tumours. Immunohistochemical analysis of adult cancers often reveal a significant infiltration of leukocytes, either intratumoral or peritumoral, at the edges of the tumour tissue between the tumour islands and their stromal component. It has been suggested that the features of the tumours microenvironment infiltration with T-cells, especially cytotoxic tumour infiltrating CD8+ T-cells (CD8+TILs) allows more powerful prognostic staging than traditional staging, and the results of the immune infiltration cells ("immunoscore") are now considered as a new component for the classification of cancer (TNM-Immune) [19, 20]. In contrast, paediatric tumours present a relative paucity of lymphocytes and dendritic cells, highlighting the potential difference in immune environment of paediatric *vs* adult tumours. Here we describe the known immune biomarkers for the most common paediatric cancers according to the source of each biomarker.

12.2 Tumor-Infiltrating Immune Cells

The immunohistochemical studies of paediatric cancers have shown that in children, the infiltrating cells are predominantly macrophages (more than twofold higher than T cells) with rare other cell types, and with almost absent dendritic cells [21]. The microenvironment in paediatric tumours might favour macrophage rather than dendritic cell differentiation from monocytes because of local signals such as hypoxia, tumour necrosis, and apoptosis [22].

12.2.1 *Tumour-Associated Macrophages (TAMs)*

The infiltrate of macrophages associates strongly with the presence of necrosis, with the exception represented by the osteosarcoma (OS), where macrophages and osteoclasts are well represented also in the non-necrotic areas of the tumours [23]. The tumour-associated macrophages (TAMs) may significantly contribute to tumour growth and metastasis and are associated with poor prognosis in various types of cancer, by promoting growth, angiogenesis and tumour cell motility [24]. In neuroblastoma (NB), the most common solid extracranial tumour in children, TAMS induce the IL-6 release in bone marrow which, in turn, induces NB growth and expansion [25]. Moreover, the high-level expression of TAM-specific genes (CD14, CD16, IL6, IL6R, and TGFB1) was associated with poor 5-year event-free survival. Song et al demonstrated that Valpha24-invariant natural killer T (NKT) cells could counter balance this immune evasion mechanism by killing TAMs directly. Also in haematological malignancies (leukaemia and lymphoma) the presence of TAMs has been associated with progressive disease by promoting and proliferation of leukemic stem cells in the bone marrow [26]. However, the presence of tumour-infiltrating macrophages at the time of diagnosis has been positively correlated with a favourable outcome of patients with osteosarcoma, thus suggesting macrophage-activating agents as an option to add to standard treatments [27].

12.2.2 *T Lymphocytes*

Infiltrating T cells in paediatric cancers are infrequent, and often functionally ineffective [28]. Lymphocytic infiltration has been described in neuroblastomas [29, 30], and some early studies have shown a positive correlation between their number and outcome [31]. In Ewing sarcoma (ES), tumour-infiltrating T-cells contain significantly higher percentages of CD8+ T-lymphocytes as compared to stroma-infiltrating cells, and they are associated to high expression of pro-inflammatory chemokines (CXCR3- and CCR5-ligands CXCL9, CXCL10, and CCL5). Survival analyses demonstrated an impact of tumour-infiltrating, and not stroma-infiltrating, CD8+ T-lymphocytes on Ewing sarcoma progression [32]. It is important to note that most of solid paediatric cancers down-regulate MHC-I expression, which means that cancer's cells are more susceptible to natural killer lymphocytes (NK) cell killing. This remark could explain why very rare naturally occurring specific T cell responses are observed against the numerous potential antigens of interest identified in paediatric solid tumours (ie GD2 in ES and NB, NY-ESO-1, IGF-1 and Her

Neu in sarcomas). On the other hand, the majority of ALL cases present class MHC –I expression [33] and some antigens have been identified as tumor antigens targeted by cytotoxic T lymphocytes-CTL (i.e. ETV6-AML1 and WT1) [34, 35]. Leukemic cells escape from CTLs killing by up-regulation of non-classical HLA-G molecules after chemotherapy [36]. Several studies have demonstrated the anti-correlation between the presence of T-regulatory cells (T-reg) at the tumour site and the survival in both solid and blood paediatric tumours [37, 38].

12.2.3 Natural Killer (NK) Cells

NK cells are a subset of innate immunity cells, capable of lysing tumor cells without prior sensitization. NK recognize target cells by the interactions between both activating and inhibitory receptors and their corresponding ligands; as mentioned before, the down regulation of the MHC class I in some paediatric cancers allow the cell can be identified as a target and then killed [39, 40]. Several biomarkers of tumoral NK sensitivity have been identified:

- Up regulation on cancer cells of the NK activating receptors ligands like B7 molecules (i.e. B7-H6), PVR (Poliovirus Receptor), Nectin-2, MICA and/or MICB. [41, 42].
- In situ NK downregulation of a specific NK activating receptor (NKp30, NKG2D) is often correlated with the specific receptor involvement and activation against cancer cells [43]
- Biomarkers of immune escape, mostly soluble forms of the already mentioned ligands (sMICA, sMICAB, sB7-H6), but also immune suppressive surface ligand like B7-H3 [44, 45].
- The presence of a KIR-mismatched donor NK cells in haematopoietic stem cell transplantation is well known to be an important biomarker to mediate a graft-versus-leukemia effect in acute myelogenous leukemia (AML) and acute lymphoblastic leukemia (ALL) [46–48].

However, despite T cell tumoral infiltration, NK cells seem to be important in antitumor response in their circulating fraction while the extravased NK cells (in situ tumour) seem to be exhausted then inactive [49].

12.3 Systemic Immune Biomarkers

Among systemic immune parameters, the total amount of lymphocyte cells has been demonstrated to be predictive of response to treatment: the prognostic value of lymphopenia has been established in advanced carcinomas, sarcomas, and lymphomas [50]. In the recent years, several studies have reported dysregulation of peripheral CD3+CD4+CXCR5+ cells in patients with breast cancer and lymphomas. A positive correlation between increased peripheral CD4+CXCR5+ T cells and tumour metastasis or high grade has been displayed in osteosarcoma, with a significantly higher proportion of Th1 and Th17 subsets in advanced stages and high grade tumours than those with localized or low grade osteosarcoma [51].

The role of NK cells seems to be crucial in several paediatric cancers, especially in neuroblastoma. The expression of NKp30 isoforms affecting the polarization of NK cell functions correlated with survival in patients with high-risk neuroblastoma in remission from metastases after induction chemotherapy. Moreover, serum concentration of soluble B7-H6 correlated with the down-regulation of NKp30, bone marrow metastases, and resistance to chemotherapy [43]. The impact of genotypes for killer immunoglobulin-like receptor (KIR), KIR ligands (HLA class I), and FCGR polymorphisms on the survival and on the response to treatment has also been reported in two cohorts of patients with relapsed/refractory neuroblastoma [39, 40, 52], thus supporting NK-cell mediated ADCC as one the main mechanism of action of anti-GD2 monoclonal antibodies.

We have already discussed the role of myeloid suppressor cells (MDSCs) in tumor infiltrate, moreover, several researches highlighted the negative prognostic impact of MDSCs increase in the peripheral blood in paediatric patients with metastatic sarcomas, high-risk neuroblastoma, non-Hodgkin lymphoma (NHL), and glioblastoma [53–55]. Elevated levels of CD14+ HLA-DRlo/neg monocytes are associated with aggressive disease and immune suppression via alteration of STAT signalling, increased IDO, arginase, iNOS, NOX2 and VEGF expression, prevention of DC maturation, and alteration of co-stimulatory and cytokine expression [56, 57].

Zhang and colleagues described a novel subset of MDSC known as fibrocytes, a unique population found circulating in the blood of patients with metastatic paediatric sarcomas, which mediate angiogenesis and do not expand T-cell populations like more typical fibrocytes involved in inflammatory responses [58].

12.4 Cytokines and Chemokines

12.4.1 Cytokines

Several studies have shown that cytokines might play important roles in regulating immune responses against cancer. Cytokines are easily measured in sera and in tumour microenvironment.

In bone sarcomas, IL-6 and IL-6 receptor interaction may contribute to the migration of tumour cells through integrin-linked kinase (ILK) and Akt, which in turn activates AP-1, resulting in the activations of ICAM-1[59]. At the genomic level also in NB and ependymoma the high expression of genes related to IL-6, IL-6R and inflammation is associated with more aggressive diseases [60, 61].

Macrophage migration inhibitory factor (MIF) is a pro-inflammatory cytokine overexpressed in a several types of cancer such as melanoma, glioblastoma, osteosarcoma and hepatocellular carcinoma. It participates to many aspects of tumour progression, including cell proliferation and survival, invasion of normal tissue, and angiogenesis [62]. Its correlation with tumour aggressiveness makes it a potential prognostic marker and may also serve as a therapeutic target. For instance, NB cells are able to produce high levels of MIF, which, in turn, cause induced T-cell death activation and contribute to NB progression by VEGF NB cell's production [63]. Furthermore NB can induce also the secretion of the pro-angiogenic chemokine IL-8 which blocks TRAIL-mediated apoptosis.

12.4.2 Chemokines

Chemokine is a type of cytokine that is produced as a "chemo-attractant molecules" mostly secreted by secreted by stromal cells, including fibroblasts and endothelial cells. Elevated chemokines levels are found in sera of paediatric cancer's patients and correlate with the clinical outcome. Among them:

- CXCL12 (CXCR4, CXCR7 ligand) is thought to mediate haematogenous metastases in several types of cancer [64, 65]. Increasing evidence indicates that CXCL12 can promote proliferation and survival in glioma [66] and glioblastoma [67] and that tumours expressing CXCR4 are more likely to migrate to organs with an abundant source of CXCL12. Previous studies have found the link between the expression of CXCR4 and an unfavourable outcome and metastasis. For instance, the high expression of the chemokine receptor CXCR4 on leukemic cells in children with ALL is strongly predictive for extramedullary organ involvement, independently of the peripheral lymphoblast count [68] or CXCR4 expression on tumoral cells is associated with poor survival of patients with bone sarcomas, such as osteosarcoma and Ewing sarcoma [69].
- CXCL4 and CXCL6 are highly expressed in osteosarcoma plasma samples and correlate with a poorer outcome [70].
- CCL2 produced by NB correlate with iNKT infiltration (positive correlation, Metelitsa 2004) and inversely correlate with N-Myc amplifications. This anti-correlation explains the different composition of tumor-infiltrating lymphocytes in MYCN amplified vs. MYCN non-amplified high risk tumors [71].
- In childhood acute lymphoblastic leukemia, the axis CXCR3-CXCL10 is involved in increased metastasis and confers resistance to chemotherapy, enhancing the chances for relapses [72].

12.5 Glycoproteins and Immune Checkpoint

- **Galectins**: Galectins belong to a family of proteins that contribute to neoplastic transformation, tumour cell survival, angiogenesis, and metastasis of tumour. Galectin-1 (Gal-1) and galectin-3 (Gal-3) are expressed by macrophages, epithelial cells, T cells, and fibroblasts. Galectin-3 has been reported to be involved in carcinogenesis, cell growth, cell adhesion, angiogenesis, and apoptosis [73]. Several studies have analysed the correlation between the expression of Gal-3 and clinicopathological parameters of different kinds of cancers [74]. With conflicting results Gal-1 expression level has been associated with tumour invasiveness and lymph node metastasis in neuroblastoma and osteosarcoma [75, 76]. In osteosarcoma, the serum level of both galectin-1 and -3 and their tissue expression were correlated with tumour stage, tumour invasion, and lymph node metastasis, suggesting that the galectin serum level might be considered as a potential marker in osteosarcoma patients. *Puchades et al.* showed a significant association between increased expression of Gal-1 in cancer cells and poor prognosis in patients with advanced-grade glioblastoma [77]. Further investigations are needed to identify molecular mechanisms of galectin-1 and -3 by targeting studies.

- **Neuropilins** (NRPs): NRP1 and NRP2 are type I transmembrane glycoproteins that have an important role in development, immunity and cancer. Their aberrant expression has been shown to promote tumorigenesis and metastasis *in vivo* in many solid tumours. The analysis of NRP1 and/or NRP2 immunostaining in patients with osteosarcoma identified NRP2 as an indicator of poor survival [78, 79], whereas results for NRP1 immunostaining value are conflicting [80]. Interestingly, patients with stage 4 and with NRP2 immunostaining in their primary tumours had a significantly shorter survival rate than patients with metastases but NRP2-negative tumours, thus underlining a potential role of NRP2 expression as a biomarker for patient's stratification at diagnosis.
- **Immune checkpoints**: With the new forthcoming era of immune checkpoint blockers (e.g. anti-CTLA-4 and anti-PD-1 monoclonal antibodies), new growing interest biomarkers are represented by the expression of inhibitory molecules CTLA-4 and PD1 [81] and by their ligands in paediatric tumors [82]. PD-1 and CTLA-4 signaling in the tumor microenvironment dampens immune responses to cancer and blocking this axis induces anti-tumor effects in several malignancies. PD1-positive lymphocytes and PD-L1 expression in tumor tissue were seen in 65% and 58% of 105 soft tissue sarcomas [83]. The positivity was also associated with worse clinical outcomes and higher clinical stage indicating a possible lead in the use of anti-PD1 in this type of sarcomas. Also in acute myeloid leukemia (AML) the expression of negative regulatory receptors like PD-1/PDL-1 correlates with a worse prognosis [84]. Investigations focusing on PD-L1 detection by immunohistochemistry have demonstrated the paediatric non-Hodgkin lymphoma (positivity: 80%), the glioblastoma (30%) and NB (14%) as positive PDL-1 target (Berghoff poster ASCO 2014 [38, 85]). Another study for PD-L1 expression has demonstrated on 115 pediatric tumors (collected at the time of diagnosis) that the proportion of PD-L1+ tumors was 86% for alveolar rhabdomyosarcoma, 72% for high-risk neuroblastoma, 57% for Ewing's sarcoma, 50% for embryonal rhabdomyosarcoma and 47% for osteosarcoma, supporting then the hypothesis that PD-1/PD-L1 blockade would be a viable treatment strategy (*Ferdousi Chowdhurya, Oncoimmunology 2015*).

12.6 Conclusion

Currently most of these biomarkers were identified retrospectively and prospectively in small cohort of patients. Prospective evaluation of large cohort of patients and development of robust technologies that can be integrated into routine clinical practice is mandatory. Techniques such as mass cytometry [86, 87], full exosome sequencing [87] TCR diversity analysis, and identification of specific activation markers will help to better characterize the immune responses. Analysis harmonization is an essential step, indeed inherent complexity of these analyses and development of immunomonitoring protocols in different laboratories are sources of the high variability and low reproducibility of data. Quality controls, publication of harmonized protocols and specific procedures [88] that could be used by different laboratories could be a way to overcome these limitations[89]. These steps will allow the comparison of data between laboratories and also facilitate the identification of relevant immune biomarkers with the ultimate goal to guide the development of new therapies.

Acknowledgements This work was supported by Gustave Roussy Cancer Campus, the Direction Générale de l'Offre de Soins (DGOS), the Institut National du Cancer (INCa), SIRIC SOCRATE (INCa DGOS INSERM 6043), Agence Régionale pour la Recherche (MMO program: ANR-10IBHU-0001). CP was sponsored by the "Etoile de Martin". MS was supported by the SIRIC-SOCRATE program.

References

1. Kalia M. Biomarkers for personalized oncology: recent advances and future challenges. Metabolism. 2015;64:S16–21.
2. Hodi FS, O'Day SJ, McDermott DF, Weber RW, Sosman JA, Haanen JB, Gonzalez R, Robert C, Schadendorf D, Hassel JC, Akerley W, van den Eertwegh AJ, Lutzky J, Lorigan P, Vaubel JM, Linette GP, Hogg D, Ottensmeier CH, Lebbe C, Peschel C, Quirt I, Clark JI, Wolchok JD, Weber JS, Tian J, Yellin MJ, Nichol GM, Hoos A, Urba WJ. Improved survival with ipilimumab in patients with metastatic melanoma. N Engl J Med. 2010;363:711–23.
3. Markiewicz K, Zeman K, Kozar A, Golebiowska-Wawrzyniak M, Wozniak W. Evaluation of selected parameters of specific immunity in children with osteosarcoma at various stages of antitumour treatment. Dev Period Med. 2014;18:155–68.
4. Pollack IF, Jakacki RI, Butterfield LH, Hamilton RL, Panigrahy A, Potter DM, Connelly AK, Dibridge SA, Whiteside TL, Okada H. Antigen-specific immune responses and clinical outcome after vaccination with glioma-associated antigen peptides and polyinosinic-polycytidylic acid stabilized by lysine and carboxymethylcellulose in children with newly diagnosed malignant brainstem and nonbrainstem gliomas. J Clin Oncol. 2014;32:2050–8.
5. Wong EC. Blood banking/immunohematology: special relevance to pediatric patients. Pediatr Clin North Am. 2013;60:1541–68.
6. Appin CL, Brat DJ. Biomarker-driven diagnosis of diffuse gliomas. Mol Aspects Med. 2015;45:87–96.
7. Weiland J, Elder A, Forster V, Heidenreich O, Koschmieder S, Vormoor J. CD19: a multifunctional immunological target molecule and its implications for Blineage acute lymphoblastic leukemia. Pediatr Blood Cancer. 2015;62:1144–8.

8. Hiroki CH, Amarante MK, Petenuci DL, Sakaguchi AY, Trigo FC, Watanabe MA, De Oliveira CE. IL-10 gene polymorphism and influence of chemotherapy on cytokine plasma levels in childhood acute lymphoblastic leukemia patients: IL-10 polymorphism and plasma levels in leukemia patients. Blood Cells Mol Dis. 2015;55:168–72.
9. Raffaghello L, Prigione I, Airoldi I, Camoriano M, Morandi F, Bocca P, Gambini C, Ferrone S, Pistoia V. Mechanisms of immune evasion of human neuroblastoma. Cancer Lett. 2005;228:155–61.
10. Hoos A, Britten CM, Huber C, O'Donnell-Tormey J. A methodological framework to enhance the clinical success of cancer immunotherapy. Nat Biotechnol. 2011;29:867–70.
11. Fei F, Lim M, George AA, Kirzner J, Lee D, Seeger R, Groffen J, Abdel-Azim H, Heisterkamp N. Cytotoxicity of CD56-positive lymphocytes against autologous B-cell precursor acute lymphoblastic leukemia cells. Leukemia. 2015;29:788–97.
12. Folgiero V, Goffredo BM, Filippini P, Masetti R, Bonanno G, Caruso R, Bertaina V, Mastronuzzi A, Gaspari S, Zecca M, Torelli GF, Testi AM, Pession A, Locatelli F, Rutella S. Indoleamine 2,3-dioxygenase 1 (IDO1) activity in leukemia blasts correlates with poor outcome in childhood acute myeloid leukemia. Oncotarget. 2014;5:2052–64.
13. Todorova R. Ewing's sarcoma cancer stem cell targeted therapy. Curr Stem Cell Res Ther. 2014;9:46–62.
14. Lea P. Multiplex planar microarrays for disease prognosis, diagnosis and theranosis. World J Exp Med. 2015;5:188–93.
15. Schumacher TN, Schreiber RD. Neoantigens in cancer immunotherapy. Science. 2015;348:69–74.
16. Capitini CM, Mackall CL, Wayne AS. Immune-based therapeutics for pediatric cancer. Expert Opin Biol Ther. 2010;10:163–78.
17. Haworth KB, Leddon JL, Chen CY, Horwitz EM, Mackall CL, Cripe TP. Going back to class I: MHC and immunotherapies for childhood cancer. Pediatr Blood Cancer. 2015;62:571–6.
18. Hochberg J, El-Mallawany NK, Cairo MS. Humoral and cellular immunotherapy in ALL in children, adolescents, and young adults. Clin Lymphoma Myeloma Leuk. 2014;14(Suppl):S6–13.
19. Galon J, Pages F, Marincola FM, Angell HK, Thurin M, Lugli A, Zlobec I, Berger A, Bifulco C, Botti G, Tatangelo F, Britten CM, Kreiter S, Chouchane L, Delrio P, Arndt H, Asslaber M, Maio M, Masucci GV, Mihm M, Vidal-Vanaclocha F, Allison JP, Gnjatic S, Hakansson L, Huber C, Singh-Jasuja H, Ottensmeier C, Zwierzina H, Laghi L, Grizzi F, Ohashi PS, Shaw PA, Clarke BA, Wouters BG, Kawakami Y, Hazama S, Okuno K, Wang E, O'Donnell-Tormey J, Lagorce C, Pawelec G, Nishimura MI, Hawkins R, Lapointe R, Lundqvist A, Khleif SN, Ogino S, Gibbs P, Waring P, Sato N, Torigoe T, Itoh K, Patel PS, Shukla SN, Palmqvist R, Nagtegaal ID, Wang Y, D'Arrigo C, Kopetz S, Sinicrope FA, Trinchieri G, Gajewski TF, Ascierto PA, Fox BA. Cancer classification using the Immunoscore: a worldwide task force. J Transl Med. 2012;10:205.
20. Mlecnik B, Tosolini M, Kirilovsky A, Berger A, Bindea G, Meatchi T, Bruneval P, Trajanoski Z, Fridman WH, Pages F, Galon J. Histopathologic-based prognostic factors of colorectal cancers are associated with the state of the local immune reaction. J Clin Oncol. 2011;29:610–8.
21. Vakkila J, Jaffe R, Michelow M, Lotze MT. Pediatric cancers are infiltrated predominantly by macrophages and contain a paucity of dendritic cells: a major nosologic difference with adult tumors. Clin Cancer Res. 2006;12:2049–54.
22. Murdoch C, Giannoudis A, Lewis CE. Mechanisms regulating the recruitment of macrophages into hypoxic areas of tumors and other ischemic tissues. Blood. 2004;104:2224–34.
23. Endo-Munoz L, Evdokiou A, Saunders NA. The role of osteoclasts and tumour-associated macrophages in osteosarcoma metastasis. Biochim Biophys Acta. 2012;1826:434–42.
24. Lin EY, Pollard JW. Role of infiltrated leucocytes in tumour growth and spread. Br J Cancer. 2004;90:2053–8.
25. Song L, Asgharzadeh S, Salo J, Engell K, Wu HW, Sposto R, Ara T, Silverman AM, Declerck YA, Seeger RC, Metelitsa LS. Valpha24-invariant NKT cells mediate antitumor activity via killing of tumor-associated macrophages. J Clin Invest. 2009;119:1524–36.

26. Gao L, Yu S, Zhang X. Hypothesis: Tim-3/galectin-9, a new pathway for leukemia stem cells survival by promoting expansion of myeloid-derived suppressor cells and differentiating into tumor-associated macrophages. Cell Biochem Biophys. 2014;70:273–7.
27. Buddingh EP, Kuijjer ML, Duim RA, Burger H, Agelopoulos K, Myklebost O, Serra M, Mertens F, Hogendoorn PC, Lankester AC, Cleton-Jansen AM. Tumor-infiltrating macrophages are associated with metastasis suppression in high-grade osteosarcoma: a rationale for treatment with macrophage activating agents. Clin Cancer Res. 2011;17:2110–9.
28. Rivoltini L, Arienti F, Orazi A, Cefalo G, Gasparini M, Gambacorti-Passerini C, Fossati-Bellani F, Parmiani G. Phenotypic and functional analysis of lymphocytes infiltrating paediatric tumours, with a characterization of the tumour phenotype. Cancer Immunol Immunother. 1992;34:241–51.
29. Facchetti P, Prigione I, Ghiotto F, Tasso P, Garaventa A, Pistoia V. Functional and molecular characterization of tumour-infiltrating lymphocytes and clones thereof from a major-histocompatibility-complex-negative human tumour: neuroblastoma. Cancer Immunol Immunother. 1996;42:170–8.
30. Kataoka Y, Matsumura T, Yamamoto S, Sugimoto T, Sawada T. Distinct cytotoxicity against neuroblastoma cells of peripheral blood and tumor-infiltrating lymphocytes from patients with neuroblastoma. Cancer Lett. 1993;73:11–21.
31. Martin RF, Beckwith JB. Lymphoid infiltrates in neuroblastomas: their occurrence and prognostic significance. J Pediatr Surg. 1968;3:161–4.
32. Berghuis D, Santos SJ, Baelde HJ, Taminiau AH, Egeler RM, Schilham MW, Hogendoorn PC, Lankester AC. Pro-inflammatory chemokine-chemokine receptor interactions within the Ewing sarcoma microenvironment determine CD8(+) T-lymphocyte infiltration and affect tumour progression. J Pathol. 2011;223:347–57.
33. Motawi TM, Zakhary NI, Salman TM, Tadros SA. Serum human leukocyte antigen-G and soluble interleukin 2 receptor levels in acute lymphoblastic leukemic pediatric patients. Asian Pac J Cancer Prev. 2012;13:5399–403.
34. Yang L, Han Y, Suarez Saiz F, Minden MD. A tumor suppressor and oncogene: the WT1 story. Leukemia. 2007;21:868–76.
35. Yotnda P, Garcia F, Peuchmaur M, Grandchamp B, Duval M, Lemonnier F, Vilmer E, Langlade-Demoyen P. Cytotoxic T cell response against the chimeric ETV6-AML1 protein in childhood acute lymphoblastic leukemia. J Clin Invest. 1998;102:455–62.
36. Pistoia V, Morandi F, Wang X, Ferrone S. Soluble HLA-G: Are they clinically relevant? Semin Cancer Biol. 2007;17:469–79.
37. Fritzsching B, Fellenberg J, Moskovszky L, Sapi Z, Krenacs T, Machado I, Poeschl J, Lehner B, Szendroi M, Bosch AL, Bernd L, Csoka M, Mechtersheimer G, Ewerbeck V, Kinscherf R, Kunz P. CD8/FOXP3-ratio in osteosarcoma microenvironment separates survivors from non-survivors: a multicenter validated retrospective study. Oncoimmunology. 2015;4:e990800.
38. Pistoia V, Morandi F, Bianchi G, Pezzolo A, Prigione I, Raffaghello L. Immunosuppressive microenvironment in neuroblastoma. Front Oncol. 2013;3:167.
39. Delgado DC, Hank JA, Kolesar J, Lorentzen D, Gan J, Seo S, Kim K, Shusterman S, Gillies SD, Reisfeld RA, Yang R, Gadbaw B, Desantes KB, London WB, Seeger RC, Maris JM, Sondel PM. Genotypes of NK cell KIR receptors, their ligands, and Fcγ receptors in the response of neuroblastoma patients to Hu14.18-IL2 immunotherapy. Cancer Res. 2010a;70:9554–61.
40. Delgado D, Webster DE, Desantes KB, Durkin ET, Shaaban AF. KIR receptor-ligand incompatibility predicts killing of osteosarcoma cell lines by allogeneic NK cells. Pediatr Blood Cancer. 2010b;55:1300–5.
41. Moretta L, Biassoni R, Bottino C, Mingari MC, Moretta A. Immunobiology of human NK cells. Transplant Proc. 2001;33:60–1.
42. Sivori S, Parolini S, Falco M, Marcenaro E, Biassoni R, Bottino C, Moretta L, Moretta A. 2B4 functions as a co-receptor in human NK cell activation. Eur J Immunol. 2000;30:787–93.
43. Semeraro M, Rusakiewicz S, Minard-Colin V, Delahaye NF, Enot D, Vely F, Marabelle A, Papoular B, Piperoglou C, Ponzoni M, Perri P, Tchirkov A, Matta J, Lapierre V, Shekarian T,

Valsesia-Wittmann S, Commo F, Prada N, Poirier-Colame V, Bressac B, Cotteret S, Brugieres L, Farace F, Chaput N, Kroemer G, Valteau-Couanet D, Zitvogel L. Clinical impact of the NKp30/B7-H6 axis in high-risk neuroblastoma patients. Sci Transl Med. 2015;7:283ra55.

44. Castriconi R, Dondero A, Augugliaro R, Cantoni C, Carnemolla B, Sementa AR, Negri F, Conte R, Corrias MV, Moretta L, Moretta A, Bottino C. Identification of 4Ig-B7-H3 as a neuroblastoma-associated molecule that exerts a protective role from an NK cell-mediated lysis. Proc Natl Acad Sci U S A. 2004;101:12640–5.
45. Wang L, Zhang Q, Chen W, Shan B, Ding Y, Zhang G, Cao N, Liu L, Zhang Y. B7-H3 is overexpressed in patients suffering osteosarcoma and associated with tumor aggressiveness and metastasis. PLoS One. 2013;8:e70689.
46. Leung W, Iyengar R, Turner V, Lang P, Bader P, Conn P, Niethammer D, Handgretinger R. Determinants of antileukemia effects of allogeneic NK cells. J Immunol. 2004;172:644–50.
47. Pende D, Marcenaro S, Falco M, Martini S, Bernardo ME, Montagna D, Romeo E, Cognet C, Martinetti M, Maccario R, Mingari MC, Vivier E, Moretta L, Locatelli F, Moretta A. Anti-leukemia activity of alloreactive NK cells in KIR ligand-mismatched haploidentical HSCT for pediatric patients: evaluation of the functional role of activating KIR and redefinition of inhibitory KIR specificity. Blood. 2009;113:3119–29.
48. Ruggeri L, Capanni M, Urbani E, Perruccio K, Shlomchik WD, Tosti A, Posati S, Rogaia D, Frassoni F, Aversa F, Martelli MF, Velardi A. Effectiveness of donor natural killer cell alloreactivity in mismatched hematopoietic transplants. Science. 2002;295:2097–100.
49. Larsen SK, Gao Y, Basse PH. NK cells in the tumor microenvironment. Crit Rev Oncog. 2014;19:91–105.
50. Ray-Coquard I, Cropet C, van Glabbeke M, Sebban C, Le Cesne A, Judson I, Tredan O, Verweij J, Biron P, Labidi I, Guastalla JP, Bachelot T, Perol D, Chabaud S, Hogendoorn PC, Cassier P, Dufresne A, Blay JY. Lymphopenia as a prognostic factor for overall survival in advanced carcinomas, sarcomas, and lymphomas. Cancer Res. 2009;69:5383–91.
51. Xiao H, Luo G, Son H, Zhou Y, Zheng W. Upregulation of peripheral CD4+CXCR5+ T cells in osteosarcoma. Tumour Biol. 2014;35:5273–9.
52. Lode HN, Jensen C, Endres S, Pill L, Siebert N, Kietz S, Ehlert K, Brock P, Valteau-Couanet D, Janzek E, Loibner H, Ladenstein R, Mueller I. Immune activation and clinical responses following long-term infusion of anti-GD_2 antibody ch14.18/CHO in combination with interleukin-2 in high-risk neuroblastoma patients. J Clin Oncol. 2014;32. 5s (suppl; abstr 10028)
53. Gowda M, Payne KK, Godder K, Manjili MH. HLA-DR expression on myeloid cells is a potential prognostic factor in patients with high-risk neuroblastoma. Oncoimmunology. 2013;2:e26616.
54. Lechner MG, Megiel C, Russell SM, Bingham B, Arger N, Woo T, Epstein AL. Functional characterization of human Cd33+ and Cd11b+ myeloid-derived suppressor cell subsets induced from peripheral blood mononuclear cells co-cultured with a diverse set of human tumor cell lines. J Transl Med. 2011;9:90.
55. Santilli G, Piotrowska I, Cantilena S, Chayka O, D'Alicarnasso M, Morgenstern DA, Himoudi N, Pearson K, Anderson J, Thrasher AJ, Sala A. Polyphenon [corrected] E enhances the antitumor immune response in neuroblastoma by inactivating myeloid suppressor cells. Clin Cancer Res. 2013;19:1116–25.
56. Hingorani P, Maas ML, Gustafson MP, Dickman P, Adams RH, Watanabe M, Eshun F, Williams J, Seidel MJ, Dietz AB. Increased CTLA-4(+) T cells and an increased ratio of monocytes with loss of class II (CD14(+) HLA-DR(lo/neg)) found in aggressive pediatric sarcoma patients. J Immunother Cancer. 2015;3:35.
57. Laborde RR, Lin Y, Gustafson MP, Bulur PA, Dietz AB. Cancer Vaccines in the World of Immune Suppressive Monocytes (CD14(+)HLA-DR(lo/neg) Cells): The Gateway to Improved Responses. Front Immunol. 2014;5:147.
58. Zhang H, Maric I, Diprima MJ, Khan J, Orentas RJ, Kaplan RN, Mackall CL. Fibrocytes represent a novel MDSC subset circulating in patients with metastatic cancer. Blood. 2013;122:1105–13.

59. Lissat A, Joerschke M, Shinde DA, Braunschweig T, Meier A, Makowska A, Bortnick R, Henneke P, Herget G, Gorr TA, Kontny U. IL6 secreted by Ewing sarcoma tumor microenvironment confers anti-apoptotic and cell-disseminating paracrine responses in Ewing sarcoma cells. BMC Cancer. 2015;15:552.
60. Griesinger AM, Josephson RJ, Donson AM, Mulcahy Levy JM, Amani V, Birks DK, Hoffman LM, Furtek SL, Reigan P, Handler MH, Vibhakar R, Foreman NK. Interleukin-6/STAT3 Pathway Signaling Drives an Inflammatory Phenotype in Group A Ependymoma. Cancer Immunol Res. 2015;3:1165–74.
61. Yang F, Jove V, Buettner R, Xin H, Wu J, Wang Y, Nam S, Xu Y, Ara T, Declerck YA, Seeger R, Yu H, Jove R. Sorafenib inhibits endogenous and IL-6/S1P induced JAK2-STAT3 signaling in human neuroblastoma, associated with growth suppression and apoptosis. Cancer Biol Ther. 2012;13:534–41.
62. Nishihira J, Ishibashi T, Fukushima T, Sun B, Sato Y, Todo S. Macrophage migration inhibitory factor (MIF): Its potential role in tumor growth and tumor-associated angiogenesis. Ann N Y Acad Sci. 2003;995:171–82.
63. Zhou Q, Yan X, Gershan J, Orentas RJ, Johnson BD. Expression of macrophage migration inhibitory factor by neuroblastoma leads to the inhibition of antitumor T cell reactivity in vivo. J Immunol. 2008;181:1877–86.
64. Li T, Li H, Wang Y, Harvard C, Tan JL, Au A, Xu Z, Jablons DM, You L. The expression of CXCR4, CXCL12 and CXCR7 in malignant pleural mesothelioma. J Pathol. 2011a;223:519–30.
65. Teicher BA, Fricker SP. CXCL12 (SDF-1)/CXCR4 pathway in cancer. Clin Cancer Res. 2010;16:2927–31.
66. Zhou Y, Larsen PH, Hao C, Yong VW. CXCR4 is a major chemokine receptor on glioma cells and mediates their survival. J Biol Chem. 2002;277:49481–7.
67. Barbero S, Bonavia R, Bajetto A, Porcile C, Pirani P, Ravetti JL, Zona GL, Spaziante R, Florio T, Schettini G. Stromal cell-derived factor 1alpha stimulates human glioblastoma cell growth through the activation of both extracellular signal-regulated kinases 1/2 and Akt. Cancer Res. 2003;63:1969–74.
68. Crazzolara R, Kreczy A, Mann G, Heitger A, Eibl G, Fink FM, Mohle R, Meister B. High expression of the chemokine receptor CXCR4 predicts extramedullary organ infiltration in childhood acute lymphoblastic leukaemia. Br J Haematol. 2001;115:545–53.
69. Sand, L. G., Scotlandi, K., Berghuis, D., Snaar-Jagalska, B. E., Picci, P., Schmidt, T., Szuhai, K. & Hogendoorn, P. C. 2015. CXCL14, CXCR7 expression and CXCR4 splice variant ratio associate with survival and metastases in Ewing sarcoma patients. Eur J Cancer.
70. Li Y, Flores R, Yu A, Okcu MF, Murray J, Chintagumpala M, Hicks J, Lau CC, Man TK. Elevated expression of CXC chemokines in pediatric osteosarcoma patients. Cancer. 2011b;117:207–17.
71. Song L, Ara T, Wu HW, Woo CW, Reynolds CP, Seeger RC, Declerck YA, Thiele CJ, Sposto R, Metelitsa LS. Oncogene MYCN regulates localization of NKT cells to the site of disease in neuroblastoma. J Clin Invest. 2007;117:2702–12.
72. Gomez AM, Martinez C, Gonzalez M, Luque A, Melen GJ, Martinez J, Hortelano S, Lassaletta A, Madero L, Ramirez M. Chemokines and relapses in childhood acute lymphoblastic leukemia: A role in migration and in resistance to antileukemic drugs. Blood Cells Mol Dis. 2015;55:220–7.
73. Fortuna-Costa A, Gomes AM, Kozlowski EO, Stelling MP, Pavao MS. Extracellular galectin-3 in tumor progression and metastasis. Front Oncol. 2014;4:138.
74. Chen HY, Liu FT, Yang RY. Roles of galectin-3 in immune responses. Arch Immunol Ther Exp (Warsz). 2005;53:497–504.
75. Cimmino F, Schulte JH, Zollo M, Koster J, Versteeg R, Iolascon A, Eggert A, Schramm A. Galectin-1 is a major effector of TrkB-mediated neuroblastoma aggressiveness. Oncogene. 2009;28:2015–23.

76. Esmailiejah, A. A., Taheriazam, A., Golbakhsh, M. R., Jamshidi, M., Shakeri, M., Yahaghi, E. & Moghtadaei, M. 2015. Analysis of serum levels and tissue expression of galectin-1 and galectin-3 as noninvasive biomarkers in osteosarcoma patients. Tumour Biol.
77. Puchades M, Nilsson CL, Emmett MR, Aldape KD, Ji Y, Lang FF, Liu TJ, Conrad CA. Proteomic investigation of glioblastoma cell lines treated with wild-type p53 and cytotoxic chemotherapy demonstrates an association between galectin-1 and p53 expression. J Proteome Res. 2007;6:869–75.
78. Boro A, Arlt MJ, Lengnick H, Robl B, Husmann M, Bertz J, Born W, Fuchs B. Prognostic value and in vitro biological relevance of Neuropilin 1 and Neuropilin 2 in osteosarcoma. Am J Transl Res. 2015;7:640–53.
79. Handa A, Tokunaga T, Tsuchida T, Lee YH, Kijima H, Yamazaki H, Ueyama Y, Fukuda H, Nakamura M. Neuropilin-2 expression affects the increased vascularization and is a prognostic factor in osteosarcoma. Int J Oncol. 2000;17:291–5.
80. Zhu H, Cai H, Tang M, Tang J. Neuropilin-1 is overexpressed in osteosarcoma and contributes to tumor progression and poor prognosis. Clin Transl Oncol. 2014;16:732–8.
81. Topalian SL, Hodi FS, Brahmer JR, Gettinger SN, Smith DC, Mcdermott DF, Powderly JD, Carvajal RD, Sosman JA, Atkins MB, Leming PD, Spigel DR, Antonia SJ, Horn L, Drake CG, Pardoll DM, Chen L, Sharfman WH, Anders RA, Taube JM, Mcmiller TL, Xu H, Korman AJ, Jure-Kunkel M, Agrawal S, Mcdonald D, Kollia GD, Gupta A, Wigginton JM, Sznol M. Safety, activity, and immune correlates of anti-PD-1 antibody in cancer. N Engl J Med. 2012;366:2443–54.
82. Mackall CL, Merchant MS, Fry TJ. Immune-based therapies for childhood cancer. Nat Rev Clin Oncol. 2014;11:693–703.
83. Kim JR, Moon YJ, Kwon KS, Bae JS, Wagle S, Kim KM, Park HS, Lee H, Moon WS, Chung MJ, Kang MJ, Jang KY. Tumor infiltrating PD1-positive lymphocytes and the expression of PD-L1 predict poor prognosis of soft tissue sarcomas. PLoS One. 2013;8:e82870.
84. Norde WJ, Maas F, Hobo W, Korman A, Quigley M, Kester MG, Hebeda K, Falkenburg JH, Schaap N, De Witte TM, van der Voort R, Dolstra H. PD-1/PD-L1 interactions contribute to functional T-cell impairment in patients who relapse with cancer after allogeneic stem cell transplantation. Cancer Res. 2011;71:5111–22.
85. Chen BJ, Chapuy B, Ouyang J, Sun HH, Roemer MG, Xu ML, Yu H, Fletcher CD, Freeman GJ, Shipp MA, Rodig SJ. PD-L1 expression is characteristic of a subset of aggressive B-cell lymphomas and virus-associated malignancies. Clin Cancer Res. 2013;19:3462–73.
86. Chang S, Kohrt H, Maecker HT. Monitoring the immune competence of cancer patients to predict outcome. Cancer Immunol Immunother. 2014;63:713–9.
87. Madhavan S, Gusev Y, Natarajan TG, Song L, Bhuvaneshwar K, Gauba R, Pandey A, Haddad BR, Goerlitz D, Cheema AK, Juhl H, Kallakury B, Marshall JL, Byers SW, Weiner LM. Genome-wide multi-omics profiling of colorectal cancer identifies immune determinants strongly associated with relapse. Front Genet. 2013;4:236.
88. Welters MJ, Gouttefangeas C, Ramwadhdoebe TH, Letsch A, Ottensmeier CH, Britten CM, van der Burg SH. Harmonization of the intracellular cytokine staining assay. Cancer Immunol Immunother. 2012;61:967–78.
89. van der Burg SH, Kalos M, Gouttefangeas C, Janetzki S, Ottensmeier C, Welters MJ, Romero P, Britten CM, Hoos A. Harmonization of immune biomarker assays for clinical studies. Sci Transl Med. 2011;3:108ps44.

Chapter 13
Future Perspectives

Aurelien Marabelle and Juliet C. Gray

Abstract Over the last 5 years, cancer immunotherapy has come of age. In particular, a new class of monoclonal antibodies has emerged, revolutionizing the treatment of many tumour types, and changing the paradigm of treatment in oncology by targeting immune cells rather than cancer cells. Antagonistic antibodies blocking immunosuppressive pathways such as PD-1/PD-L1 have shown anti-tumor activity in patients with advanced relapsed and refractory cancers that have failed conventional treatments. By enhancing their anti-tumor immunity, these drugs can help the patient's own immune system to take control of their cancer. Although this new class of antibodies has already show considerable benefit in adult cancers, their role in treating paediatric malignancies is as yet relatively unexplored and uncertain. In principle these antibodies are a 'generic' immunotherapy, and the same mechanisms of action should be applicable in paediatric and adult cancers. However, although the PD-1 and PD-L1 pathway is clearly active in paediatric cancers, there are other differences in the paediatric immune environment compared to cancers, which may make it more challenging to establish therapeutic immune responses. Realizing the full benefit of these exciting agents, as well as that of other cancer immunotherapeutics, in the paediatric population will depend on a number of factors, including identification of biomarkers and establishing how best to use these agents in combination with other therapies.

Keywords Checkpoint blockade • Monoclonal antibody • PD-1 • Immunotherapy • Paediatric cancer

---

A. Marabelle, M.D., Ph.D.
Département d'Innovation Thérapeutique et d'Essais Précoces, INSERM Lab U1015, Gustave Roussy, Université Paris-Saclay,
114, rue Édouard-Vaillant, Villejuif Cedex 94805, France
e-mail: aurelien.marabelle@gustaveroussy.fr

J.C. Gray, M.A., FRCPCH, Ph.D. (✉)
Cancer Sciences Unit, University of Southampton, Southampton, UK
e-mail: j.c.gray@soton.ac.uk

J.C. Gray, A. Marabelle (eds.), *Immunotherapy for Pediatric Malignancies*,
https://doi.org/10.1007/978-3-319-43486-5_13

13.1 Introduction

Over the last 5 years, cancer immunotherapy has come of age [1–4]. A new class of monoclonal antibodies has emerged, revolutionizing the treatment of many tumour types, and changing the paradigm of treatment in oncology by targeting immune cells rather than cancer cells. These immune-targeted therapies are designed to block immune checkpoint molecules expressed by immune cells. Antagonistic antibodies blocking immunosuppressive pathways such as CTLA-4/B7.1 and PD-1/PD-L1 have shown anti-tumor activity in patients with advanced relapsed and refractory cancers that have failed conventional treatments [5–10]. By enhancing their anti-tumor immunity, these drugs can help the patient's own immune system to take control of their cancer. The single blockade of the PD-1/PD-L1 pathway has shown a broad spectrum of activity across more than 20 cancer types (Fig. 13.1). Of course, not all patients respond to an anti-PD-1/PD-L1 monotherapy, but in those who do, the anti-tumor immune response developed can generate long lasting tumor responses which eventually turn into sustained benefits in overall survival for many cancer patients [11–14]. Although this new class of antibodies has already show considerable benefit in adult cancers, their role in treating paediatric malignancies is as yet relatively unexplored and uncertain. In principle these antibodies are a 'generic' immunotherapy, and the same mechanisms of action should be applicable in paediatric and adult cancers. However, although the PD-1 and PD-L1 pathway is clearly active in paediatric cancers [1], there are other differences in the paediatric immune environment compared to cancers which may make it more challenging to establish therapeutic immune responses [2]. Realizing the full benefit of these exciting agents, as well as that of other cancer immunotherapeutics, in the paediatric population will depend on a number of factors:

13.2 Identification of Predictive Biomarkers

Because the majority of patients do not develop objective tumor responses to immunotherapy, predictive biomarkers of response could help to stratify patients with good chances of responding to a monotherapy and intensify or the treatment of patients with low or no chance of responses. This is essential to avoid delivering potentially toxic treatments to children where there is little chance of response, and also to focus the use of these highly expensive agents on those patients who are likely to derive benefit.

One of the first proposed biomarkers of response to an anti-PD-1/PD-L1 monotherapy has been the level of expression of PD-L1 in the tumor micro-environment [6] and the level of tumor infiltrative CD8+ T-cells [15]. Stratification of patients based on the immune contexture of their tumor is therefore one promising way for the very near future [16, 17].

Also, within a cancer type, it seems that patients with the biggest number of somatic point mutation in their cancer cells DNA have a higher likelihood of

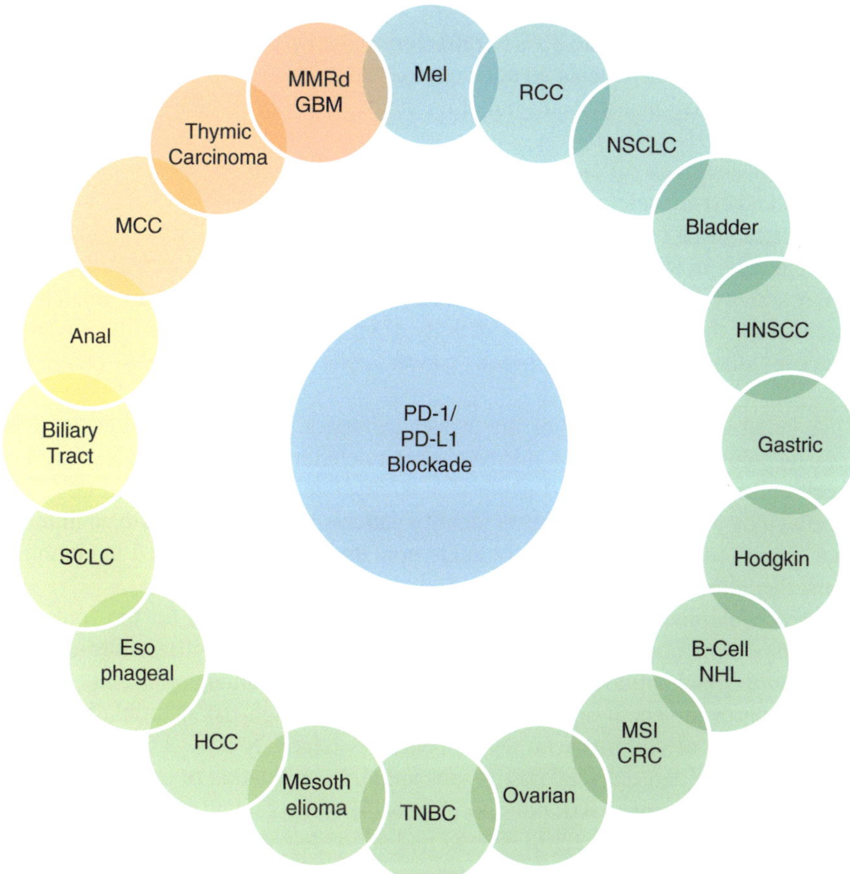

Fig. 13.1 Spectrum of activity of anti-PD-1/PD-L1 monoclonal antibodies. From 10% and up to 80% of patients can respond to an anti-PD-1/PD-L1 monotherapy depending on the cancer type. *Mel* melanoma, *RCC* Renal Cell Cancer, *NSCLC* Non-small cell lung cancer, *HNSC* Head and neck squamous cell carcinoma, *NHL* non hodgkin lymphoma, *MSI CRC* microsatellite instable colorectal cancers, *TNBC* Triple negative breast cancers, *HCC* Hepatocarcinoma, SCLC: Small cell lung cancers, *MCC* Merckel Cell Carcinoma, *MMRd GBM* Mismatch repair deficient glioblastoma

response to immune checkpoint blockade antibodies [18, 19]. This observation could be the consequence of the generation of immunogenic neoepitopes [20–22]. This hypothesis is currently supported by the high level of activity of anti-PD-1 therapy in patients bearing tumors with DNA mismatch repair deficiencies [23–26].

However, it is not understood why for the same level of somatic mutations, the immunogenicity of cancers varies across cancer types [27]. Also it is not clear why highly mutated cancers such as colo-rectal cancers do not respond to anti-PD-1/PD-L1 antibodies, whereas medium/low mutated cancers such as B-cell lymphomas respond well. Neither is it understood why anti-PD-1/PD-L1 antibodies can generate tumor responses in up to 80% of refractory stage IV Hodgkin lymphoma, where around 70% of these patients do not express MHC I on their cancer cells, while the common explanation is that anti-tumor immunity is driven by a CD8+/MHC-I pathway [10, 28, 29].

The mechanisms of action of these immunomodulatory antibodies remain unclear and do not solely rely on their antagonistic or agonistic properties. Indeed, the cells targeted by these antibodies, and the Fc-gamma receptors expressed on myeloid cells in the tumor microenvironment seems critical for their in vivo anti-tumor activity [30–34]. Also the presence and type of the host microbiota seems essential for the in vivo anti-tumor activity of immune checkpoint antibodies, with possible shared epitopes between cancer cells neoepitopes and pathogens [35–40].

A better characterization of the cancer cells (e.g. PD-L1 expression, level of somatic point mutations, DNA mismatch repair deficiency) and the host (e.g. level of T-cell infiltrate, level of PD-L1 expression on myeloid cells, level of PD-1 on CD8+ T-cells) may provide ways to better identify patients likely to respond to an immune checkpoint targeted, and rationally guide how they may be best used in combinational therapies.

The development of predictive biomarkers will also be vital for the continued development of other immunotherapies, including the now well-established anti-GD2 monoclonal antibody therapies in neuroblastoma. Although this class of antibody has proven benefit on outcome in children with high-risk neuroblastoma [3], the proportion of children who derive benefit is relatively low, and the treatment burden, toxicity and financial cost is substantial. Identification of biomarkers, such as Fc gamma receptor or KIR polymorphisms [4] will potentially restrict delivery to those children who are likely to benefit, and allow delivery of alternative therapies to children with unfavorable phenotypes.

Ultimately, it may be hoped that detailed immune profiling of the patient's tumour microenvironment will allow immunotherapy to be tailored accordingly. It may be possible, for instance, to identify those patients in whom it may be feasible to boost an endogenous anti-tumour response with check point blockade antibodies, and those in whom passive immunotherapies may be more beneficial, as well as for instance selecting immune adjuvants to co-administer that will best complement the patient's immune environment.

13.3 Synergistic Combinations

It is highly likely that the true benefit of most immunotherapies will not be as single agents, but through their use in combinational therapies, either with other immunotherapies, or combined with conventional therapies such as chemotherapy or radiotherapy.

13.3.1 *Combining Other Therapies with Checkpoint Blockade*

The concept of synergistic combinations of immunotherapies has been most widely investigated with respect to the checkpoint blockade agents. There is extensive preclinical data showing improved efficacy when used with other agents, through a variety of synergistic mechanisms. There are currently over 200 clinical trials in adult cancer patients involving the anti-PD-1 antibody Nivolumab, the majority of which are investigating it in combination with other agents. Of the combinations investigated clinically to date, perhaps the most impressive results have been seen by combining the two different checkpoint blockade antibodies, anti-CTLA-4 and anti-PD-1. This combination has already been approved in the USA for the treatment of metastatic melanoma [11], and also shows synergistic activity in SCLC and NSCLC [41–43]. It is perhaps surprising that two antibodies with apparently broadly similar mechanisms of action show such synergy, but this perhaps highlights that there is still a lot that we have to understand about these agents.

Other clinical trials are combining checkpoint blockade antibodies with chemotherapy, radiotherapy or with other immunotherapies. The huge number of potential combinations of agents that could be used, brings with it challenges, particularly in the paediatric population. It will not be feasible to test all potentially synergistic combinations in the relatively small numbers of children who are available to participate in early phase clinical trials. It is therefore important that data from preclinical models and adult patients is maximally used to identify combinations most relevant to paediatric tumours, to elucidate mechanisms of action and to identify potential biomarkers. This will allow prioritization of agents for testing in paediatric clinical trial as well as the design of early phase trials with pharmacodynamics and biomarker endpoints, which provide a signal of immune 'efficacy' at an early stage.

Many other immune checkpoint targeted antibodies are currently in clinical development, not only targeting co-inhibitory signals, but also targeting co-stimulatory signals with the aim of modulating T-cells (e.g. OX40, GITR), but also NK cells (e.g. NKG2A, CD137), dendritic cells (CD40), and macrophages (e.g. CD47, CSF1R). Many of these new immune targeted antibodies are already being investigated in combination with anti-PD-1/PD-L1 or anti-CTLA-4 antibodies with the hope that the synergistic activity seen in mouse tumor models will translate into patients with cancers.

Other potential strategies include combining with:

(a) Bispecific T-Cell Engagers
Besides immune checkpoint targeted antibodies, a new generation of immunomodulatory antibodies is in active development: the bispecific T-cell engager antibodies. These antibodies have two different arms: one arm directed at a tumor specific antigen, and one arm with agonistic properties to stimulate CD3. The aim of these antibodies is to directly activate any T-cell in the tumor microenvironment against the cancer cell. The advantage of such therapy is that it bypasses the need of a pre-existing antigen specific T-cell response, and an

expression of MHC expression. However, it is not known if they can work in tumors that are not infiltrated by T-cells, and if a tumor-specific memory immune response can be eventually generated by tumor antigen spreading. This type of immunotherapy has already become a clinical reality with the approval of blinatumomab, an anti-CD19xanti-CD3 bispecific T-cell engager, for the treatment of relapsing/refractory B-cell lymphoblastic leukemia (including in children). Several other compounds from the same class are currently in clinical development in acute myeloid leukemia and solid tumors. Most interestingly, some of these antibodies are already developed in combination with immune checkpoint targeted antibodies with the aim of boosting the anti-tumor response that is artificially generated with the bispecific compound (e.g. the anti-CEAxanti-CD3 antibody RO6958688 currently tested in combination with the anti-PD-L1 atezolizumab; NCT NCT02650713).

(b) Anti-angiogenic Compounds

Anti-angiogenic drugs, either monoclonal antibodies or tyrosine kinase inhibitors (TKI), blocking the VEGF/VEGFR pathway, have been shown preclinically to enhance immune cell trafficking into tumors and to synergize when used in combination with immune checkpoint blockades [44–47]. The combination of anti-PD-1/PD-L1 antibodies with anti-VEGF/VEGFR antibodies seems tolerable and is currently in development in many cancer indications (see clinicaltrials.gov). The combination of anti-PD-1/PD-L1 antibodies with anti-VEGF/VEGFR TKIs seems more difficult to develop. Indeed, depending on the TKI used, the level of treatment-related grade 3/4 adverse events might compromise such combination development [48].

(c) In situ Immunization

Preclinical model have shown that intratumoral injections of immunostimulatory products can overcome resistance to immune checkpoint blockade therapy. These immunostimulatory products of interest are mainly pattern recognition receptor agonists (such as agonists for Toll-like receptor 4 or 9) and oncolytic viruses [34, 49]. This type of strategy is coined intra-tumoral or "in situ" immunization because it aims at priming the anti-tumor immune response directly into the tumor where all the tumor antigens and immune effectors are present (or need to be attracted) [50].

Intra-tumoral toll-like receptors (TLR) have shown their ability to induce objective tumor responses both in injected and non-injected lesions (so called abscopal effect) [51, 52]. The combination of TLR agonists with immune checkpoint targeted antibodies is ongoing (NCT02501473, NCT02254772, NCT02680184).

Oncolytic viruses are common viruses (such as herpes or vaccinia virus) that have been selected and modified to preferentially infect and destroy cancer cells over healthy cells. These viruses can be injected either intra-venously or intra-tumorally. Some of them have also been genetically engineered to express a human pro-inflammatory cytokine to enhance the tumor inflammation and recruit new immune effectors in the tumor micro-environment. The first in class T-VEC, an herpes virus modified to express GM-CSF, has been recently approved for the intra-tumoral treatment of metastatic melanoma [53]. Most interestingly, T-VEC has shown promising synergistic activity when used in combination with anti-CTLA-4 or anti-PD-1 antibodies [54, 55]. A phase 3 clinical trial is currently testing the combination of T-VEC with pembrolizumab for patients with metastatic melanoma (NCT02263508).

(d) Oral Immunomodulators

Oral immunomodulators are also in clinical development with the aim of overcoming anti-PD-1/PD-L1 resistance. IDO (Indoleamine-pyrrole 2,3-dioxygenase) is an enzyme often expressed by cancer cells and which degrades tryptophan in the tumor microenvironment. Tryptophan being critical for the biology of T-cells, its depletion in the vicinity of tumors hampers the ability of anti-tumor T-cells to be fully functional [56]. Several IDO inhibitors are currently in clinical development in combination with anti-CTLA-4 or anti-PD-1/PD-L1. Preliminary results have shown promising synergistic activity in metastatic melanoma, RCC and NSCLC [57, 58].

Although anti-PD-1 have shown no activity in multiple myeloma, it has shown surprising activity in combination with IMIDs and dexamethasone, including in IMIDs refractory patients. Indeed, combinations of anti-PD-1 with either lenalidomide or pomalidomide and dexamethasone have shown objective responses in more than one patient out of two [59, 60]. Both combinations are actively pursued in phase 3 clinical trials in myeloma (NCT02579863, NCT02576977) but are also currently extended to other tumors types.

The examples of combinations mentioned above are the most innovative that are currently in active development. However, more incremental approaches are also currently studied in clinical trials testing immune checkpoint blockades with chemotherapy, radiotherapy, cytokines or tumor adapted therapies (e.g. everolimus, oncogene inhibitors, hormonotherapy) (Fig. 13.2). These combinations also have strong pre-clinical rationale, and some of these combinations have already shown preliminary promising synergistic activity. For instance, the anti-PD-L1 atezolizumab is currently developed in combination with chemotherapy in multiple phase 3 trials in first line NSCLC and TNBC (e.g. NCT02657434 and NCT02425891 respectively).

13.3.2 Other Immunotherapy Combinations

There has also been recent data suggesting synergy between the directly tumour targeting anti-GD2 monoclonal antibody and conventional chemotherapy. The US COG reported at ASCO in 2016 of response rate of 55% (9/17) in children with relapsed/refractory neuroblastoma receiving temozolamide and irinotecan in conjunction with dinutuxiamb (anti-GD2) and GM-CSF, as compared to a 5% objective response rate in the control arm (chemotherapy alone) [61]. In addition, Furman et al recently enhanced responses in children with recently diagnosed high risk

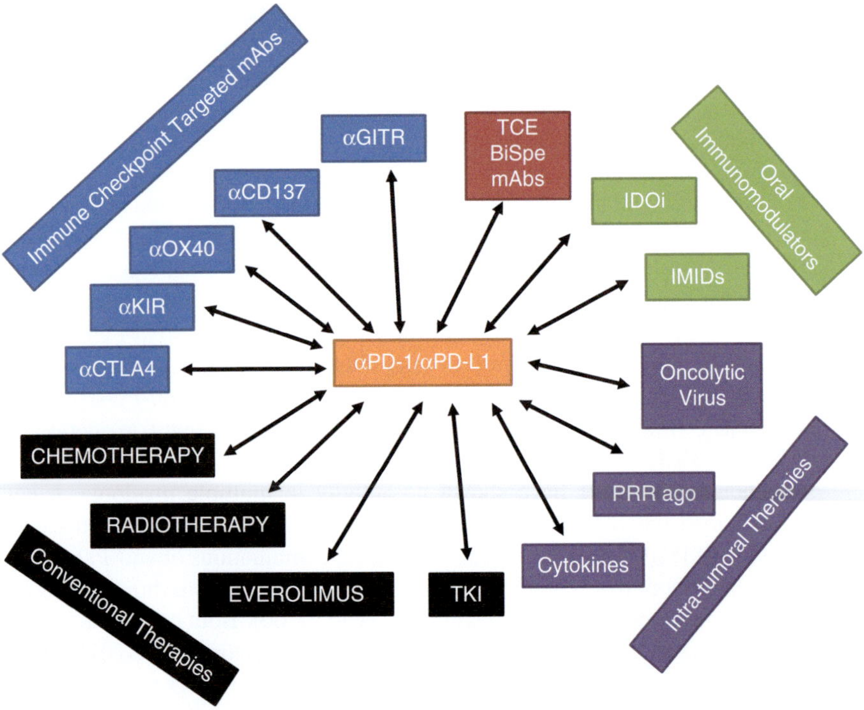

Fig. 13.2 Ongoing immunotherapy combinations

neuroblastoma receiving the humanized anti-GD2 antibody hu14.18K322A, GM-CSF and low dose IL-2, in conjunction with cyclophosphamide and topotecan induction chemotherapy [62]. The mechanism of this apparent synergy is not clear, but it again opens up the possibility of large numbers of potential combinational therapies, with an even larger range of possible dosing and scheduling possibilities. As a result of these studies, it is likely that anti-GD2 immunotherapies will be tested further in combination with chemotherapy, and explored further in the upfront setting, rather than in the context of minimal residual disease. The feasibility and toxicity of delivering this on a wider scale is unclear, but this will need careful monitoring.

13.4 Management of Immune-Related Toxicities

Because these novel immunotherapies are potently stimulating the immune system of cancer patients, they can be also responsible for auto-immune types of adverse events (Fig. 13.3). These so called "immune-related adverse events" (irAEs) can be either mild (CTCAE grade 1–2) or severe (CTCAE grade 3–4). Anti-PD-1/PD-L1 monotherapy only generate severe irAEs in about 10% of cancer patients treated,

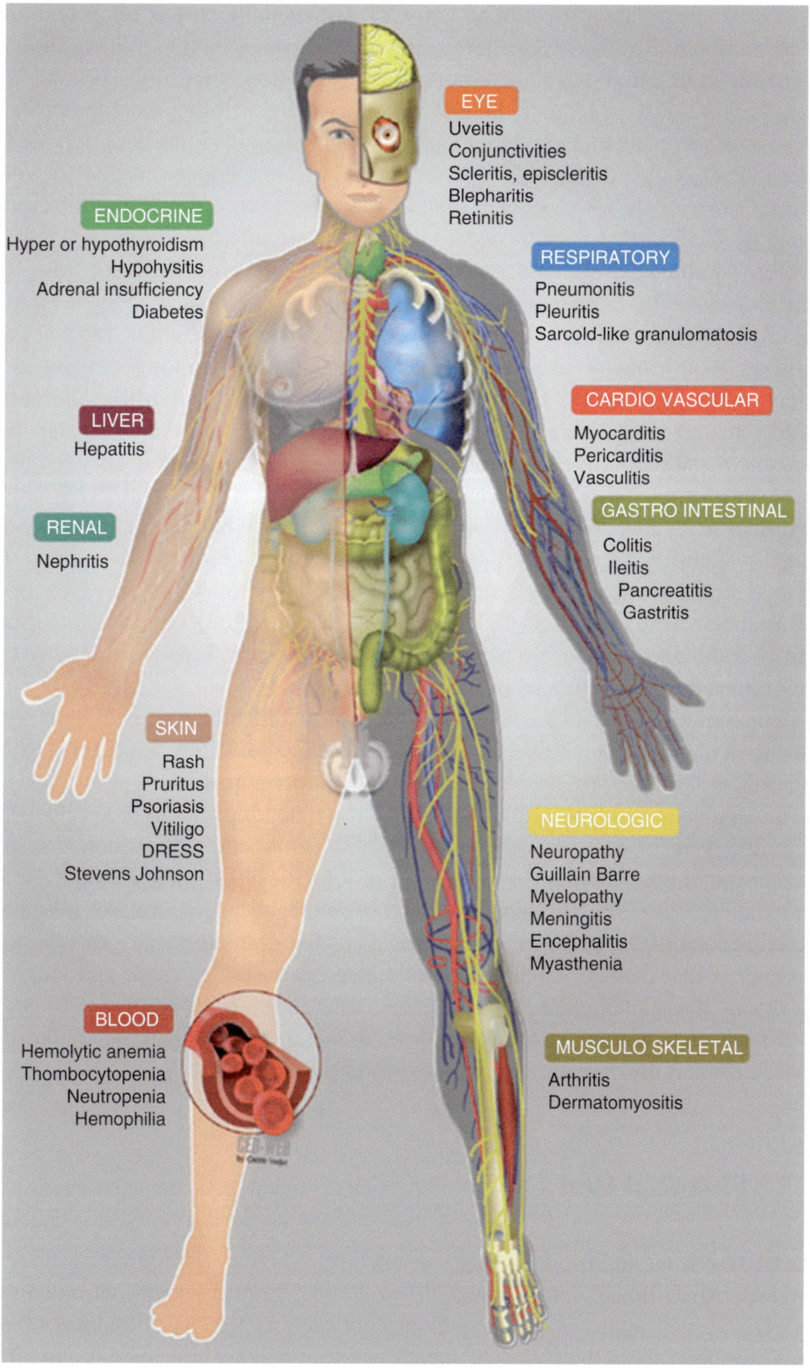

Fig. 13.3 Novel immunotherapy toxicities. Copyright: Annals of Oncology. *Champiat S, Lambotte O, Barreau E, Belkhir R, Berdelou A, Carbonnel F, et al. Management of Immune Checkpoint Blockade Dysimmune Toxicities: a collaborative position paper. Ann Oncol. 2015*

the most frequent being thyoiditis. Anti-CTLA-4 monotherapy is more toxic and generates about 20% of severe irAEs, the more frequent being colitis. Although synergistic in its activity against tumors, the combination of anti-PD-1/PD-L1 with anti-CTLA-4 is also synergistic in terms of toxicities, generating more than 50% of severe irAEs in patients [63]. Only anti-CTLA-4 safety data has been reported in children [64]. An incidence of 27% severe irAEs was reported in this pediatric population. However, the lower level of toxicity seen here in comparison to adults might be due by the fact that these phase 1 children are usually heavily pre-treated and therefore significantly immunocompromised with low levels of lymphocytes.

One of the major hurdles with the implementation of these new therapies in routine oncology practice is the education of the medical and nurse staffs. Indeed, these irAEs are new types of toxicities in oncology and the symptoms developed by patients can be misleading. For instance, a thrombopenia or a diarrhea in immunotherapy treated patients should be seriously considered rather than treated with usual oncology supportive care. Indeed, immunotherapy induced irAEs have been responsible for toxic deaths in the early trials of anti-CTLA-4 and anti-PD-1, mostly because of delayed diagnosis of colitis or pneumonitis. When teams are aware and trained to identify and treat adequately irAEs, then toxic death can be avoided. For instance, in the randomized phase 3 trial of anti-PD-1+anti-CTLA-4 where about 1,000 patients were treated, no toxic deaths were reported [63]. Guidelines to timely identify and manage irAEs are now implemented by cancer centers in order to take care of immunotherapy treated patients adequately [65].

Most immune toxicities are reversible, especially if identified early in their onset. Some toxicities are irreversible, notably the endocrine toxicities. Luckily, hormone replacement therapies are now available for all endocrinopathies.

The incidence and type of toxicities might be much higher and diverse depending on the types of combinations tested. Indeed, combination of immunotherapies together might not generate the same types of toxicities than when they are used in combination with anti-angiogenic drugs or with oncogene kinase inhibitors. Therefore, one of the practical consequences of the immunotherapy revolution in oncology is that cancer patient supportive care has to be rewritten and taught to accompany the implementation of these new treatments. Also, predictive biomarkers of response are urgently needed in order to avoid exposing patients to unnecessary toxicities if they are not likely to respond to immunotherapy.

13.5 Financial Cost

Like all new drugs approved nowadays in oncology, these new immunotherapies are very expensive. Taking into account the wide spectrum of activity of anti-PD-1/PD-L1, and their approval in frequent cancers such as NSCLC, this level of cost raises questions about the ability of social securities and health insurances to afford their reimbursement in the medium term [66, 67]. The UK National Institute for Health and Care Excellence (NICE) recently reviewed Dinutuximab (anti-GD2 monoclonal antibody) therapy for children with high risk neuroblastoma, and concluded that although it extended life expectancy by 2.81 years, it did not offer value for money to the UK National Health System. The antibody therefore had marketing authorization within the UK, but it was not possible for clinicians to prescribe because of the cost. Potential costs are likely to increase as more new immunotherapy agents are developed, and particularly as more combinational therapies are explored. In order to make funding such therapies affordable, the cost needs to come down, the efficacy needs to be improved, or we need to have better biomarkers to identify which children are most likely to benefit.

13.6 Accelerating Pediatric Clinical Translation

The development of pediatric cancer immunotherapy will rely on three critical aspects. First, it will need an access to clinical grade new immunotherapies, either translated from the adult development or specifically developed for pediatric cancers. Second, it will need dedicated funding in order to be able to run these trials, either through academic or industrial sponsorship. Third, this clinical development will need to be done within a dedicated network of Pediatric Phase I units with immunology, immunotherapy, and immune monitoring expertise. These three conditions will efficiently develop our knowledge of the immune contexture of pediatric cancers, their sensitivity to specific types of immunotherapies, and their short/long term tolerance by children. In addition, it may be necessary to re-think the paradigm of how we test new cancer therapeutics, which has historically been largely restricted to those patients with end-stage disease, who have failed all established therapies. Such heavily pre-treated patients are unlikely to be in optimal condition to respond to an immunotherapy, and early phase trials may therefore fail to detect any signal of efficacy, or indeed immune response. The challenge will be to identify how experimental immunotherapies can be tested at an earlier stage. It may be that in some disease subgroups where prognosis is extremely poor despite intensive conventional therapies, that we can consider up front window studies. At the other end of the spectrum, for instance patients with Hodgkin's disease and an excellent prognosis, it may be possible to contemplate reducing the chemotherapy and/or radiotherapy burden to patients and adding an immunotherapy such as anti-PD-1 antibodies.

References

1. Couzin-Frankel J. Breakthrough of the year 2013: cancer immunotherapy. Science. 2013;342:1432–3.
2. Mellman I, Coukos G, Dranoff G. Cancer immunotherapy comes of age. Nature. 2011;480:480–9.
3. Topalian SL, Weiner GJ, Pardoll DM. Cancer immunotherapy comes of age. J Clin Oncol. 2011;29:4828–36.

4. Sharma P, Wagner K, Wolchok J, Allison J. Novel cancer immunotherapy agents with survival benefit: recent successes and next steps. Nat Rev Cancer. 2011;11:805–12.
5. Hamid O, Robert C, Daud A, Hodi FS, Hwu W-J, Kefford R, et al. Safety and tumor responses with lambrolizumab (anti–PD-1) in melanoma. N Engl J Med. 2013;2013(369):134–44.
6. Topalian SL, Hodi FS, Brahmer JR, Gettinger SN, Smith DC, McDermott DF, et al. Safety, activity, and immune correlates of anti-PD-1 antibody in cancer. N Engl J Med. 2012;366:2443–54.
7. Brahmer JR, Tykodi SS, Chow LQM, Hwu W-J, Topalian SL, Hwu P, et al. Safety and activity of anti-PD-L1 antibody in patients with advanced cancer. N Engl J Med. 2012;366:2455–65.
8. Herbst RS, Soria J-C, Kowanetz M, Fine GD, Hamid O, Gordon MS, et al. Predictive correlates of response to the anti-PD-L1 antibody MPDL3280A in cancer patients. Nature. 2014;515:563–7.
9. Herbst RS, Gordon MS, Fine GD, Sosman JA, Soria J-C, Hamid O, et al. A study of MPDL3280A, an engineered PD-L1 antibody in patients with locally advanced or metastatic tumors. J Clin Oncol. 2013;31(15):3000.
10. Ansell SM, Lesokhin AM, Borrello I, Halwani A, Scott EC, Gutierrez M, et al. PD-1 blockade with nivolumab in relapsed or refractory hodgkin's lymphoma. N Engl J Med. 2014;372(4):311–9.
11. Postow MA, Chesney J, Pavlick AC, Robert C, Grossmann K, McDermott D, et al. Nivolumab and ipilimumab versus ipilimumab in untreated melanoma. N Engl J Med. 2015;372:2006–17.
12. Garon EB, Rizvi NA, Hui R, Leighl N, Balmanoukian AS, Eder JP, et al. Pembrolizumab for the treatment of non–small-cell lung cancer. N Engl J Med. 2015;372:2018–28.
13. Robert C, Schachter J, Long GV, Arance A, Grob JJ, Mortier L, et al. Pembrolizumab versus ipilimumab in advanced melanoma. N Engl J Med. 2015;372:2521–32.
14. Brahmer J, Reckamp KL, Baas P, Crinò L, Eberhardt WEE, Poddubskaya E, et al. Nivolumab versus docetaxel in advanced squamous-cell non–small-cell lung cancer. N Engl J Med. 2015;373(2):123-135.
15. Tumeh PC, Harview CL, Yearley JH, Shintaku IP, Taylor EJM, Robert L, et al. PD-1 blockade induces responses by inhibiting adaptive immune resistance. Nature. 2015;515:568–71.
16. Blank CU, Haanen JB, Ribas A, Schumacher TN. The "cancer immunogram". Science. 2016;352:658–60.
17. Teng MWL, Ngiow SF, Ribas A, Smyth MJ. Classifying cancers based on T-cell infiltration and PD-L1. Cancer Res. 2015;75:2139–45.
18. Snyder A, Makarov V, Merghoub T, Yuan J, Zaretsky JM, Desrichard A, et al. Genetic basis for clinical response to CTLA-4 blockade in melanoma. N Engl J Med. 2014;371(23):2189–99.
19. Rizvi NA, Hellmann MD, Snyder A, Kvistborg P, Makarov V, Havel JJ, et al. Mutational landscape determines sensitivity to PD-1 blockade in non-small cell lung cancer. Science. 2015;348(6230):124–8.
20. Kreiter S, Vormehr M, van de Roemer N, Diken M, Löwer M, Diekmann J, et al. Mutant MHC class II epitopes drive therapeutic immune responses to cancer. Nature. 2015;520(7549):692–6.
21. Brown SD, Warren RL, Gibb EA, Martin SD, Spinelli JJ, Nelson BH, et al. Neo-antigens predicted by tumor genome meta-analysis correlate with increased patient survival. Genome Res. 2014;24:743–50.
22. Schumacher TN, Schreiber RD. Neoantigens in cancer immunotherapy. Science. 2015;348:69–74.
23. Bouffet E, Larouche V, Campbell BB, Merico D, de Borja R, Aronson M, et al. Immune checkpoint inhibition for hypermutant glioblastoma multiforme resulting from germline biallelic mismatch repair deficiency. J Clin Oncol. 2016;34(19):2206–11.
24. Dudley JC, Lin MT, Le DT, Eshleman JR. Microsatellite instability as a biomarker for PD-1 blockade. Clin Cancer Res. 2016;22(4):813–20.
25. Maby P, Tougeron D, Hamieh M, Mlecnik B, Kora H, Bindea G, et al. Correlation between density of CD8+ T-cell infiltrate in microsatellite unstable colorectal cancers and frameshift mutations: a rationale for personalized immunotherapy. Cancer Res. 2015;75:3446–55.

26. Le DT, Uram JN, Wang H, Bartlett BR, Kemberling H, Eyring AD, et al. PD-1 Blockade in tumors with mismatch-repair deficiency. N Engl J Med. 2015;372:2509–20.
27. Rooney MS, Shukla SA, Wu CJ, Getz G, Hacohen N. Molecular and genetic properties of tumors associated with local immune cytolytic activity. Cell. 2015;160:48–61.
28. Moskowitz CH. PD-1 Blockade with the monoclonal antibody pembrolizumab (MK-3475) in patients with classical hodgkin lymphoma after brentuximab vedotin failure: preliminary results from a phase 1b study (KEYNOTE-013). ASH Annu Meet Abstr. 2014; session 624, abstract 290.
29. Reichel J, Chadburn A, Rubinstein PG, Giulino-Roth L, Tam W, Liu Y, et al. Flow-sorting and exome sequencing reveals the oncogenome of primary Hodgkin and Reed-Sternberg cells. Blood. 2015;12:1061–72.
30. Selby MJ, Engelhardt JJ, Quigley M, Henning KA, Chen T, Srinivasan M, et al. Anti-CTLA-4 antibodies of IgG2a isotype enhance antitumor activity through reduction of intratumoral regulatory T cells. Cancer Immunol Res. 2013;1(1):32–42.
31. Simpson TR, Li F, Montalvo-Ortiz W, Sepulveda MA, Bergerhoff K, Arce F, et al. Fc-dependent depletion of tumor-infiltrating regulatory T cells co-defines the efficacy of anti-CTLA-4 therapy against melanoma. J Exp Med. 2013;210:1695–710.
32. Bulliard Y, Jolicoeur R, Windman M, Rue SM, Ettenberg S, Knee DA, et al. Activating Fc γ receptors contribute to the antitumor activities of immunoregulatory receptor-targeting antibodies. J Exp Med. 2013;210:1685–93.
33. Bulliard Y, Jolicoeur R, Zhang J, Dranoff G, Wilson NS, Brogdon JL. OX40 engagement depletes intratumoral Tregs via activating FcγRs, leading to antitumor efficacy. Immunol Cell Biol. 2014;
34. Marabelle A, Kohrt H, Sagiv-Barfi I, Ajami B, Axtell R, Zhou G, et al. Depleting tumor-specific Tregs at a single site eradicates disseminated tumors. J Clin Invest. 2013;123:2447–63.
35. Garrett WS. Cancer and the microbiota. Science. 2015;348:80–6.
36. Zitvogel L, Galluzzi L, Viaud S, Vetizou M, Daillere R, Merad M, et al. Cancer and the gut microbiota: an unexpected link. Sci Transl Med. 2015;7:271ps1.
37. Viaud S, Saccheri F, Mignot G, Yamazaki T, Daillère R, Hannani D, et al. The intestinal microbiota modulates the anticancer immune effects of cyclophosphamide. Science. 2013;342:971–6.
38. Iida N, Dzutsev A, Stewart CA, Smith L, Bouladoux N, Weingarten RA, et al. Commensal bacteria control cancer response to therapy by modulating the tumor microenvironment. Science. 2013;342:967–70.
39. Uncovering microbes' role in tumor progression. Cancer Discov. 2015; doi: 10.1158/2159-8290.CD-NB2015-009.
40. Rutkowski MR, Stephen TL, Svoronos N, Allegrezza MJ, Tesone AJ, Perales-Puchalt A, et al. Microbially driven TLR5-dependent signaling governs distal malignant progression through tumor-promoting inflammation. Cancer Cell. 2014;27:27–40.
41. Antonia SJ, Lopez-Martin JA, Bendell JC, Ott PA, Taylor MH, Eder JP, et al. Checkmate 032: Nivolumab (N) alone or in combination with ipilimumab (I) for the treatment of recurrent small cell lung cancer (SCLC). ASCO Meet Abstr., vol. 34, 2016, p 100.
42. Hellmann MD, Gettinger SN, Goldman JW, Brahmer JR, Borghaei H, Chow LQ, et al. CheckMate 012: safety and efficacy of first-line (1L) nivolumab (nivo; N) and ipilimumab (ipi; I) in advanced (adv) NSCLC. ASCO Meet Abstr. 2016;34, p. 3001.
43. Antonia S, Goldberg SB, Balmanoukian A, Chaft JE, Sanborn RE, Gupta A, et al. Safety and antitumour activity of durvalumab plus tremelimumab in non-small cell lung cancer: a multicentre, phase 1b study. Lancet Oncol. 2016;17:299–308.
44. Voron T, Colussi O, Marcheteau E, Pernot S, Nizard M, Pointet A-L, et al. VEGF-A modulates expression of inhibitory checkpoints on CD8+ T cells in tumors. J Exp Med. 2015;212(2):139–48.
45. Terme M, Pernot S, Marcheteau E, Sandoval F, Benhamouda N, Colussi O, et al. VEGFA-VEGFR pathway blockade inhibits tumor-induced regulatory T-cell proliferation in colorectal cancer. Cancer Res. 2013;73:539–49.

46. Olsson A-K, Dimberg A, Kreuger J, Claesson-Welsh L. VEGF receptor signalling—in control of vascular function. Nat Rev Mol Cell Biol. 2006;7:359–71.
47. Motz GT, Santoro SP, Wang L-P, Garrabrant T, Lastra RR, Hagemann IS, et al. Tumor endothelium FasL establishes a selective immune barrier promoting tolerance in tumors. Nat Med. 2014;20:607–15.
48. Amin A, Plimack ER, Infante J. Nivolumab (anti-PD-1; BMS-936558, ONO-4538) in combination with sunitinib or pazopanib in patients (pts) with metastatic renal cell carcinoma (mRCC). J Clin Oncol. 2014;32:5010.
49. Zamarin D, Holmgaard RB, Subudhi SK, Park JS, Mansour M, Palese P, et al. localized oncolytic virotherapy overcomes systemic tumor resistance to immune checkpoint blockade immunotherapy. Sci Transl Med. 2014;6:226ra32.
50. Marabelle A, Kohrt HE, Caux C, Levy R. Intra-tumoral Immunization: a new paradigm for cancer therapy. Clin Cancer Res. 2014;20:1747–56.
51. Kim YH, Gratzinger D, Harrison C, Brody JD, Czerwinski DK, Ai WZ, et al. In situ vaccination against mycosis fungoides by intratumoral injection of a TLR9 agonist combined with radiation: a phase 1/2 study. Blood. 2012;119:355–63.
52. Brody JD, Ai WZ, Czerwinski DK, Torchia JA, Levy M, Advani RH, et al. In situ vaccination with a TLR9 agonist induces systemic lymphoma regression: a phase I/II study. J Clin Oncol. 2010;28:4324–32.
53. Andtbacka RHI, Kaufman HL, Collichio F, Amatruda T, Senzer N, Chesney J, et al. Talimogene laherparepvec improves durable response rate in patients with advanced melanoma. J Clin Oncol. 2015;33:2780–8.
54. Puzanov I, Milhem MM, Minor D, Hamid O, Li A, Chen L, et al. Talimogene laherparepvec in combination with ipilimumab in previously untreated, unresectable stage IIIB-IV melanoma. J Clin Oncol. 2016;34(22):2619–26.
55. Long G V, Dummer R, Ribas A, Puzanov I, VanderWalde A, Andtbacka RHI, et al. Efficacy analysis of MASTERKEY-265 phase 1b study of talimogene laherparepvec (T-VEC) and pembrolizumab (pembro) for unresectable stage IIIB-IV melanoma. ASCO Meet Abstr., 2016, vol. 34, p 9568.
56. Platten M, Wick W, Van den Eynde BJ. Tryptophan catabolism in cancer: beyond IDO and tryptophan depletion. Cancer Res. 2012;72:5435–40.
57. Gangadhar TC, Hamid O, Smith DC, Bauer TM, Wasser JS, Luke JJ, et al. Preliminary results from a phase I/II study of epacadostat (incb024360) in combination with pembrolizumab in patients with selected advanced cancers. J Immunother Cancer. 2015;3:1–2.
58. Gibney G, Hamid O, Lutzky J, Olszanski A, Gangadhar T, Gajewski T, et al. 511 Updated results from a phase 1/2 study of epacadostat (INCB024360) in combination with ipilimumab in patients with metastatic melanoma. Eur J Cancer Elsevier. 2016;51:S106–7.
59. Badros AZ. A phase II study of anti PD-1 antibody pembrolizumab, pomalidomide and dexamethasone in patients with relapsed/refractory multiple myeloma (RRMM). ASH Annu Meet Abstr. 2015: page session 653, abstract 506.
60. San Miguel J. Pembrolizumab in combination with lenalidomide and low-dose dexamethasone for relapsed/refractory multiple myeloma (RRMM): keynote-023. ASH Annu Meet Abstr. 2015: page session 653, abstract 505.
61. Mody R Lancet Oncology 2017; doi: http://dx.doi.org/10.1016/S1470-2045(17)30355-8.
62. Furman W et al; Improved clinical responses with the concomitant use of an anti-GD2 monoclonal antibody and chemotherapy in newly diagnosed children with high risk neuroblastoma. Preliminary results of St Judes Phase II study NB2012. ASCO abstract. 2016.
63. Larkin J, Chiarion-Sileni V, Gonzalez R, Grob JJ, Cowey CL, Lao CD, et al. Combined nivolumab and ipilimumab or monotherapy in untreated melanoma. N Engl J Med. 2015;373:23–34.
64. Merchant MS, Wright M, Baird K, Wexler LH, Rodriguez-Galindo C, Bernstein D, et al. Phase I clinical trial of ipilimumab in pediatric patients with advanced solid tumors. Clin Cancer Res. 2016;22(6):1364–70.

65. Champiat S, Lambotte O, Barreau E, Belkhir R, Berdelou A, Carbonnel F, et al. Management of immune checkpoint blockade dysimmune toxicities: a collaborative position paper. Ann Oncol 2015;27(4):559-74
66. Tartari F, Santoni M, Burattini L, Mazzanti P, Onofri A, Berardi R. Economic sustainability of anti-PD-1 agents nivolumab and pembrolizumab in cancer patients: recent insights and future challenges. Cancer Treat Rev. 2016;48:20–4.
67. Ledford H. Immunotherapy's cancer remit widens. Nature. 2013;497:544.
68. Chowdhury FDS, Mitchell S, Mellows S, Ashton-Keyes M, Gray JC. PD-L1 and CD8+ PD1+ lymphocytes exist as targets in the paediatric tumour microenvironment for immunomodulatory therapy. OncoImmunology. 2015;4(10):e1029701.
69. Vakkila J, Jaffe R, Michelow M, Lotze MT. Pediatric cancers are infiltrated predominantly by macrophages and contain a paucity of dendritic cells: a major nosologic difference with adult tumors. Clin Cancer Res. 2006;12(7 Pt 1):2049–54.
70. Yu AL, Gilman AL, Ozkaynak MF, London WB, Kreissman SG, Chen HX, et al. Anti-GD2 antibody with GM-CSF, interleukin-2, and isotretinoin for neuroblastoma. N Engl J Med. 2010;363(14):1324–34.
71. Siebert N, Jensen C, Troschke-Meurer S, Zumpe M, Juttner M, Ehlert K, et al. Neuroblastoma patients with high-affinity FCGR2A, -3A and stimulatory KIR 2DS2 treated by long-term infusion of anti-GD2 antibody ch14.18/CHO show higher ADCC levels and improved event-free survival. Oncoimmunology. 2016;5(11):e1235108.

Index

J.C. Gray, A. Marabelle (eds.), *Immunotherapy for Pediatric Malignancies*,
https://doi.org/10.1007/978-3-319-43486-5

MIX
Papier aus verantwortungsvollen Quellen
Paper from responsible sources
FSC® C105338

If you have any concerns about our products,
you can contact us on
ProductSafety@springernature.com

In case Publisher is established outside the EU,
the EU authorized representative is:
Springer Nature Customer Service Center GmbH
Europaplatz 3, 69115 Heidelberg, Germany

Printed by Libri Plureos GmbH
in Hamburg, Germany